Arthroscopic Shoulder Surgery
Complications and Management

Arthroscopic Shoulder Surgery
Complications and Management

Editor

Terry L. Thompson, MD
Howard University College of Medicine
Washington, District of Columbia

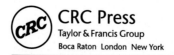

CRC Press is an imprint of the
Taylor & Francis Group, an **informa** business

First published 2022 by SLACK Incorporated

Published 2024 by CRC Press
2385 NW Executive Center Drive, Suite 320, Boca Raton FL 33431

and by CRC Press
4 Park Square, Milton Park, Abingdon, Oxon, OX14 4RN

CRC Press is an imprint of Taylor & Francis Group, LLC

Cover Artist: Lori Shields

Library of Congress Control Number: 2021948768

ISBN: 9781630917050 (pbk)
ISBN: 9781003522614 (ebk)

DOI: 10.1201/9781003522614

DEDICATION

To my wife, Audrey.

Contents

ACKNOWLEDGMENTS

First and foremost, I must thank my wife, Audrey, for her patience, insight, and encouragement throughout the writing project.

I thank my residents and medical students who performed much of the research that added depth to the chapters.

I must thank Julia Dolinger, Acquisitions Editor at SLACK Incorporated, for her guidance and support in bringing this project to fruition during an unprecedented public health crisis.

I received inspiration from my mentors Charles H. Epps Jr, E. Anthony Rankin, and Richard E. Grant. Such has been the case throughout my career.

Finally, I am extremely grateful for my contributing authors who committed their time, effort, and expertise to writing this book.

ABOUT THE EDITOR

Terry L. Thompson, MD, is the Charles H. Epps Jr Professor and Chairman of the Department of Orthopaedic Surgery and Rehabilitation at Howard University College of Medicine in Washington, District of Columbia. He served as Program Director for the orthopaedic surgery residency program at Howard University Hospital from 2001 to 2014. He has been a member of the full-time faculty since 1989.

Dr. Thompson is a native of South Carolina. He graduated with honors from South Carolina State University in 1979. He received the Doctor of Medicine degree from Howard University in 1983. Dr. Thompson took an internship in surgery and residency in orthopaedic surgery at Howard University Hospital from 1983 to 1988. He received fellowship training in sports medicine at Lenox Hill Hospital in New York City from 1988 to 1989. Dr. Thompson holds certification by the American Board of Orthopaedic Surgery in Orthopaedic Surgery and Orthopaedic Sports Medicine.

Dr. Thompson has held leadership positions in professional organizations. He is past Vice President of the American Board of Orthopaedic Surgery. He has served on the Board of Directors of the J. Robert Gladden Orthopaedic Society. Dr. Thompson has served as Vice Chairman of the Residency Review Committee for Orthopaedic Surgery of the Accreditation Council for Graduate Medical Education. He has served as Orthopaedic Section Chairman of the National Medical Association and the Medical Society of the District of Columbia.

Dr. Thompson has written and lectured in the areas of sports medicine and management of knee and shoulder injuries. He is a reviewer for *Clinical Orthopaedics and Related Research* and *Sports Health*. He is Associate Editor for *Orthopedics*.

Dr. Thompson has received several honors. He is a member of the Alpha Omega Alpha Honor Medical Society. He was selected to the inaugural class of Leadership Fellows of the American Academy of Orthopaedic Surgeons in 2001. Dr. Thompson was the 2003 recipient of the Medical Staff Leadership Award for Howard University Hospital. He received the Special Recognition Award from the District of Columbia Public Schools in 2005 for service to interscholastic sports. He was awarded Honorary Membership in the National Athletic Trainers' Association in 2016 for his strong devotion to sports medicine and the athletic training profession. Dr. Thompson has received citations for excellence in teaching.

Among his many professional activities, Dr. Thompson serves as Head Team Physician for Howard University Department of Intercollegiate Athletics. He is Team Physician for the District of Columbia Public Schools. He is a Neutral Physician for the National Football League Player Benefits Plan.

CONTRIBUTING AUTHORS

Benjamin Albertson, MD (Chapter 4)
Department of Orthopaedics and Rehabilitation
University of New Mexico
Albuquerque, New Mexico

Answorth Allen, MD (Chapter 13)
Attending Physician
Hospital for Special Surgery
Professor
Clinical Orthopedic Surgery
Weill Cornell Medical College
New York, New York

Akhil Andrews, MD (Chapter 9)
Fellow
Orthopaedic Sports Medicine
Allegheny General Hospital
Pittsburgh, Pennsylvania

Craig Bennett, MD (Chapter 8)
Co-Founder and Medical Director
Lifebridge Health Sportsmedicine Institute
Baltimore, Maryland

Alexander R. M. Bitzer, MD (Chapter 12)
Assistant Professor
Orthopedic Surgery
Sports Medicine & Shoulder/Elbow
West Virginia University–East
Martinsburg, West Virginia

James E. Carpenter, MD, MHSA (Chapter 11)
Professor
Department of Orthopaedic Surgery
University of Michigan
Ann Arbor, Michigan

Ferdinand J. Chan, MD (Chapter 14)
Montefiore Medical Center
The University Hospital for Albert Einstein College of Medicine
Bronx, New York

Filippo Familiari, MD (Chapter 6)
Associate Professor of Orthopaedic and Trauma Surgery
Department of Orthopaedic and Trauma Surgery
Magna Graecia
University of Catanzaro
Catanzaro, Italy

Gazi Huri, MD (Chapter 6)
Orthopaedica and Traumatology Department
Hacettepe University
Ankara, Turkey

Timothy S. Johnson, MD (Chapter 12)
National Sports Medicine Institute
Lansdowne, Virginia

Ibrahim M. Khaleel, MD (Chapter 2)
Michigan Medicine
Ann Arbor, Michigan

Stephanie L. Logterman, MD (Chapter 1)
Orthopedic Sports Medicine Fellow
Emory University School of Medicine
Atlanta, Georgia

Eric C. McCarty, MD (Chapter 1)
Professor and Chief of Sports Medicine and Shoulder Surgery
Department of Orthopaedics
University of Colorado School of Medicine
Denver, Colorado
Associate Professor Adjunct
Department of Integrative Physiology
University of Colorado, Boulder
Boulder, Colorado
Director of Sports Medicine
University of Colorado Department of Athletics
Head Team Physician
Colorado Avalanche Hockey Club
Fellowship Director
University of Colorado Sports Medicine and Shoulder Fellowship

Edward G. McFarland, MD (Chapter 6)
The Wayne H. Lewis Professor of Shoulder Surgery
Director, Division of Shoulder Surgery
Department of Orthopedic Surgery
Johns Hopkins University School of Medicine
Baltimore, Maryland

Prashant Meshram, MS, DNB (Chapter 6)
Department of Orthopedics
Shoulder Division
Johns Hopkins University
Baltimore, Maryland

Jerome Colin Murray, BS (Chapter 8)
Georgetown University
Washington, District of Columbia

Abbas Naqvi, MD (Chapter 10)
Resident Physician
Department of Orthopaedic Surgery and Rehabilitation
Howard University Hospital
Washington, District of Columbia

Thomas X. Nguyen, MD (Chapter 10)
Resident Physician
Department of Orthopaedic Surgery and Rehabilitation
Howard University Hospital
Washington, District of Columbia

Stephen J. Nicholas, MD (Chapter 14)
Founder and Director
NY Orthopedics
Director
Nicholas Institute of Sports Medicine and Athletic Trauma
Lenox Hill Hospital
New York, New York

Jane H. O'Connor, MD (Chapter 2)
Department of Orthopaedic Surgery
Howard University Hospital
Washington, District of Columbia

Gabriella Ode, MD (Chapter 13)
Department of Orthopaedic Surgery
Prisma Health–Upstate
Greenville, South Carolina

Emmanuel N. Osadebey, MD (Chapters 2 and 5)
Howard University Hospital
Washington, District of Columbia

Benjamin Packard, MD, MS (Chapter 3)
Department of Orthopedics
University of New Mexico
Albuquerque, New Mexico

Rajeev Pandarinath, MD (Chapter 7)
Precision Orthopedics and Sports Medicine
Falls Church, Virginia

Marc E. Rankin, MD (Chapter 9)
Clinical Associate Professor
Department of Orthopaedic Surgery and Rehabilitation
Howard University College of Medicine
Washington, District of Columbia

Dustin L. Richter, MD (Chapters 3 and 4)
Assistant Professor
Sports Medicine
Director
Sports Medicine Fellowship Program
Department of Orthopaedic Surgery
University of New Mexico Health Sciences Center
Albuquerque, New Mexico

Jorge Rojas, MD (Chapter 6)
Mayo Clinic
Rochester, Minnesota

Christopher G. Salib, MD, MS (Chapter 5)
Rubin Institute of Advanced Orthopaedics
Sinai Hospital of Baltimore
Baltimore, Maryland

Robert C. Schenck Jr, MD (Chapters 3 and 4)
Professor and Chair
Orthopaedics and Rehabilitation
Sports Medicine and Complex Knee
Team Physicians for UNM Lobo Athletics
UNM Health Sciences
The University of New Mexico
Albuquerque, New Mexico

Christopher Shultz, MD (Chapters 3 and 4)
Department of Orthopaedics and Rehabilitation
University of New Mexico
Albuquerque, New Mexico

Seth Stake, MD (Chapter 7)
George Washington University Hospital
Washington, District of Columbia

Taylor Swansen, MD, MS (Chapter 7)
George Washington University Hospital
Washington, District of Columbia

Daniel C. Wascher, MD (Chapter 3)
Professor of Orthopaedic Surgery
University of New Mexico
Albuquerque, New Mexico

Rolanda A. Willacy, MD (Chapter 2)
Department of Orthopaedic Surgery
Howard University Hospital
Washington, District of Columbia

Robert H. Wilson, MD (Chapter 2)
Associate Professor
Department of Orthopaedic Surgery and Rehabilitation
Howard University College of Medicine
Washington, District of Columbia

INTRODUCTION

Shoulder arthroscopy has been one of the great innovations in modern orthopedic surgery (Figure I-1). Improvements in our knowledge and understanding of shoulder biomechanics and pathology along with refinements in arthroscopic implants and techniques have made shoulder arthroscopy more accessible to a growing number of surgeons and has led to expanded indications for treating patients with shoulder injuries and conditions. The procedure can be used for diagnosis and treatment of a variety of conditions, including rotator cuff tears, instability, and cartilage lesions. The ability to look inside the shoulder through a tiny incision without opening the joint has greatly expanded our understanding of many shoulder problems and has given shoulder surgeons the ability to provide minimally invasive solutions to treat pathology that previously required open surgery.

Historically, advancements in shoulder arthroscopy have lagged behind knee arthroscopy. Beginning in the 1980s, rapid progress in surgical techniques was made possible by some of the great innovators in the field of shoulder arthroscopy. Ellman[1] described the management of subacromial impingement by arthroscopic decompression. Morgan and Bodenstab[2] pioneered arthroscopic Bankart repair. Snyder et al[3] advanced the diagnosis and arthroscopic treatment of superior labrum anterior to posterior (SLAP) tears, a previously poorly understood lesion. Gartsman et al[4] and Burkhart et al[5] were among the first to report results of arthroscopic rotator cuff repair.

Complications of shoulder arthroscopy differ in some ways from open surgery owing to its minimally invasive approach, unique instruments, and implants and requirement to distend the joint with fluid. Like any evolving technique, the nature of complications associated with shoulder arthroscopy has evolved with improvements in implants and techniques. Neurovascular injury was among the early reported complications as surgeons learned arthroscopic anatomy and portal placement.[6,7] Instrument and implant breakage was once the bane of the shoulder arthroscopist.[8-10] As implant and instrument design evolved, these problems became less frequent.

Complications can come in various forms, including operative, medical, and anesthetic related. Shin et al[11] reported complication rates for arthroscopic shoulder surgery among candidates for Part II of the American Board of Orthopaedic Surgery Certifying Examination. A total of 27,072 procedures were reviewed. Surgical complications (7.9%) were more common than anesthetic (1.0%) or medical (2.2%) complications. Intraoperative complications include neurovascular injury, instrument and implant breakage, and fluid extravasation. Medical complications are rare but may include stroke, pulmonary embolism, and deep vein thrombosis. Anesthetic

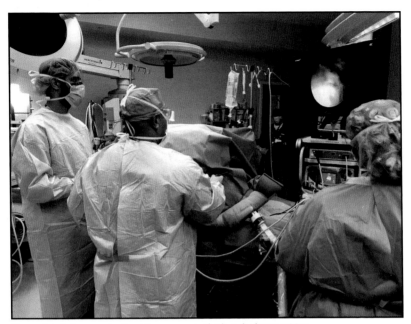

Figure I-1. Arthroscopic shoulder surgery in the beach chair position.

complications are largely related to regional anesthesia. Other complications that become apparent in the postoperative period include nerve injury from positioning, septic arthritis, arthrofibrosis, and failure of repair. Complication rates are higher when more complex procedures are performed arthroscopically.[11]

It is widely known that surgeons are more enthusiastic about reporting their successes than their complications. However, most surgeons do not hesitate to seek help from a colleague or search the literature when faced with a challenging complication. While there are several useful books on complications in shoulder surgery, there is currently no resource that focuses on arthroscopic shoulder surgery and its unique challenges in a comprehensive manner. With this work, we offer a reference that brings together the current literature and provides expert opinion on the management of commonly encountered and unusual complications.

—Terry L. Thompson, MD

References

1. Ellman H. Arthroscopic subacromial decompression: analysis of one- to three-year results. *Arthroscopy*. 1987;3(3):173–181.
2. Morgan CD, Bodenstab AB. Arthroscopic Bankart suture repair: technique and early results. *Arthroscopy*. 1987;3(2):111–122.
3. Snyder SJ, Karzel RP, Del Pizzo W, Ferkel RD, Friedman MJ. SLAP lesions of the shoulder. *Arthroscopy*. 1990;6(4):274–279.
4. Gartsman GM, Khan M, Hammerman SM. Arthroscopic repair of full-thickness tears of the rotator cuff. *J Bone Joint Surg Am*. 1998;80(6):832–840.
5. Burkhart SS, Danaceau SM, Pearce CE Jr. Arthroscopic rotator cuff repair: analysis of results by tear size and by repair technique-margin convergence versus direct tendon-to-bone repair. *Arthroscopy*. 2001;17(9):905–912.
6. Cameron SE. Venous pseudoaneurysm as a complication of shoulder arthroscopy. *J Shoulder Elbow Surg*. 1996;5(5):404–406.
7. Paulos LE, Franklin JL. Arthroscopic shoulder decompression development and application: a five year experience. *Am J Sports Med*. 1990;18(3):235–244.
8. Song HS, Ramsey ML. Suture passing needle breakage during arthroscopic rotator cuff repair: a complication report. *Arthroscopy*. 2008;24(12):1430–1432.
9. Wilkerson JP, Zvijac JE, Uribe JW, Schürhoff MR, Green JB. Failure of polymerized lactic acid tacks in shoulder surgery. *J Shoulder Elbow Surg*. 2003;12(2):117–121.
10. Kaar TK, Schenck RC Jr, Wirth MA, Rockwood CA Jr. Complications of metallic suture anchors in shoulder surgery: a report of 8 cases. *Arthroscopy*. 2001;17(1):31–37.
11. Shin JJ, Popchak AJ, Musahl V, Irrgang JJ, Lin A. Complications after arthroscopic shoulder surgery: a review of the American Board of Orthopaedic Surgery Database. *J Am Acad Orthop Surg Glob Res Rev*. 2018;2(12):e093.

1

Complications of Positioning in Arthroscopic Shoulder Surgery

Stephanie L. Logterman, MD
and Eric C. McCarty, MD

INTRODUCTION

Shoulder arthroscopy is one of the most common orthopedic procedures, with more than 500,000 being performed annually in the United States.[1] The beach chair and lateral decubitus positions are the most common patient positions for shoulder arthroscopy. In the United States, roughly two-thirds of all arthroscopic shoulder surgeries are performed in the beach chair position.[2,3] Each position has its own advantages and disadvantages, with visualization, ease of setup, access to certain parts of the shoulder, and risks to patients being the frequent subjects of controversy (Table 1-1). The primary advantages of the lateral decubitus position are the larger working space within the glenohumeral joint and improved visualization. The upright, anatomic position of the beach chair position makes orientation easier, plus the upright position allows for easy conversion to an open procedure such as a biceps tenodesis. Finally, cost of setup for each position varies based on equipment and surgeon preference. The cost for

Thompson TL, ed.
Arthroscopic Shoulder Surgery:
Complications and Management (pp 1-20).
© 2022 Taylor & Francis Group.

TABLE 1-1. ADVANTAGES AND DISADVANTAGES OF BEACH CHAIR AND LATERAL DECUBITUS POSITIONS		
	BEACH CHAIR	LATERAL DECUBITUS
ADVANTAGES	• Anatomic position • Ease of exam under anesthesia • Easily convert to open with no need to redrape or reposition • Arm not blocking anterior portal • Can use regional anesthesia with sedation • Intraoperative arm mobility	• Traction increases space in glenohumeral joint and subacromial space • Traction accentuates labral tears • Patient's head/operating room bed not in way of posterior or superior portals • Cautery bubbles out of view • No increased risk of hypotension/bradycardia • Better cerebral perfusion
DISADVANTAGES	• Potential mechanical blocks of posterior or superior portals • Increased risk of hypotension/bradycardia causing cardiovascular complications • Cautery bubbles obscure view in subacromial space • Fluid can fog camera • Increased risk air embolus • Expensive equipment: beach chair attachment and/or mechanical arm holder	• Nonanatomic orientation • Reach around arm for anterior portal • Need to reposition or redrape to convert to open • Cannot use regional anesthesia • Traction can cause neurovascular or soft tissue injuries • Potential risk to axillary and musculocutaneous nerves when placing anteroinferior portal

beach chair attachments and arm holders ranges from \$12,000 to \$20,500. Equipment for the lateral decubitus position ranges from \$9,000 to \$11,500.[4]

With regard to complications, each position has specific risks associated with it. Nerve injuries are most often related to positioning, traction, or portal placement. For the beach chair position, the ulnar and common peroneal nerves are most often injured, which are due to arm and leg positioning, respectively.[5] Brachial plexus and peripheral nerve traction palsies have been documented at 10% to 30%, respectively, in the literature.[6,7] Peroneal nerve injuries can also occur in the lateral decubitus position due to failure to pad the fibular head during positioning. Furthermore, compared to the beach chair, the axillary and musculocutaneous nerves are at increased risk with the anterolateral portal placement.[8] While the majority of neurologic injuries reported have been transient, permanent nerve damage due to shoulder arthroscopy also has been documented.[9] Furthermore, malpositioning in the beach chair position can lead to reduced vertebral artery blood flow or restriction of cerebral venous drainage, which can have devastating consequences in the form of posterior brain infarcts.[10] Thus, proper positioning for shoulder arthroscopy, either the lateral decubitus or beach chair, is imperative to prevent complications and to improve the ease of surgical intervention.

EPIDEMIOLOGY

The complication rate for arthroscopic shoulder surgery is cited in the literature as anywhere from 5.8% to 9.5%.[11] For neurapraxia in particular, the reported incidence ranges from 0% to 30%.[12-16] The rate of venous thromboembolism following arthroscopic shoulder surgery is 0.15% to 0.31%.[17,18] The incidence of cerebrovascular events during shoulder surgery is reported as 0.00291%, with all of these events occurring in patients in the beach chair position; however, once these data were adjusted for confounding variables, no difference was found in the rate of cardiovascular events between beach chair and lateral decubitus positions.[2] Overall, complications following shoulder arthroscopy, regardless of position used, are very rare (Table 1-2).

REVIEW OF LITERATURE

Complications From Beach Chair

Neurapraxia and nerve palsies have both been documented in the literature as complications resulting from shoulder arthroscopy in the beach chair position. The ulnar and common peroneal nerves are most often

TABLE 1-2. INCIDENCE OF COMPLICATIONS FOLLOWING SHOULDER ARTHROSCOPY

COMPLICATION	INCIDENCE, %
Neurapraxia	0 to 30
DVT/PE	0.15 to 0.31
Cerebrovascular event	0.00291

injured, which are due to arm and leg positioning, respectively.[5] Park and Kim[19] reported neurapraxia of not only the lesser occipital nerve but also the greater auricular nerve that occurred from inadequate padding around the head. Furthermore, Ng and Page[20] noted greater auricular nerve neurapraxia in 3 patients resulting from use of a horseshoe headrest. Finally, one case of hypoglossal nerve palsy was recorded in a case report by Mullins et al,[21] who attributed the complication to nerve compression due to a mid-procedure position change. Nerve injuries due to the beach chair position are rare as Small[15] reported no instances of nerve palsy in a sample of 1184 shoulder arthroscopies performed by experienced surgeons. Levy et al[22] reported 6 cases of lateral femoral cutaneous nerve (LFCN) palsy (prevalence of 1.5%) in a retrospective chart review of 400 patients who underwent arthroscopic shoulder surgery in the beach chair position. All LFCN neurapraxia symptoms resolved within 6 months of surgery. In addition, Satin et al[23] also documented 4 cases of LFCN neurapraxia following shoulder arthroscopy in the beach chair position, with all cases occurring patients with a body mass index (BMI) >30 kg/m^2.

Deep vein thrombosis (DVT) and pulmonary embolus have also been documented after arthroscopic shoulder surgery performed in the beach chair position. In one case series, Bongiovanni et al[24] reported 3 patients developed a DVT after shoulder arthroscopy; however, upon further investigation, all 3 patients were noted to have a heritable thrombophilia. Furthermore, Creighton and Cole[25] and Cortes et al[26] each reported one patient with a DVT after shoulder arthroscopy. Creighton and Cole[25] noted one upper extremity DVT while Cortes et al[26] documented a lower extremity DVT with subsequent pulmonary embolus.

Other uncommon complications from the beach chair position have also been reported in the literature. Bhatti and Enneking[27] noted a case of unilateral vision loss with associated ophthalmoplegia after shoulder arthroscopy in the beach chair position. Twenty cases of profound hypotension and bradycardia, one of which resulted in asystolic cardiac arrest, were reported by D'Alessio et al[28] in a retrospective chart review of

116 patients undergoing arthroscopic shoulder surgery in the beach chair position. The authors suspect these events were due to activation of the Bezold-Jarisch reflex due to high circulating epinephrine levels after interscalene block combined with the patient in a sitting position. In a case series, Cho et al[29] documented 2 patients who developed ventricular tachycardia and subsequent cardiogenic shock due to the patients receiving an infusion of solution containing epinephrine. Pulmonary complications have also been reported in the literature. Lee et al[30] reported 3 cases of subcutaneous emphysema, pneumomediastinum, and tension pneumothorax. Finally, reports of sudden, profound hypotension and bradycardic events have been documented in greater than 20% of patients intraoperatively during shoulder arthroscopy in the beach chair position.[31,32] Liguori et al[32] found that administration of metoprolol could decrease the incidence of these hypotensive/bradycardic events.

One of the more severe yet rare complications from the beach chair position is cerebral hypoperfusion and subsequent neurologic injury. The estimated incidence cited in the literature is less than 0.005%.[2] Near-infrared spectroscopy has been employed as a noninvasive method to continuously monitor cerebral oxygenation (regional oxygen saturation [rSO_2]) intraoperatively. A cerebral desaturation event (CDE) is defined as a drop of 20% or greater from baseline readings on the near-infrared spectroscopy monitor.[33,34] Salazar et al[34] found that increased BMI has a statistically significant ($P < .001$) association with intraoperative CDEs. In their 50-patient series, they had an 18% incidence of intraoperative CDE and calculated an odds ratio of 12.4 for patients with a BMI more than 34 kg/m[2] experiencing a CDE. Songy et al[35] examined whether beach chair position angle had an effect on cerebral oxygenation as a prior study on the subject by Pant et al[33] had been inconclusive. In their prospective cohort study of 50 patients, Songy et al[35] demonstrated a linear decrease in rSO_2 with increasing beach chair angles from 0 to 60 degrees; however, the average drop in rSO_2 was significantly less than the threshold of 20%. One case series noted 4 instances of ischemic brain and spinal cord injury after both open and arthroscopic shoulder surgeries with patients in the beach chair position.[36] It should be noted, however, that many of the ischemic events reported for beach chair positioning are attributed to errors in interpretation of blood pressure readings.[3,36] Since hypotensive anesthesia is used intraoperatively to minimize bleeding, accurate measuring of blood pressure is necessary. It is recommended to place the blood pressure cuff at the level of the heart rather than placing it on the calf.[4] Furthermore, it is also recommended to aggressively treat perioperative blood pressures less than 80% of preoperative resting values in order to avoid ischemic complications.[3]

Complications From Lateral Decubitus

Neurapraxias and nerve palsies with patients in the lateral decubitus position have been reported in the literature. Peroneal nerve injuries occur due to failure to pad the fibular head of the "down leg" or bottom leg during positioning. In a retrospective review, Ellman[37] documented 3 cases of neurapraxia of the dorsal sensory branch of the radial nerve, which was attributed to inadequate padding of the extremity at the wrist. Andrews et al[12] noted 2 ulnar nerve neurapraxias and one musculocutaneous nerve neurapraxia in their 120-patient retrospective chart review. One case of musculocutaneous nerve palsy was reported by Ogilvie-Harris and Wiley.[13] Gartsman[38] reported a case of lateral femoral cutaneous nerve neurapraxia following arthroscopic shoulder surgery in the lateral decubitus position. Finally, Paulos and Franklin[39] noted one case of axillary nerve neurapraxia with associated deltoid dysfunction in their retrospective chart review of 76 patients undergoing shoulder arthroscopy in the lateral decubitus position.

Hynson et al[40] noted a case of airway obstruction resulting from extra-articular spread of arthroscopy fluid while the patient was placed in the lateral decubitus position.

DVT and/or pulmonary embolus (PE) are associated with both the beach chair and lateral decubitus positions. Edgar et al[41] reported 3 non-fatal pulmonary emboli after arthroscopic shoulder surgery in the lateral decubitus position, with 2 of the 3 patients having a risk factor for DVT/PE. Burkhart[42] documented one case of postoperative DVT in a patient with a history of Hodgkin lymphoma, while Garofalo et al[43] noted 2 patients with DVTs following shoulder surgery in the lateral decubitus position. Finally, Kuremsky et al[18] performed a large retrospective review of nearly 2000 patients and found 6 patients who developed a total of 5 DVTs and 4 PEs after arthroscopic shoulder surgery in the lateral decubitus position. All 6 patients required hospitalization for treatment of their DVT/PE, and 3 of the 6 patients had risk factors.

Last, an extremely rare, yet devastating, complication from the lateral decubitus position is a stroke. Zeidan et al[44] had one case report of a postoperative brain stroke following arthroscopic shoulder surgery performed in the lateral decubitus position.

Please refer to Table 1-3 for a list of complications from the beach chair and lateral decubitus positions.

TABLE 1-3. COMPLICATIONS OF BEACH CHAIR AND LATERAL DECUBITUS POSITIONS (NUMBER OF CASES DOCUMENTED IN LITERATURE)		
	BEACH CHAIR	**LATERAL DECUBITUS**
COMPLICATIONS	• Neurapraxia: lesser occipital (1), great auricular (4), hypoglossal (1), LFCN (4), ulnar, and common peroneal nerve • DVT (5) • PE (1) • Ischemic brain/ spinal cord injury • Asystolic cardiac arrest • Ventricular tachycardia and cardiogenic shock • Unilateral vision loss and ophthalmoplegia • Subcutaneous emphysema, pneumomediastinum, and tension pneumothorax	• Neurapraxia: dorsal sensory branch radial (3), musculocutaneous (2), ulnar (1), axillary (1), and common peroneal nerves • Contralateral brachial plexus neurapraxia (1) • Stroke (1) • DVT (8) • PE (5) • Airway obstruction

ETIOLOGY

The etiology of complications due to positioning is often known; however, the cause of some complications remains unknown. There were 15 total cases of DVT reported following shoulder arthroscopy. Of those, 10 where in patients placed in the lateral decubitus position while 5 occurred in patients placed in the beach chair position. Ten patients or 67% of documented cases had known risk factors (7 of 10 in lateral decubitus and 3 of 5 in beach chair position). Pohl and Cullen[36] found that for patients undergoing arthroscopic shoulder surgery in the beach chair position, infarcts of the posterior cerebral circulation were caused by neck rotation or hyperextension that reduced vertebral artery blood flow. Neurapraxias following arthroscopic shoulder surgery usually have an identifiable cause such as malpositioning, traction, and/or portal placement. The use of both longitudinal and vertical traction can cause decreased limb perfusion.[6,45] Klein et al[46] found that 45 degrees of forward flexion combined with either 90 degrees or 0 degrees of abduction allowed for maximal intra-articular visibility while minimizing strain on the brachial plexus. To further minimize strain on the brachial plexus, it is recommended that no more than 15 to 20 pounds of traction be used.[47,48] Three cases of neurapraxia of the dorsal sensory branch of the radial nerve were caused by inadequate padding of the extremity at the wrist.[37] Peroneal nerve injuries can be attributed to failure to adequately pad the fibular head. Ulnar nerve injuries in the beach chair position are due to inadequate padding of the contralateral elbow during positioning. LFCN palsy can occur in either the beach chair or lateral decubitus position and is due to inadequate padding during positioning. Specifically, in the beach chair position, LFCN neurapraxia is due to excessive hip flexion. Patients with a BMI more than 30 kg/m^2 have a statistically significant higher risk for developing a LFCN palsy.[49] Levy et al[50] recommend 45 degrees of hip flexion with thick foam padding between the abdominal pannus and the thigh plus an additional foam pad underneath a wide restraining belt to prevent LFCN palsy in patients undergoing shoulder arthroscopy in the beach chair position. Three cases of great auricular nerve neurapraxia were due to the use of a horseshoe headrest while another case of dual great auricular plus lesser occipital nerve neurapraxia was attributed to a combination of head and neck rotation in addition to compression by the head strap. With patients in the lateral decubitus position, the axillary and musculocutaneous nerves are at increased risk for injury with the anterolateral portal placement.[8]

The 2 cases of sudden ventricular tachycardia and subsequent development of cardiogenic shock occurred following an infusion of irrigation that contained epinephrine. The documented case of airway obstruction occurred due to extra-articular spread of arthroscopic irrigation fluid while the patient was in the lateral decubitus position. Furthermore, individuals with abdominal obesity are at increased risk of hypotension as compression of the vena cava while in the upright position will cause decreased venous return.[51]

AUTHORS' PREFERRED TREATMENT WITH PEARLS

The authors' preferred technique for shoulder arthroscopy depends on the procedure. For patients undergoing rotator cuff repair, the senior author prefers the beach chair position, while for patients needing a labral repair, he prefers to use the lateral decubitus position.

Beach Chair Positioning

Prior to the patient being brought back to the operating room, the anesthesia team performs an interscalene nerve block in the preoperative holding area. The patient is placed supine on the operating table. General endotracheal anesthesia is induced with the endotracheal tube taped to the opposite side of the mouth as the surgical shoulder. A foam face mask is then placed over the patient's forehead and chin, and the straps are then affixed to the operating table headrest. Sequential compression devices are also placed on the patient's legs to help prevent DVT. A pillow is placed beneath the patient's knees in the popliteal fossa. The patient is adjusted on the table such that the hip joint is at the level of the break in the bed and the shoulders are slightly above the shoulder pad. The shoulder pad part of the table is then slid toward the contralateral shoulder. The operating table is next adjusted using the controller. The bed is placed into the Trendelenburg position and the knees are flexed to about 30 degrees. The patient is then raised into the upright beach chair position. This is done with the help of the anesthesia team to ensure the patient does not become hypotensive and to protect the endotracheal tube. The patient's head is then adjusted in the head holder such that the head and neck are in a neutral position. The contralateral arm is placed on an armrest with the wrist in neutral position and extra padding placed at the elbow to protect the ulnar nerve. A safety belt is placed over the patient's legs with a blanket or foam padding first placed between the legs and the belt. A lower extremity inflatable warming blanket is placed over the patient's legs. An arm holder is then affixed to the ipsilateral side of the operating table. The arm is then prepped and draped in the usual sterile fashion. Key steps for positioning are listed in Table 1-4 while pictures of key steps are placed in Figure 1-1. Pearls and pitfalls of beach chair positioning are included in Table 1-5 with associated pictures in Figure 1-2.

TABLE 1-4. KEY POSITIONING STEPS FOR THE BEACH CHAIR POSITION
1. Position patient on bed with shoulders at level with the top of the bed
2. Place side boards to secure the patient on the table
3. Place foam mask over forehead and chin
4. Have anesthesia secure endotracheal tube on contralateral side of mouth
5. Place pillow beneath knees and sequential compression devices on patient's legs
6. Place bed in Trendelenburg and drop foot of bed 30 degrees
7. Sit patient upright and adjust head/neck to a neutral position
8. Place arm board under nonoperative arm and pad the ulnar nerve
9. Turn bed 90 degrees
10. Attach arm holder to operative side of bed
11. Prep and drape extremity with standard sterile technique

Lateral Decubitus Positioning

Prior to the patient being brought back to the operating room, the anesthesia team performs an interscalene nerve block in the preoperative holding area. The patient is placed supine on the operating table with a beanbag placed beneath the patient's torso, and general endotracheal anesthesia is induced. Sequential compression devices are placed on the patient's legs to help prevent DVT. With coordination from anesthesia, the patient is then turned onto their nonoperative side. Blankets are placed beneath the head to ensure the neck is in neutral. The contralateral arm is forward flexed so that it is not compressed and it is placed on an arm board. An axillary roll is then placed under chest wall. The edges of the beanbag are then lifted up to cover the front and back of the patient to maintain stability in the lateral position. The breasts, genitals, and other bony prominences are then checked to ensure that they are not compressed from the beanbag. The beanbag is then attached to vacuum suction to stabilize both the beanbag and the patient. Attention is next turned to the legs. The bottom leg is slightly flexed at the hip and knee. Foam padding is placed beneath the bottom leg at the knee (to protect the common peroneal nerve) and at the ankle to decrease pressure on the bony prominences. A pillow is next placed between the legs. A blanket is then placed over the torso, and 2 to 3 pieces of heavy cloth tape are placed over the torso to secure the patient in place. A lower extremity

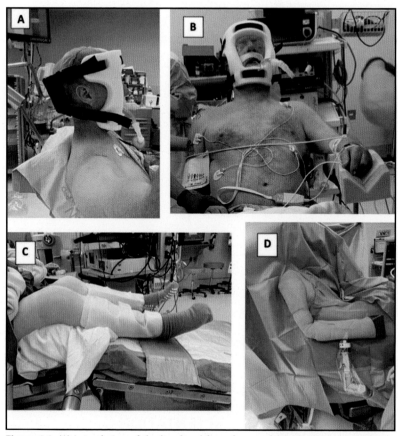

Figure 1-1. (A) Lateral view of the head and foam face mask. Notice how the neck is in neutral and the head holder is securing the occiput. (B) The foam face holder is placed over the chin and forehead, and the endotracheal tube is taped to the contralateral side of the mouth by anesthesia. Also notice that the nonoperative arm is gently resting in an arm holder with a foam cushion protecting the ulnar nerve. (C) A pillow is placed beneath the knees, and sequential compression devices are placed on both legs. (D) The operative arm is placed into a foam arm holder after the extremity is prepped with ChloraPrep (BD). The arm holder then articulates with the shoulder positioner. Coban (3M) is then used to wrap the arm in the foam holder with care taken to place the Coban around the arm proximal to the foam arm holder to ensure that the arm does not fall out of the arm holder.

TABLE 1-5. PEARLS AND PITFALLS OF THE BEACH CHAIR POSITION

PEARLS	PITFALLS
• Position patients the same way each case to avoid variability between cases • Adequately pad the elbows to avoid ulnar nerve injury • Keep the head and neck in neutral to prevent cervical neurapraxia • Flex hips to 45 degrees and pad the thighs to prevent LFCN nerve injury (especially important in patients with obesity)	• Cerebral hypoperfusion is a rare but known risk—consider monitoring cerebral oxygenation intraoperatively • Expensive equipment • Setup time-consuming

inflatable warming blanket is placed over the patient's legs. An "A-frame" pulley system is then affixed to the contralateral side of the bed at the level of the feet. The arm is then prepped and draped in the usual sterile fashion. Key steps for positioning are listed in Table 1-6, while pictures of key steps are placed in Figure 1-3. Pearls and pitfalls of beach chair positioning are included in Table 1-7 with associated pictures in Figure 1-4.

CASE PRESENTATION

A 50-year-old right-hand–dominant woman was seen in the sports medicine clinic for evaluation of right shoulder pain. She reports her pain began 9 months prior to presentation in clinic while she was horseback riding. She states that the jolting of the right shoulder for many hours caused acute pain. While doing yoga the following day, she developed sharp pain in the shoulder during a plank. Since then, the pain has been progressively worsening. She localizes the pain to the area anterior aspect of the shoulder that is made worse with behind-the-back movement and swimming. Her pain is improved with rest and minimal motion. The patient underwent a course of formal physical therapy for 3 months with minimal relief of her pain. She denied any prior injury or surgery to the right shoulder. She works as an operating room nurse. The patient is also a triathlete and is eager to get back to her races.

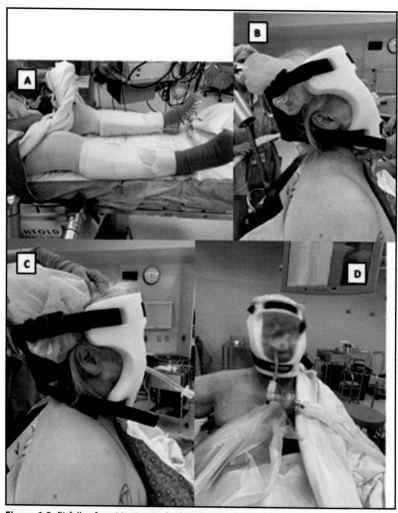

Figure 1-2. Pitfalls of positioning in the beach chair. (A) Do not leave the knees extended. They need to be flexed about 45 degrees. Padding should be placed under the heels. (B, C) Do not flex or extend the neck. It should be in neutral position when visualizing the patient from the side. (D) The white foam padding should rest on the forehead and chin, not below the chin. Ensure anesthesia secures the endotracheal tube on the contralateral side from the operative extremity.

TABLE 1-6. KEY POSITIONING STEPS FOR THE LATERAL DECUBITUS POSITION

1. Place beanbag properly on operating table
2. Synchronize effort to roll patient into lateral decubitus position with anesthesia stabilizing the head
3. Extend nonoperative arm and place axillary roll
4. Slightly flex bottom and place padding beneath both the bottom leg and between the legs
5. Inflate beanbag
6. Place blanket over patient followed by tape to secure patient
7. Turn bed 90 degrees
8. Affix traction device to the bed
9. Prep and drape extremity with standard sterile technique

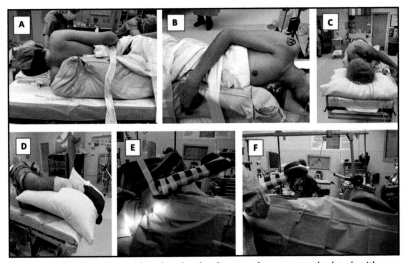

Figure 1-3. (A) Blankets are placed under the donut pad to support the head, with care taken to ensure the neck is at neutral. (B) A blanket is placed over the patient's torso and cloth tape is then used to secure the patient within the beanbag. (C) The ideal position of the patient is leaning 30 degrees posterior from upright. (D) The fibular head is padded with a soft gel pad or egg crate, and pillows are placed between the knees. (E, F) After the operative arm is prepped, a sterile stockinette is placed and wrapped with Coban. The patient's operative arm is then placed into a foam arm holder and attached to the traction tower with no more than 10 to 15 pounds of traction applied.

TABLE 1-7. PEARLS AND PITFALLS OF THE LATERAL DECUBITUS POSITION

PEARLS	PITFALLS
• Ensure adequate padding of genitals, areolae, and all bony prominences to avoid pressure injuries from beanbag • Pad the lateral knee of the "down leg" to protect the common peroneal nerve • Do not use more than 10 to 15 pounds of traction • Place portals under direct visualization to prevent neurovascular injury • Position patients the same way each case to avoid variability between cases	• DVT—use SCDs • Compression neurapraxias can occur from failure to pad nerves • Pressure injuries to soft tissues are possible from failure to pad bony prominences • Traction neurapraxia

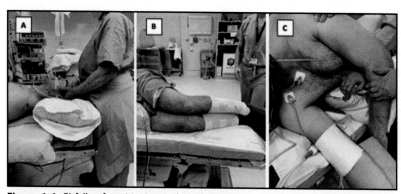

Figure 1-4. Pitfalls of positioning in lateral decubitus. (A) The beanbag is improperly placed. The top of the beanbag should not be placed more proximal than the axilla. (B) The fibular head is unpadded, and there is no padding between the legs. Padding needs to be placed under the fibular head to protect the common peroneal nerve. Furthermore, pillows need to be placed between the legs. (C) The axillary roll should be placed under the chest wall, not beneath the down arm or axilla.

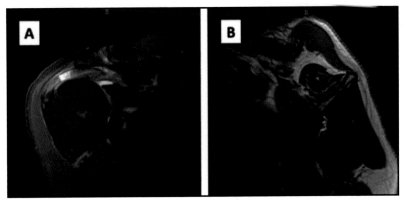

Figure 1-5. (A) Coronal T2 magnetic resonance imaging (MRI) of the right shoulder demonstrating a full-thickness supraspinatus tear at the musculotendinous junction. (B) Sagittal T1 MRI of the right shoulder demonstrating Goutallier grade II fatty degeneration of the supraspinatus muscle.

On physical exam, the patient had pain and weakness with empty can testing in addition to difficulty with forward flexion, abduction, and external rotation of the right arm. Magnetic resonance imaging of the right shoulder (Figure 1-5) demonstrated a full-thickness supraspinatus tear at the musculotendinous junction. The patient underwent an arthroscopic rotator cuff repair in the beach chair position. She was seen at her 2-week postoperative visit and found to have right ear numbness. She was diagnosed with right great auricular nerve palsy likely due to the head straps (Figure 1-6). At her 3-month follow-up appointment, her ear numbness had fully resolved.

CONCLUSION

When comparing patient positioning for shoulder arthroscopy, the data regarding efficacy, efficiency of setup, and risks of beach chair and lateral decubitus positioning fail to demonstrate superiority of one position over another. The advantages and disadvantages of both positions have been described. The decision to perform shoulder arthroscopy in either the beach chair or lateral decubitus position is often based on surgeon preference, including the purpose of the procedure (ie, rotator cuff repair vs Bankart repair) and surgeon level of comfort with each patient position.

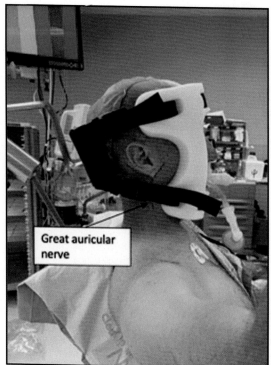

Figure 1-6. Diagram of the great auricular nerve and its branches (red lines). The great auricular nerve is derived from the cervical plexus, specifically branches of C2 and C3. It becomes superficial at the Erbs point just posterior to the sternocleidomastoid muscle, where it then proceeds to travel proximally up the neck toward the skull. It provides sensation to the outer ear.

Great auricular nerve

Complications due to patient positioning in shoulder arthroscopy are very rare. Known complications from arthroscopic shoulder surgery include neurapraxias, DVT, and cerebral hypoperfusion. When complications due occur, they are usually transient issues that fully resolve; however, serious complications can occur. Specific to the lateral decubitus position, complications include traction injuries, anesthesia airway difficulties, and thromboembolic events. The beach chair position also has known complications ranging from neurapraxias to cerebral hypoperfusion and even infarct. During the positioning process, it is imperative to adequately pad all nerves and bony prominences to prevent injury. Furthermore, cerebral oxygenation monitoring is recommended for high-risk patients undergoing arthroscopic shoulder surgery in the beach chair position. Overall, arthroscopic shoulder surgery is a safe procedure regardless if performed in the beach chair or lateral position.

REFERENCES

1. Jain NB, Higgins LD, Losina E, Collins J, Blazar PE, Katz JN. Epidemiology of musculoskeletal upper extremity ambulatory surgery in the United States. *BMC Musculoskeletal Disorders.* 2014;15:4.

2. Friedman DJ, Parnes NZ, Zimmer Z, Higgins LD, Warner JJ. Prevalence of cerebrovascular events during shoulder surgery and association with patient position. *Orthopedics.* 2009;32(4):256-260.

3. Papadonikolakis A, Wiesler ER, Olympio MA, Poehling GG. Avoiding catastrophic complications of stroke and death related to shoulder surgery in the sitting position. *Arthroscopy.* 2008;24:481-482.

4. Peruto CM, Ciccotti MG, Cohen SB. Shoulder arthroscopy positioning: lateral decubitus versus beach chair. *Arthroscopy.* 2009;25(8):891-896.

5. Li X, Eichinger JK, Hartshorn T, Zhou H, Matzkin EG, Warner JP. A comparison of the lateral decubitus and beach-chair positions for shoulder surgery: advantages and complications. *J Am Acad Orthop Surg.* 2015;23:18-28.

6. Phillips BB. Arthroscopy of the upper extremity. In: Canale ST, Beaty JH, eds. *Campbell's Operative Orthopaedics.* 11th ed. CV Mosby Elsevier; 2008:2923-2926.

7. Skyhar MJ, Altchek DW, Warren RF, Wickiewicz TL, O'Brien SJ. Shoulder arthroscopy with the patient in the beach-chair position. *Arthroscopy.* 1988;4:256-259.

8. Gelber PE, Reina F, Caceres E, Monllau JC. A comparison of risk between the lateral decubitus and the beach-chair position when establishing an anteroinferior shoulder portal: a cadaveric study. *Arthroscopy.* 2007;23:522-528.

9. Matthews LS, Zarins B, Michael RH, Helfet DL. Anterior portal selection for shoulder arthroscopy. *Arthroscopy.* 1985;1:33-39.

10. Cullen D, Kirby R. Beach chair position may decrease cerebral perfusion: catastrophic outcomes have occurred. *APSF Newsletter.* 2007;22(2):25-27.

11. Weber SC, Abrams JS, Nottage WM. Complications associated with arthroscopic shoulder surgery. *Arthroscopy.* 2002;18(2)(suppl 1):88-95.

12. Andrews JR, Carson WG Jr, Ortega K. Arthroscopy of the shoulder: technique and normal anatomy. *Am J Sports Med.* 1984;12(1):1-7.

13. Ogilvie-Harris DJ, Wiley AM. Arthroscopic surgery of the shoulder: a general appraisal. *J Bone Joint Surg Br.* 1986;68(2):201-207.

14. Pitman MI, Nainzadeh N, Ergas E, Springer S. The use of somatosensory evoked potentials for detection of neuropraxia during shoulder arthroscopy. *Arthroscopy.* 1988;4:250-255.

15. Small NC. Complications in arthroscopic surgery performed by experienced arthroscopists. *Arthroscopy.* 1988;4:215-221.

16. Small NC. Complications in arthroscopy: the knee and other joints. *Arthroscopy.* 1986;2:253-258.

17. Schick CW, Westermann RW, Gao Y, ACESS Group, Wolf BR. Thromboembolism following shoulder arthroscopy. *Orthop J Sports Med.* 2014;2(11):2325967114559506.

18. Kuremsky MA, Cain EL Jr, Fleischli JE. Thromboembolic phenomena after arthroscopic shoulder surgery. *Arthroscopy.* 2011;27(12):1614-1619.

19. Park TS, Kim YS. Neuropraxia of the cutaneous nerve of the cervical plexus after shoulder arthroscopy. *Arthroscopy.* 2005;21(5):631.

20. Ng Ak, Page RS. Greater auricular nerve neuropraxia with beach chair positioning during shoulder surgery. *Int J Shoulder Surg.* 2010;4(2):48-50.

21. Mullins RC, Drez D Jr, Cooper J. Hypoglossal nerve palsy after arthroscopy of the shoulder and open operation with the patient in the beach-chair position: a case report. *J Bone Joint Surg Am.* 1992;74(1):137–139.
22. Levy BJ, Tauberg BM, Holtzman AJ, Gruson KI. Reducing lateral femoral cutaneous nerve palsy in obese patients in the beach chair position: effect of a standardized positioning and padding protocol. *J Am Acad Orthop Surg.* 2019;27:437–443.
23. Satin AM, DePalma AA, Cuellar J, Gruson KI. Lateral femoral cutaneous nerve palsy following shoulder surgery in the beach chair position: a report of 4 cases. *Am J Orthop.* 2014;43:e206–e209.
24. Bongiovanni SL, Ranalletta M, Guala A, Maignon GD. Case reports: heritable thrombophilia associated with deep venous thrombosis after shoulder arthroscopy. *Clin Orthop Relat Res.* 2009;467(8):2196–2199.
25. Creighton RA, Cole BJ. Upper extremity deep vein thrombosis after shoulder arthroscopy: a case report. *J Shoulder Elbow Surg.* 2007;16(1):e20–e22.
26. Cortes ZE, Hammerman SM, Gartsman GM. Pulmonary embolism after shoulder arthroscopy: could patient positioning and traction make a difference? *J Shoulder Elbow Surg.* 2007;16(2):e16–e17.
27. Bhatti MT, Enneking FK. Visual loss and ophthalmoplegia after shoulder surgery. *Anesth Analg.* 2003;96(3):899–902.
28. D'Alessio JG, Weller RS, Rosenblum M. Activation of the Bezold-Jarish reflex in the sitting position for shoulder arthroscopy using interscalene block. *Anesth Analg.* 1995;80(6):1158–1162.
29. Cho SH, Yi JW, Kwack YH, Park SW, Kim MK, Rhee YG. Ventricular tachycardia during arthroscopic shoulder surgery: a report of two cases. *Arch Orthop Trauma Surg.* 2010;130(3):353–356.
30. Lee HC, Dewan N, Crosby L. Subcutaneous emphysema, pneumomediastinum, and potentially life-threatening tension pneumothorax: pulmonary complications from arthroscopic shoulder decompression. *Chest.* 1992;101(5):1256–1267.
31. Terry MA, Altchek DW. Diagnostic shoulder arthroscopy technique: beach chair position. In: Tibone JE, Savoie FH III, Shaffer BS, eds. *Shoulder Arthroscopy.* Springer-Verlag; 2003:9–15.
32. Liguori GA, Kahn RL, Gordon J, Gordan MA, Urban MK. The use of metoprolol and glycopyrrolate to prevent hypotensive/bradycardic events during shoulder arthroscopy in the sitting position under interscalene block. *Anesth Analg.* 1998;87:1320–1325.
33. Pant S, Bokor DJ, Low AK. Cerebral oxygenation using near-infrared spectroscopy in the beach-chair position during shoulder arthroscopy under general anesthesia. *Arthroscopy.* 2014;30:1520–1527.
34. Salazar D, Sears BW, Aghdasi B, et al. Cerebral desaturation events during shoulder arthroscopy in the beach chair position: patient risk factors and neurocognitive effects. *J Shoulder Elbow Surg.* 2013;22:1228–1235.
35. Songy CE, Seigel ER, Stevens M, Wilkinson JT, Ahmadi S. The effect of beach-chair position angle on cerebral oxygenation during shoulder surgery. *J Shoulder Elbow Surg.* 2017;26:1670–1675.
36. Pohl A, Cullen DJ. Cerebral ischemia during shoulder surgery in the upright position: a case series. *J Clin Anesth.* 2005;17(6):463–469.
37. Ellman H. Arthroscopic subacromial decompression: analysis of one- to three-year results. *Arthroscopy.* 1987;3(3):173–181.
38. Gartsman GM. Arthroscopic acromioplasty for lesions of the rotator cuff. *J Bone Joint Surg Am.* 1990;72:169–180.
39. Paulos LE, Franklin JL. Arthroscopic shoulder decompression development and application: a five year experience. *Am J Sports Med.* 1990;18(3):235–244.

40. Hynson JM, Tung A, Guevara JE, Katz JA, Glick JM, Shapiro WA. Complete airway obstruction during arthroscopic shoulder surgery. *Anesth Analg.* 1993;76(4):875–878.
41. Edgar R, Nagda S, Huffman R, Namdari S. Pulmonary embolism after shoulder arthroscopy. *Orthopedics.* 2012;35(11):e1673–e1676.
42. Burkhart SS. Deep venous thrombosis after shoulder arthroscopy. *Arthroscopy.* 1990;6(1):61–63.
43. Garofalo R, Notarnicola A, Moretti L, Moretti B, Marini S, Castagna A. Deep vein thromboembolism after arthroscopy of the shoulder: two case reports and a review of the literature. *BMC Musculoskelet Disord.* 2010;11:65.
44. Zeidan A, Bluwi M, Elshamaa K. Postoperative brain stroke after shoulder arthroscopy in the lateral decubitus position. *J Stroke Cerebrovasc Dis.* 2014;23(2):384–386.
45. Hennrikus WL, Mapes RC, Bratton MW, Lapoint JM. Lateral traction during shoulder arthroscopy: its effect on tissue perfusion measured by pulse oximetry. *Am J Sports Med.* 1995;23:444–446.
46. Klein AH, France JC, Mutschler TA, Fu FH. Measurement of brachial plexus strain in arthroscopy of the shoulder. *Arthroscopy.* 1987;3:45–52.
47. Jinnah AH, Mannava S, Plate JF, Stone AV, Freehill MT. Basic shoulder arthroscopy: lateral decubitus patient positioning. *Arthroscopy Techniques.* 2016;5(5):e1069–e1075.
48. Hamamoto JT, Frank RM, Higgins JD, Provencher MT, Romeo AA, Verma NN. Shoulder arthroscopy in the lateral decubitus position. *Arthroscopy Techniques.* 2017;6(4):e1169–e1175.
49. Holtzman AJ, Glezos CD, Feit EJ, Gruson KI. Prevalence and risk factors for lateral femoral cutaneous nerve palsy in the beach chair position. *Arthroscopy.* 2017;33:1958–1962.
50. Levy BJ, Tauberg BM, Holtzman AJ, Gruson KI. Reducing lateral femoral cutaneous nerve palsy in obese patients in the beach chair position: effect of a standardized positioning and padding protocol. *J Am Acad Orthop Surg.* 2019;27(12):437–443.
51. Bonner KF. Patient positioning, portal placement, normal arthroscopic anatomy, and diagnostic arthroscopy. In: Cole BJ, Sekiya JK, eds. *Surgical Techniques of the Shoulder, Elbow, and Knee in Sports Medicine.* WB Saunders Elsevier; 2008:3–5.

2

Fluid Extravasation

Jane H. O'Connor, MD; Emmanuel N. Osadebey, MD;
Rolanda A. Willacy, MD; Ibrahim M. Khaleel, MD;
and Robert H. Wilson, MD

INTRODUCTION

Arthroscopy involves the infusion of water-based fluid into a joint or potential space in order for enhanced visualization and surgical procedures. Fluid extravasation is the flow or injection of fluid into undesired areas, such as the interstitial spaces or beyond the surgical environment. This can be fairly common, but resultant complications related to this are rare. Fluid extravasation as a complication of arthroscopic shoulder surgery was first described in 1990.[1-4] As stated, it may result in edema to the chest wall, neck, and face, which could result in respiratory compromise. Also, an excess amount of fluid injected into tissues may lead to electrolyte imbalance and hematologic abnormalities. The sequelae could result in potential organ dysfunction, failure, and possibly death, if not managed expeditiously, although a catastrophic event or death resulting from fluid extravasation after shoulder arthroscopy has not yet been described in current literature.

Thompson TL, ed.
Arthroscopic Shoulder Surgery:
Complications and Management (pp 21-32).
© 2022 Taylor & Francis Group.

As fluid extravasation is a common, well-documented phenomenon of shoulder arthroscopy, it is mostly asymptomatic and resolves within 12 hours.[5] Patients may experience minor residual effects such as mild weight gain or a drop in hematocrit as the extravasated fluid is absorbed slowly into the circulatory system and eventually excreted.[6] Uncommonly, however, fluid extravasation resulting from shoulder arthroscopy may cause multiple complications. Airway compromise, rhabdomyolysis, neurovascular injury, and iatrogenic tendon or cartilage injury have been described in the current literature.[4] The incidence of these complications varies depending on their clinical recognition, and a number of procedure-specific (surgery complexity, irrigation fluid pressure, etc), surgeon-specific (surgeon experience, patient positioning, etc), and patient-specific factors should be considered. In turn, the prognosis and management of these complications vary widely based on the severity of symptoms.

ETIOLOGY

Extravasation is the leakage of fluid out of its intended space, that is, in shoulder arthroscopy—outside of the joint space and into the interstitial and potential spaces. As pressurized fluid is introduced into the surgical space, the excess volume and pressure force the fluid into cells for absorption in the patient's tissues. And as irrigation continues, cells reach their maximum absorptive rate and the tissues are overwhelmed, which results in edema, as shown in Figure 2-1. The swelling collapses the spaces the fluid was initially intended to inflate, which then interferes with the procedure. Therefore, shoulder arthroscopy is typically limited to approximately 90 to 120 minutes.[7]

Extravasation injuries are caused by an efflux of fluid, mostly saline, leading to damage of the surrounding tissue spaces. Shoulder arthroscopy has grown in its popularity and is being performed more than ever before for a variety of indications.[8] While many complications associated with shoulder arthroscopy are procedure specific (eg, capsular necrosis following a thermal capsulorrhaphy), fluid extravasation exists as an uncommon, but potentially severe complication generalized to any procedure performed arthroscopically.[5] This surgery is "minimally invasive," wherein incisions are created to allow for introduction of surgical instruments to allow for visualization. Once inserted, pressurized fluid is used to inflate the area to improve visualization and allow for greater surgical exposure for the procedure. This pressurized fluid, however, can leak around surgical portals and collect in extracapsular soft tissue, resulting in edema.[6]

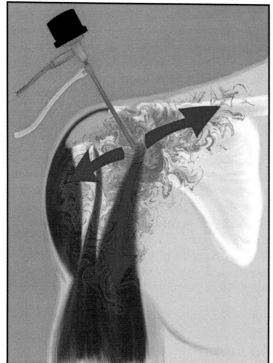

Figure 2-1. Illustration showing potential directions of fluid extravasation. (Illustrated by and reproduced with permission from Tiffany M. O'Connor.)

Edema can be problematic for a number of reasons. Most immediately of which, the resultant swelling can interfere with the ongoing procedure— oftentimes limiting the time allowed within the joint space for surgical intervention. As such, many studies point to a correlation between factors that increase surgical duration (including procedure complexity and surgeon experience) and complication rates.[9] In addition, postoperative tissue swelling can compress local structures and give rise to long-term complications. Significant weight gain (correlated to the amount of arthroscopy fluid used), compartment syndrome and resultant rhabdomyolysis (from compression of adjacent muscle microcirculation), and airway compromise are just a few of these complications described in the current literature.[5,10,11]

Anatomy-Based Etiology

The glenohumeral joint is encompassed by a capsule that protects and stabilizes the joint. Surgical procedures that involve altering the integrity of the capsule, such as partial resection of the capsule, allow for fluid to dissect into the surrounding extra-articular tissues.[12] Additionally, the subacromial space also allows for fluid extravasation. The morphology of the subacromial space contains incomplete encapsulation, resulting in communication between the surrounding tissues in various anatomic planes.[13,14]

Anatomic variants in the shoulder involving the neck, thorax, and infraspinous fossa have been described as causes of extravasation. A report by Edwards et al[12] described a patient with an abnormal communication between the shoulder joint and the supraspinatus, allowing for fluid to travel via the spinoglenoid notch and suprascapular notch to the infraspinous fossa and neck. *Gray's Anatomy* describes anatomic variants in the shoulder that augment fluid dissection from the shoulder joint due to increased patency.[12] Other reported suppositions include pathologic tears in the parascapular musculature, "loose subcutaneous tissue," and iatrogenic lesions.[13,15]

Procedural-Based Etiology

The very nature of arthroscopy allows for the opportunity for a surplus of fluid to accumulate in the surrounding tissues. Overuse of these fluids due to high pump pressures, prolonged surgical time, and/or limited surgeon experience portends possible fluid extravasation. As such, a number of procedural-based mechanisms can potentiate fluid extravasation, which can lead to further complication. An example of the equipment setup is shown in Figure 2-2.

Factors Prognosticating Arthroscopic Complications

Fluid extravasation and its resultant complications occur depending on a number of factors both procedure and surgeon specific. The current research, however, consistently identifies high irrigation fluid pressures, large volumes of arthroscopic fluid used, and extended operative times as the most significant factors in predicting a high risk of these complications.[16]

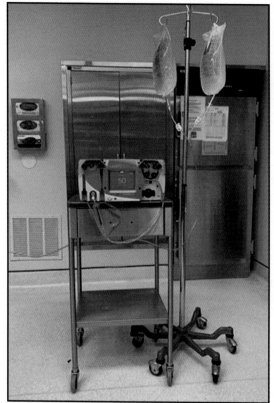

Figure 2-2. Arthroscopy pump with safety features to minimize risk of extravasation, including presets to maintain optimal joint distension and real-time pressure readings.

In a study reviewing 22 cases of arthroscopic subacromial decompression, Morrison et al[16] found a direct correlation between systolic blood pressure, subacromial space pressure, and surgical field clarity. They observed that maintaining an average pressure difference of 49 mm Hg or less between systolic and subacromial space pressures both prevented bleeding and permitted good visualization; greater pressure differences resulted in significant bleeding. The study further advocated the use of hypotensive anesthetics to allow for lower irrigation pressures, thus reducing the risk of fluid extravasation.[16]

A subsequent study performed by Sperber and Wredmark[10] found that irrigation pump and resultant bursal pressures of 150 mm Hg yielded intramuscular pressures of 40 to 60 mm Hg in the supraspinatus and deltoid muscles. The study found that these values, being nearly equal to critical muscle perfusion pressures, resulted in an increased risk of affecting muscle microcirculation in procedures exceeding 25 minutes.[10] Given these findings, 150 mm Hg has resultantly been observed as a maximum for irrigation pump pressures in an effort to avoid compromising extracapsular muscle perfusion.[10]

Despite the extensive investigation on this subject, there remains no definitive upper limit to the amount of irrigation fluid to be used during shoulder arthroscopy to prevent fluid extravasation. However, studies exploring this phenomenon and its complications in symptomatic patients report volumes typically ranging from 20 to 36 L.[2,18,19] Through these previous reports, it can be extrapolated that surgeons should attempt to use irrigation fluid volumes less than 20 L when performing shoulder arthroscopic procedures as an added precaution until more definitive limits can be determined. Operative times should also be curtailed without compromising surgical accuracy in an attempt to reduce the total amount of irrigation fluid used.

Patient Positioning

During an arthroscopic shoulder procedure, patients can be situated in a variety of positions based on the surgeon's preference and/or the nature of the procedure. Positioning of the patient can provide challenges in maneuvering and visualization during the procedure, which in turn can lead to overinflation of the potential space with pressurized fluid. Memon et al[13] investigated patient positioning during shoulder arthroscopy procedures and reported that fluid extravasation occurred in patients positioned in the lateral decubitus position and the beach chair position. Of the 205 patients included in the study, 134 were placed in the lateral decubitus position vs 63 patients placed in the beach chair position. The fluid extravasation rate was noted to be higher in the lateral decubitus position, possibly due to the gravity-assisted movement of fluid, although superiority of one method of positioning over the other is still under debate.[19,20] Also, placement of surgical pads around the neck has been reported as possibly causing large amounts of fluid extravasation in the neck as well.[13,15,18]

Regional Block

There is no specific literature regarding the correlation of regional anesthesia and fluid extravasation. Clearly, the application of a regional block should have an effect on the soft tissue response to arthroscopic fluid infusion. However, the combination of excessive fluid extravasation on the anesthetized brachial plexus should be considered. Conclusions about problems related to regional anesthesia are speculative and require more serious investigation.

Fluid Pressure

As it is pressurized fluid that is introduced into the joint, this increased pressure could predicate the resultant edema, which can further lead to fluid extravasation. Memon et al[13] noted that patients with a large range of pump pressure (29 to 150 mm Hg) during their procedures were found to have a larger rate of fluid extravasation as a complication. Thus, the accurate measurement of the intra-articular fluid pressure is vital in controlling this outcome. While a variety of fluid pumps are available, the accuracy of these pumps comes into question. Mayo et al[21] compared a number of commercial arthroscopic pumps vs a gravity feed system to measure joint compliance and found that the gravity feed system was the most accurate modality.

With continued irrigation of the joint space during arthroscopy, the postoperative fluid that may collect or extravasate is usually absorbed slowly into the circulatory system and eventually excreted. While this process oftentimes proceeds without complication, it may result in weight gain or a drop in the patient's hematocrit. Lo et al[5] evaluated which factors affect this phenomenon in a cohort study of patients undergoing shoulder arthroscopy for various shoulder conditions. The study consisted of 53 patients with a mean volume of irrigation fluid of 30 ± 24 L and a mean surgical time of 91.2 ± 45 minutes and revealed any tense swelling that developed after surgery resolved within 30 to 45 minutes, and there was a net weight gain of 8.7 ± 3.9 pounds of which 4.2 ± 3.8 pounds was attributable to the fluid from the procedure. Factors affecting weight gain were identified as surgical time, amount of arthroscopy fluid used, rotator cuff tear size, number of procedures, and total number of anchors used.[5] Of these factors, surgical time and volume of fluid used were most easily controlled by the surgeon.

In addition to weight gain, there was also a question as to whether postoperative fluid absorption could affect a patient's cardiovascular physiology. Smith and Shah[6] investigated this relationship in 40 patients undergoing shoulder arthroscopy. With a mean time for surgery of 27.4 minutes (11 ± 2) and a mean fluid use of 3.2 ± 2.2 L, patients exhibited a hemoglobin and hematocrit decrement of 0.6 ± 0.5 g/dL and $1.5\% \pm 1.5\%$, respectively. While this study did not find a significant change in circulating volume following arthroscopic surgery, further research is needed to assess the effect extravasated fluid reabsorption has on older patients and when using greater volumes of arthroscopic fluid.[6]

POTENTIAL COMPLICATIONS

During an arthroscopic procedure, as fluid is pumped into the shoulder, the surplus of fluid by nature of gravity and vascularity has the potential to collect in the neck and arm. Excess fluid collecting in the neck, arm, and shoulder itself can result in a plethora of muscular, arterial, and neurologic manifestations and complications.

Increase in Neck, Chest, and Midarm Circumference

An overall increase in circumference of the neck, chest, and midarm has been noted, and Chiplonkar et al[1] investigated neck circumference of patients undergoing elective shoulder arthroscopy. This observational study focused on the changes in neck circumference of a total of 32 patients between 18 and 70 years old following an arthroscopic shoulder procedure. Neck circumference was measured at the level of the thyroid cartilage in the supine position before the administration of local anesthetic (combination of the 10 mL 2% lidocaine and 15 mL 0.5% bupivacaine).[1] The neck circumference was then measured again following the block and after the procedure, and the leak test was used to evaluate if there was airway edema. A negative leak test indicated extensive airway edema. Out of the 32 patients included in the study, only 2 patients displayed an average increase in neck circumference and a negative leak test and were thus kept intubated.[1]

Additionally, a prospective observational study was conducted by Bomberg[22] with 36 patients aged 15 to 60 years undergoing shoulder arthroscopy under general anesthesia. The patients were monitored with pulse oximeter (SpO_2), noninvasive blood pressure, and electrocardiograph, along with the temperature and endotracheal tube cuff pressure. The variables (neck, chest, midarm, and midthigh) were measured preoperatively for baseline values and following surgery. No patients demonstrated respiratory failure, but there were significant increases observed in the mean values of the neck, chest, midarm, and midthigh circumferences and weight.[22] The study concluded that regional and systemic absorption of irrigation fluid in arthroscopic shoulder surgery was reflected in the change in the variables and hemoglobin, despite not resulting in airway/respiratory compromise.[22]

Airway Compromise

A feared complication of fluid extravasation is airway compromise following shoulder arthroscopy, which can prove life-threatening if managed improperly. A majority of the literature surrounding this topic points to extracapsular tissue swelling leading to compression of the airway. Blumenthal[23] described one such case report wherein a patient undergoing arthroscopic repair of a rotator cuff rupture began to complain of breathing difficulties 110 minutes into the procedure. The patient displayed massive swelling of the left chest and anterior portion of neck, and oxygen saturation dropped below 50%. Resultant swelling prevented emergency intubation, and a cricothyroidotomy was performed to allow for orotracheal intubation.[23] Manjuladevi[11] described 3 separate case studies with similar complications. These studies involved repair of a subscapular tear and arthroscopic rotator cuff repair, which lasted a minimum of 4 hours with a minimum of 60 L of irrigation fluid. Each case resulted in edema of the chest and neck, airway compromise, and initial difficulty with intubation.[11]

As intubation difficulty appears as a recurring hindrance to rapid patient resuscitation, subsequent literature proposes preemptive measures such as the initial use of general anesthesia and endotracheal intubation to ensure a secure airway, as well as the use of hypotensive anesthetic agents to minimize the use of irrigation fluid intraoperatively in an effort to prevent this complication.[2] Additionally, if the patient is already intubated prior to surgery, the patency of the patient's airway should be assessed before extubation, as the airway can become obstructed after extubation.[15]

Rhabdomyolysis

Compartment syndrome due to fluid extravasation may arise as a complication from arthroscopic procedures. There are a few reported cases on the development of compartment syndrome following lower extremity arthroscopy using a mechanical fluid irrigation system. Bomberg[22] described 4 complicated cases of knee arthroscopy due to irrigation fluid extravasation, 2 of which developed symptoms of compartment syndrome that were subsequently treated with drainage. While this is an uncommon complication, compartment syndrome may develop in the upper extremity following shoulder arthroscopy. One such unique case was reported by Lim,[24] wherein a patient underwent arthroscopic shoulder stabilization and intraoperatively showed significant extravasation involving the right shoulder girdle and right hemithorax. The patient's condition declined. Urinary output decreased and creatine kinase levels elevated, consistent with rhabdomyolysis during the first postoperative day. Magnetic resonance imaging revealed diffuse swelling throughout the entire deltoid muscle as well as changes in proximal biceps, triceps, and brachialis muscles. The patient was subsequently treated with fluid management, electrolyte correction, intravenous furosemide, and hemodialysis.[24] Consequent cadaveric studies revealed that the deltoid is covered by a thin fascial layer in which extravasation fluid may accumulate subcutaneously, leading to significant muscular compression and myonecrosis.[23] Such cases draw attention to a need for close monitoring of the upper extremity and surrounding chest wall for signs of fluid accumulation as well as a judicious use of high-pressure infusion pumps when performing shoulder arthroscopy.

Arterial

There are no reports of arterial compromise, injury, or compression from excessive fluid extravasation. The ample arterial flow to the shoulder is via multiple conduits. The distal upper extremity arterial flow is provided through the axillary artery. It is well protected regardless of the surgical position of the patient. A great deal of fluid is required in order to compress the artery. Nevertheless, blood flow to the shoulder is abundant. Theoretically, compression could lead to a distal ischemic event. A remarkable injury to the axillary artery would require a significant deviation from the standard surgical approach.

Cerebral Edema and Brain Death

During arthroscopy, a 1.5% solution of glycine irrigation fluid is commonly used. The intravascular absorption of this solution may cause cardiovascular, neurologic, and visual disorders. Additionally, water intoxication also may lead to a fatal outcome as a result of cerebral edema. A rare case of unexplained death due to cerebral edema was reported in the literature in a patient who underwent shoulder arthroscopy, indicated for chronic pain of the shoulder.[25] Preoperatively, the patient's physical examination and routine laboratory measurements were normal (sodium: 141 mmol/L; potassium: 4.9 mmol/L; chloride: 104 mmol/L, protein: 75 g/L; hematocrit: 41%). During this procedure, 18 L of 1.5% glycine was infused during the 90-minute surgery and 500 mL of 10% glucose was administered. It was documented that subsequent to tracheal extubation, the patient complained of nausea. Physical examination yielded unremarkable results regarding cardiovascular instability or altered consciousness. However, examination of the shoulder demonstrated a significant increase in volume. However, 7.5 hours postoperatively, the patient developed severe bradypnea and lost consciousness. The patient recorded a Glasgow Coma Scale score of 3. Cerebral angiography confirmed the diagnosis of brain death, and autopsy demonstrated severe cerebral edema.[25]

CONCLUSION

It is clear that fluid extravasation is one of the most common consequences of shoulder arthroscopic surgery. The question remains, when does the consequence become a complication? A surgical complication is defined as an adverse event after a surgical procedure. That definition is quite ambiguous in the context of fluid extravasation. Fluid extravasation is nearly ubiquitous. The treatment for fluid extravasation effects is usually observation or respiratory support until the problem dissipates. The requirement for intervention is uncommon. For the purposes of this chapter, we have concluded fluid extravasation is a relevant complication when an intervention is documented in order to monitor or mitigate its effects.

We must consider the possibility that patients may have adverse effects that are not recognized. Therefore, we must be diligent to pay more attention to this surgical consequence and identify possible effects that may improve more rapidly with aggressive management. In the past, techniques have been devised in order to avoid such occurrences. For the future, we should consider even further what can be done in order to avoid any chance of fluid extravasation complications.

REFERENCES

1. Chiplonkar S, Pathak K, Chellam S. Change in neck circumference after shoulder arthroscopy: an observational study. *Indian J Anaesth.* 2015;59(6):365.
2. Gogia A, Bajaj J, Sahni A, Saigal D. Negative-pressure pulmonary edema in a patient undergoing shoulder arthroscopy. *Indian J Anaesth.* 2012;56(1):62.
3. Gupta S, Manjuladevi M, Vasudeva Upadhyaya KS, Kutappa AM, Amaravathi R, Arpana J. Effects of irrigation fluid in shoulder arthroscopy. *Indian J Anaesth.* 2016;60(3):194–198.
4. Ozhan MO, Suzer MA, Cekmen N, Caparlar CO, Eskin MB. Tracheal compression during shoulder arthroscopy in the beach-chair position. *Curr Ther Res Clin Exp.* 2010;71(6):408–415.
5. Lo IKY, Burkhart SS. Immediate postoperative fluid retention and weight gain after shoulder arthroscopy. *Arthroscopy.* 2005;21(5):605–610.
6. Smith CD, Shah MM. Fluid gain during routine shoulder arthroscopy. *J Shoulder Elbow Surg.* 2008;17(3):415–417.
7. Duralde XA. *Complications in Orthopaedics: Shoulder Arthroscopy, Severe Edema During Shoulder Arthroscopy.* American Academy of Orthopaedic Surgeons; 2008.

8. Vitale MA, Arons RR, Hurwitz S, Ahmad CS, Levine WN. The rising incidence of acromioplasty. *J Bone Joint Surg Am.* 2010;92:1842–1850.
9. Antonucci S, Orlandi P, Mattei P, Amato F. Airway obstruction during arthroscopic shoulder surgery: anesthesia for the patient or for the surgeon? *Minerva Anestesiol.* 2006;72(12):995–1000.
10. Sperber A, Wredmark T. Intramuscular pressure and fluid absorption during arthroscopic acromioplasty. *J Shoulder Elbow Surg.* 1999;8(5):414–418.
11. Manjuladevi M. Postoperative airway compromise in shoulder arthroscopy: a case series. *Indian J Anaesth.* 2013;57(1):52.
12. Edwards DS, Davis I, Jones NA, Simon DW. Rapid tracheal deviation and airway compromise due to fluid extravasation during shoulder arthroscopy. *J Shoulder Elbow Surg.* 2014;23(7):e163–e165.
13. Memon M, Kay J, Gholami A, Simunovic N, Ayeni OR. Fluid extravasation in shoulder arthroscopic surgery: a systematic review. *Orthop J Sports Med.* 2018;6(5):2325967118771616.
14. Khan F, Padmanabha S, Shantaram M, Aravind M. Airway compromise due to irrigation fluid extravasation following shoulder arthroscopy. *J Anaesthesiol Clin Pharmacol.* 2013;29(4):578–579.
15. Saeki N, Kawamoto M. Tracheal obstruction caused by fluid extravasation during shoulder arthroscopy. *Anaesth Intensive Care.* 2011;39(2):317.
16. Morrison DS, Schaefer RK, Friedman RL. The relationship between subacromial space pressure, blood pressure, and visual clarity during arthroscopic subacromial decompression. *Arthroscopy.* 1995;11:557–560.
17. Errando CL. Ultrasound observation of tissue fluid infiltration causing stridor in a woman undergoing shoulder arthroscopy. *Rev Esp Anestesiol Reanim.* 2011;58(9):582–584.
18. Ercin E, Bilgili MG, Ones HN, Kural C. Postoperative pectoral swelling after shoulder arthroscopy. *Joints.* 2016;3(3):158–160.
19. Hynson JM, Tung A, Guevara JE, Katz JA, Glick JM, Shapiro WA. Complete airway obstruction during arthroscopic shoulder surgery. *Anesth Analg.* 1993;76(4):875–878.
20. Rains DD, Rooke GA, Wahl CJ. Pathomechanisms and complications related to patient positioning and anesthesia during shoulder arthroscopy. *Arthroscopy.* 2011;27(4):532–554.
21. Mayo M, Wolsky R, Baldini T, Vezeridis PS, Bravman JT. Gravity fluid flow more accurately reflects joint fluid pressure compared with commercial peristaltic pump systems in a cadaveric model. *Arthroscopy.* 2018;34(12):3132–3138.
22. Bomberg BC. Complications associated with the use of an infusion pump during knee arthroscopy. *Arthroscopy.* 1992;8(2):224–228.
23. Blumenthal S. Severe airway obstruction during arthroscopic shoulder surgery. *Anesthesiology.* 2003;99(6):1455–1456.
24. Lim JK. Rhabdomyolysis following shoulder arthroscopy. *Arthroscopy.* 2006;22(12):1366–e1.
25. Ichai C, Ciais JF, Roussel LJ. Intravascular absorption of glycine irrigating solution during shoulder arthroscopy: a case report and follow-up study. *Anesthesiology.* 1996;85(6):1481–1485.

3

Broken Instruments

Benjamin Packard, MD, MS; Christopher Shultz, MD;
Dustin L. Richter, MD; Daniel C. Wascher, MD;
and Robert C. Schenck Jr, MD

INTRODUCTION

When Dr. Michael Burman[1] initially described arthroscopy for the shoulder in 1931, he likely did not appreciate the positive consequences his work would have on surgeons and patients today. Since then, orthopedic surgeons have enjoyed the improved visualization and relatively low complication rates associated with employing arthroscopic techniques for treating various shoulder pathologies. With the development of more advanced arthroscopic instrumentation, even advanced shoulder arthroscopic procedures can be performed safely without complications. However, surgeons should be aware of the risk of broken instrumentation.[2-5] A broken instrument or device can quickly turn a routine arthroscopy into a complicated case. In this chapter, we will review the epidemiology and etiology of broken instruments, summarize the current literature, and present representative cases and techniques to manage this anxiety-provoking and hopefully avoidable complication.

33

Thompson TL, ed.
Arthroscopic Shoulder Surgery:
Complications and Management (pp 33-43).
© 2022 Taylor & Francis Group.

EPIDEMIOLOGY

Comparing open and arthroscopic surgical techniques, complication rates are not significantly different, yet the types of complications vary.[6] Numerous complications of shoulder arthroscopy include portal fistula formation, iatrogenic chondral and rotator cuff injury, neurologic impairment (transient or permanent), infection (including *Propionibacterium acnes*), arthofibrosis, severe postoperative pain, acromial fracture, subcutaneous emphysema, pneumothorax, pneumomediastinum, and instrument breakage.[7] Although exceedingly rare in shoulder arthroscopy, instrument breakage is reported to occur in 0.18% to 0.35% of cases.[8] As arthroscopic shoulder instrumentation and suture passing devices become more complex, and the volume of arthroscopic procedures increases, the reported rate of instrument breakage may in fact be higher. With the advent of thermal ablators, arthroscopic suture passers, and myriad intra-articular instrumentation, these rates are potentially higher since Price et al[8] published their findings in 2002.

ETIOLOGY OF BROKEN INSTRUMENTS

All instruments passed into the shoulder joint are at risk of failing. These include arthroscopic graspers, shavers, scissors, thermal ablators, drills, anchor insertors, suture passers, and even cannulas. The etiology of broken instruments is multifactorial. The limited space within the joint and the fine nature of arthroscopic instrumentation lend to increased risk of breakage, both new and consistently used instruments. Furthermore, most arthroscopic instruments tend to be long and narrow, which results in increased torque across a relatively thin strut. Arthroscopic instruments also tend to have finer articulating couplings, which may be more prone to early metal fatigue stress. The challenges of placing instruments in hard-to-reach areas of the shoulder can cause the surgeon to apply excessive stress to instruments. Instrument breakage can also be caused by inappropriate use of instruments or using an instrument outside the limits for which it was designed.[9] However, the most common cause of instrument breakage is overuse leading to bending and eventual catastrophic failure.[10] For example, Song and Ramsey[11] showed, after inspection of a broken flexible nitinol needle, failure occurred 4 mm from the tip of the needle, likely from fatigue failure secondary to numerous abutments with the acromion. Öztekin[12] also determined that the probe that had broken in the case occurred from metal fatigue. Based on these reports of failure methods, it is critical to regularly inspect instrumentation prior to use. Metal instruments, although very strong, can break after numerous cycles. Even more at risk of breakage are disposable instruments, such as an arthroscopic rotator cuff passing needle, which has a finite number of cycles prior to instrument weakening and breakage. Manufacturers rarely provide the material wear and fatigue properties of their instrumentation. They do, however, provide clear instructions for use and reuse of instrumentation and equipment. Per the Arthrex brochure, the Scorpion passing needle should not be resterilized or reused and should be changed after every case.[13]

REVIEW OF LITERATURE

Broken instrumentation in shoulder arthroscopy is quite rare and therefore sparsely reported. Concerns regarding litigation may also dampen enthusiasm for reporting these complications.

The limited literature on the topic mainly consists of case reports. Additionally, much of the literature regarding broken arthroscopic instrumentation is described in knee arthroscopy; however, generalities, tips, pitfalls, and pearls can still be learned with regard to the glenohumeral joint and subacromial space.

Broken instruments can be inconspicuous, and the team may be unaware of an instrument breaking during the case. As a result, it may not be determined that an instrument has broken until the patient arrives in the recovery area, the first follow-up visit, or even further down the road when imaging is first obtained. Oldenburg and Mueller[14] reported a 33-year-old male patient who had a piece of an arthroscope shaft break in the left knee during debridement and partial meniscectomy. The patient had bloody effusions with pain that resolved with corticosteroid injections. He was counseled that the low level of persistent knee pain was secondary to the degenerative nature of his knee. Fourteen months later, the knee pain began to worsen. Radiographs were performed, demonstrating an intra-articular metallic object. The piece was identified, and the patient returned to the operating room (OR) for removal and subsequently made a full recovery. This case exemplifies the recommended course of action; once it is determined a piece of an instrument is broken in the patient, full disclosure and honesty should be conveyed to the patient. If there is continued trust in the patient–physician relationship, then a plan can be formulated to retrieve the broken instrument, if indicated, through a second surgery. The patient should always be given the option to seek a second opinion or care from another surgeon if trust does not exist. Instruments may be removed years down the road, as shown by Rajadhyaksha et al,[15] who presented a case of a scalpel blade retained in a knee for 10 years after the index surgery. It was subsequently removed, and the patient's vague sense of pain finally subsided in the knee.

Nevertheless, clinical judgment should be used as the broken piece does not have to be retrieved. Song and Ramsey[11] demonstrated leaving a broken instrument in a 59-year-old female patient without significant long-term sequelae. She had undergone shoulder arthroscopy in the lateral position. A large, full-thickness tear of the supraspinatus tendon and a partial-thickness tear of the subscapularis tendon were found and repaired with bioabsorbable anchors. The surgery was completed uneventfully. At her postoperative visit, radiographs demonstrated a metallic object in the superior aspect of the shoulder joint, later discovered to be a flexible nitinol needle. It was decided to observe the patient and follow her clinically without a return to the OR. At the patient's 2-year follow-up, radiographs showed the particle in the same position, and her pain was well controlled and she was satisfied. No reoperation was performed. Still, the patient must be appraised of the risks as the literature clearly documents migration of broken metallic surgical pins and devices, which can migrate to the central venous system and in particular to the heart.[16] A smooth pin or object should be removed if deemed at risk for migration or is seen to migrate on subsequent radiographs.[15] Although the patient ultimately had a good clinical outcome, it provides an excellent example that instruments should be carefully examined prior to and after each case to ensure no breakage or failure.

While some case reports have demonstrated satisfactory outcomes with leaving broken instrumentation in the joint, ideally a broken instrument is quickly identified during the case and retrieved. Even with prompt recognition, removal can at times be very difficult. Öztekin[12] presented an 18-year-old female patient who underwent a left knee diagnostic arthroscopy. During the procedure, the probe broke and was recognized; however, it was unable to be retrieved despite the surgeon's best efforts. The team decided to close, as the risks of anesthesia and prolonged arthroscopy outweighed retrieving the probe at that moment. The situation was explained in detail to the patient, yet she and her family initially refused a second surgery. The broken probe tip was eventually removed 5 years later due to persistent shoulder pain.

Yewlett et al[17] described a case to remove a broken metal probe in a shoulder of a 47-year-old man treated in a beach chair position. While probing a calcium deposit, the tip of the arthroscopic probe fractured off. The authors attempted arthroscopic removal techniques but found it difficult to remove the object as the shoulder was stiff and the object moved to the axillary pouch. Eventually, the patient was moved to a head-down position (Trendelenburg) from the beach chair, and the fragment was able to be removed. At this point, the remainder of the surgery was terminated as the shoulder was too edematous to finish.

These last 2 cases raise several important points. First, retrieving a broken instrument can be technically challenging. Second, one must recognize when persistent attempts to retrieve the instrument increase the risk to the patient after several failed attempts. The surgeon must either change their strategy (eg, convert to an open procedure) or abandon the attempt, close the wound, and plan to return at a later date after further evaluation and discussion. Prolonged arthroscopy and anesthesia are not benign and should be avoided after several failed removal attempts.[17]

Surgical judgment is critical for a safe outcome and may involve leaving the broken instrument in place, at least temporarily. Alternatively, attempts to retrieve failed instrumentation may be better suited by opening the joint and using fluoroscopy. Salami et al[2] presented a 28-year-old male football player undergoing knee arthroscopy for medial meniscectomy and debridement. Upon using grasping forceps, the forceps broke and were quickly lost on visualization. After failed attempts at arthroscopic retrieval, the authors proceeded with a mini open arthrotomy. Using fluoroscopy, they were able to remove the broken instrument and complete the planned procedure. Gambardella et al[18] operated on a 50-year-old man to repair a torn meniscus. A number 11 blade was used to make the portals. After making the anterolateral portal and returning the blade to the scrub tech, it was determined the tip of the blade was in the knee. Thirty minutes was spent attempting to locate the blade tip using a 30-degree arthroscope; however, after numerous failed attempts, a mini-C arm was employed. The fragment was identified on fluoroscopy and then localized using the arthroscope. The fragment was removed without an arthrotomy.

Management of Broken Instrumentation

The first step in managing broken arthroscopic instrumentation is prevention. We recommend systematically examining instrumentation prior to entering the joint, and any bent or cracked instrument should be removed from the field and a well-maintained replacement obtained. Proper location of arthroscopic portals or placing additional portals will help the surgeon avoid placing undue stress on instruments. After instruments are removed from the joint, they should be inspected by the surgeon and scrub tech for any missing pieces or other damage. In the authors' experience, the instruments most prone to failure are arthroscopic probes and insertion devices for suture anchors. Ideally, a broken instrument is identified intraoperatively, prior to leaving the OR.

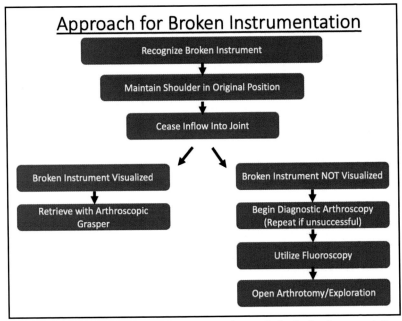

Figure 3-1. Flowchart depicting systematic approach to retrieving broken instrumentation.

Broken instrumentation in general can be identified immediately intraoperatively, delayed intraoperatively, or postoperatively. Each of these scenarios will be discussed in detail.

When a broken instrument is immediately identified, it is crucial to attempt retrieval in a systematic fashion (Figure 3-1). The first step is to maintain the shoulder in the position it was held when the instrument was broken.[19] Immediately after, we recommend ceasing inflow and outflow into the shoulder to lessen the chance of a broken instrument flowing into an undesirable or irretrievable location. These initial steps are crucial to keeping the broken instrument in a known, visible location in the joint.[19] We recommend proceeding next with a diagnostic arthroscopy, starting in the location where the surgeon was most recently using the broken instrument. Trial with a 70-degree scope can also be considered. If at this point the instrument is not visualized, it is likely that the broken piece has migrated elsewhere in the joint. One should then proceed with a diagnostic arthroscopy in the order they are most familiar with. A trial of switching inflow and outflow portals may also be used. If the instrument is not identified after 2 sequences of diagnostic arthroscopy, we recommend using fluoroscopy to assess if the broken instrument has migrated into the soft tissues around the joint. A small arthroscopic grasper is typically sufficient for retrieving the broken instrument. Magnetic graspers or suctions have historically been used to aid in retrieval; however, many of these are no longer manufactured. Nonmagnetic arthroscopic instruments should not be employed as magnetic retrievers cannot be used on them.[19] If the broken instrument piece cannot be retained in the joint without significant harm to the joint and adjacent cartilage, then an open arthrotomy may be necessary.

In some cases, a broken instrument may be identified intraoperatively but not immediately, after inspection of instrumentation. In these cases, it may be preferable to immediately utilize fluoroscopy to identify the region where the broken instrumentation is suspected (ie, glenohumeral vs subacromial). Following fluoroscopic localization, diagnostic arthroscopy can be employed until the broken instrument is located.

In rare circumstances, a broken instrument may not be retrievable or the risks associated with retrieval, such as removing excess bone or tissue, may be too high. If multiple attempts at localizing and removing a broken instrument have failed, a surgeon may consider aborting further attempts to minimize further damage. In some cases, the prolonged arthroscopic time, resultant shoulder edema, and extended anesthesia may result in more harm that benefit.[18] Hariri et al[20] presented a case of a 25-year-old undergoing a posterior labral repair: the case was 150 minutes, and the patient had a brachial vein deep venous thrombus leading to eventual pulmonary embolus. Lee et al[21] presented 3 cases of patients undergoing shoulder arthroscopy that ended in complications of extensive subcutaneous emphysema and pneumomediastinum in all 3 cases and tension pneumothorax in 2. In these cases, abandoning retrieval may still result in satisfactory outcomes.[21]

However, returning to the OR at a later time may prove even more challenging. In cases in which a broken instrument is recognized only after leaving the OR, the patient and family should be notified immediately. In the authors' experience, returning to the OR for retrieval within weeks after soft tissue swelling has subsided is preferable.

CASE PRESENTATIONS

Case 1

A 48-year-old man presented with a several-month history of progressive right shoulder pain and weakness. He underwent open rotator cuff repair with biceps tenodesis. There were no noted complications during the surgery. He was doing well at his 2- and 6-week follow-ups and then was lost to follow-up after. He returned to a separate provider after falling 2 years later

Figure 3-2. Anteroposterior radiograph depicting an arthroscopic suture passing needle tip embedded in the undersurface of the acromion.

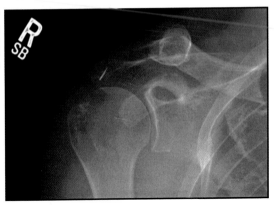

and, unfortunately, had new-onset pain and weakness in his right shoulder. Radiographs taken at that time demonstrated a radio-opaque material seated on the undersurface of the acromion (Figure 3-2). A review of the operative instrumentation suggested that the foreign object was most likely the tip of an arthroscopic suture passing device. This device can be used even in open rotator cuff repairs to more easily facilitate suture passage. The patient underwent magnetic resonance imaging demonstrating questionable rotator cuff tear, but the magnetic resonance imaging was limited by metal artifact. A computed tomography arthrogram was obtained and again demonstrated the broken suture passer tip (Figure 3-3). The patient returned to the OR for diagnostic arthroscopy. The broken suture passer tip was covered in bone and unable to be retrieved, and his rotator cuff repair remained intact.

Case 2

JD is a 50-year-old man who underwent arthroscopic rotator cuff repair. During the case, a suture anchor inserter was noted to have broken off. This was recognized intraoperatively and fluoroscopic images were obtained, but the broken piece could not be located arthroscopically. At that point, the surgeon decided to leave the broken inserter in place. The patient was not initially informed of the retained broken instrument. The patient had persistent pain with forward shoulder elevation despite physical therapy. After 4 months of persistent symptoms, repeat radiographs again revealed the broken inserter, and the patient was informed of the complication. The patient then elected to undergo repeat surgery. The broken instrument was retrieved using a mini-open approach with fluoroscopic guidance. Following removal, the patient had improvement in his motion and pain, but he chose to file a legal complaint against the surgeon (Figure 3-4).

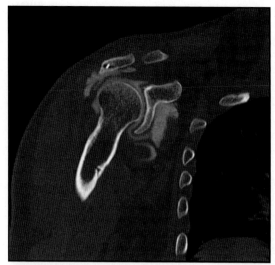

Figure 3-3. Parasagittal computed tomography arthrogram revealing broken suture passer tip embedded in the acromion.

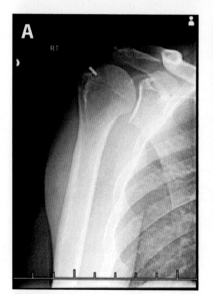

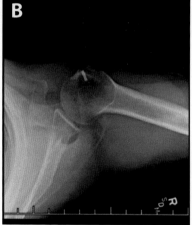

Figure 3-4. (A) AP and (B) lateral radiographs demonstrating a broken suture anchor inserter lodged in the footprint of the supraspinatus tendon on the proximal humerus.

CONCLUSION

Although instrument breakage during shoulder arthroscopy is rare, the arthroscopic surgeon should have a plan and stepwise approach to address the problem. Although it can be embarrassing, it is critical to "do the right thing." Management of instrument breakage begins with prevention. The surgeon and staff should inspect instrumentation before and after use, be cautious with disposable products that may be more prone to breakage, and avoid excess force or torque when performing arthroscopic procedures. Last, when the unfortunate event of breakage occurs, the ideal scenario identifies the instrument breakage before the patient leaves the OR. Identifying and removing broken instruments can be challenging intraoperatively, and the surgeon must maintain composure. Use of fluoroscopy, change of patient position, or an open procedure may be required for successful removal. The surgeon should use judgment to avoid prolonging the procedure based on patient safety and may need to close, discuss with patient, and possibly reoperate based on patient wishes. Patient involvement is of upmost importance. The unexpected complication should be fully disclosed to the patient and family. Leaving broken instrumentation in place around the shoulder entails risk of potential migration or structural damage. Decisions regarding clinical management should be made with patient education and shared decision making.

REFERENCES

1. Burman MS. Arthroscopy or the direct visualization of joints: an experimental cadaver study. *JBJS*. 1931;13(4):669.
2. Onimisi Salami S. Broken grasping forceps in during knee arthroscopy: a case report. *MOJ Orthop Rheumatol*. 2015;3(1):231-232.
3. Carlson MJ, Ferkel RD. Complications in ankle and foot arthroscopy. *Sports Med Arthrosc Rev*. 2013;21(2):135-139.
4. Allum R. Complications of arthroscopy of the knee. *J Bone Joint Surg Br*. 2002;84(7):937-945.
5. Sherman OH, Fox JM, Snyder SJ, et al. Arthroscopy—"no-problem surgery": an analysis of complications in two thousand six hundred and forty cases. *J Bone Joint Surg Am*. 1986;68(2):256-265.
6. Moen TC, Rudolph GH, Caswell K, Espinoza C, Burkhead WZ, Krishnan SG. Complications of shoulder arthroscopy. *J Am Acad Orthop Surg*. 2014;22(7):410-419.
7. Small NC. Complications in arthroscopic surgery performed by experienced arthroscopists. *Arthroscopy*. 1988;4(3):215-221.
8. Price M, Molloy S, Solan M, Sutton A, Ricketts D. The rate of instrument breakage during orthopaedic procedures. *Int Orthop*. 2002;26(3):185-187.
9. Gruson KI, Ilalov K, Youm T. A broken scalpel blade tip: an unusual complication of knee arthroscopy. *Bull NYU Hosp Jt Dis*. 2008;66(1):54.

10. Thomas Byrd JW. Complications associated with hip arthroscopy. In: Thomas Byrd JW, ed. *Operative Hip Arthroscopy*. Springer-Verlag; 2005:229–235.
11. Song HS, Ramsey ML. Suture passing needle breakage during arthroscopic rotator cuff repair: a complication report. *Arthroscopy*. 2008;24(12):1430–1432.
12. Öztekin HH. An unusual complication of knee arthroscopy: an extra-articular migrated asymptomatic broken probe from the knee joint. *Arch Orthop Trauma Surg*. 2005;125(4):285–287.
13. Arthrex. Scorpion Suture Passers. https://www.arthrex.com/shoulder/scorpion#:~:text=The%20Scorpion%E2%84%A2%20suture%20passers,supporting%20more%20successful%20suture%20passes. Accessed May 19, 2021.
14. Oldenburg M, Mueller RT. Intra-articular foreign body after arthroscopy. *Arthroscopy*. 2003;19(9):1012–1014.
15. Rajadhyaksha AD, Mont MA, Becker L. An unusual cause of knee pain 10 years after arthroscopy. *Arthroscopy*. 2006;22(11):1253.e1–3.
16. Tan L, Sun D-H, Yu T, Wang L, Zhu D, Li Y-H. Death due to intra-aortic migration of Kirschner wire from the clavicle: a case report and review of the literature. *Medicine (Baltimore)*. 2016;95(21):e3741.
17. Yewlett A, Bhattacharjee A, Mehta H, Kulkarni R. A technique to retrieve a broken probe during shoulder arthroscopy: a technical tip. *Internet J Orthop Surg*. 2014;22(1). http://ispub.com/IJOS/22/1/14721. Accessed March 13, 2019.
18. Gambardella RA, Tibone JE. Knife blade in the knee joint: a complication of arthroscopic surgery: a case report. *Am J Sports Med*. 1983;11(4):267–268.
19. Ward CG, Eckenhoff RG. Neurocognitive adverse effects of anesthesia in adults and children: gaps in knowledge. *Drug Saf*. 2016;39(7):613–626.
20. Hariri A, Nourissat G, Dumontier C, Doursounian L. Pulmonary embolism following thrombosis of the brachial vein after shoulder arthroscopy: a case report. *Orthop Traumatol Surg Res*. 2009;95(5):377–379.
21. Lee H-C, Dewan N, Crosby L. Subcutaneous emphysema, pneumomediastinum, and potentially life-threatening tension pneumothorax: pulmonary complications from arthroscopic shoulder decompression. *Chest*. 1992;101(5):1265–1267.

4

Protruding and Dislodged Implants

Benjamin Albertson, MD; Christopher Shultz, MD;
Dustin L. Richter, MD; and Robert C. Schenck Jr, MD

INTRODUCTION

Current arthroscopic shoulder techniques require soft tissue stabilization with some form of anchor use. Proper understanding of anchor function and insertion technique is paramount to appropriate placement and eventual stabilization of soft tissue structures. Different anchors have different modes of failure and associated complications; thus, it is important that arthroscopic surgeons understand these potential issues to minimize complications. Potential complications of soft tissue stabilization with anchors in the shoulder include osteolysis, synovitis, articular cartilage damage, and failure of fixation with formation of loose bodies or implant fragments as well as protruding implants. This chapter will discuss the epidemiology of these complications, review the literature as it relates to the many different forms of implants available for shoulder arthroscopy and their associated potential complications, discuss proper surgical technique for avoiding these complications, detail strategies for retrieval and/or removal of protruding or dislodged implants during shoulder arthroscopy, and provide case examples of these strategies in use.

Thompson TL, ed.
Arthroscopic Shoulder Surgery:
Complications and Management (pp 45-62).
© 2022 Taylor & Francis Group.

EPIDEMIOLOGY

Rates of implant failure following arthroscopic shoulder stabilization procedures such as rotator cuff, Bankart, and superior labrum anterior to posterior (SLAP) repairs are poorly defined in the literature but thought to be rare occurrences. Rates of prominent anchors, loose or dislodged anchors, or anchor failure with fragmentation and loose body formation are primarily described in small case series within the literature, and these rates vary considerably based on the type of implant used and surgery performed. One study quotes the complication rate for loose hardware associated with arthroscopic rotator cuff repair at 0.75% and repair failure at 3%.[1]

LITERATURE REVIEW

Suture Anchor Design Rationale

A variety of suture anchor designs have been developed to maximize stabilizing soft tissue to bone to allow approximation and healing of rotator cuff and labral tears. These have evolved over time and transitioned from initial tacks and staples to more modern implants such as screws and impaction anchors.

Initial tacks and staples were limited by complications such as tack breakage and loss of fixation with loose body formation, as well as inferior load-to-failure rates as compared with more modern screw and impaction suture anchors. The main benefit of staple and tack fixation was obviating arthroscopic knot tying, but this was negated by complication rates as high as 30%.[2] The primary mechanism of failure of staple and tack fixation is often loss of fixation at the tissue–implant interface, both through tissue pullout as well as anchor failure. With bioabsorbable tacks, the most common site of failure of the anchor has been shown to be just below the head of the tack at the transition point between the bone and soft tissue fixation. This is thought to represent a point of high-stress concentration as well as a change in microenvironments between the bony fixation and the soft tissue fixation. Potential differences in implant degradation rates are hypothesized to explain the high failure rate at this junction.[3]

Staples and tacks have largely been abandoned secondary to these complications associated with their use, and currently, available anchors for fixation of soft tissue to bone within the shoulder primarily involve screw and impaction-type anchors with associated sutures for soft tissue fixation (Figure 4-1). Composition of these implants includes the suture, which is generally either a braided polyester suture or, more recently, a hybrid suture

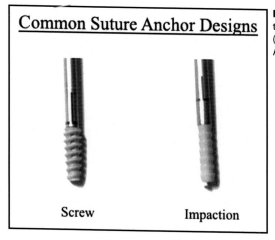

Figure 4-1. Screw and impaction suture anchor designs (corkscrew, suturetack; Arthrex).

reinforced with ultra-high molecular weight polyethylene; the suture eyelet, which is either composed of the anchor material or a loop of suture that is then attached to the base of the anchor; and the anchor itself, with its mechanism of fixation to bone. Potential sites of repair failure include at the soft tissue–suture interface, the suture–anchor interface, and the anchor-bone interface.

For rotator cuff repair surgery, the soft tissue–suture interface has been shown to be the primary site of repair failure.[4] Patient-specific factors such as tissue quality and mobility of tissue are largely implicated in this, as well as surgical technique factors such as suture configuration and anchor configuration (single row vs double row), which are beyond the scope of this chapter and are discussed elsewhere in this textbook.

The suture–anchor interface is another site where potential failure can occur (Figure 4-2), and this has been described in case reports and biomechanical studies in the literature. Initial metal suture anchors consisted of a metal eyelet through which the suture was passed. Biomechanical studies have shown that the orientation of this eyelet with respect to the suture vector and the axis of the anchor affect the failure strength of the suture. Meyer et al[5] found that suture anchors positioned at 45 degrees to the suture vector showed significant lower force to failure rates with an average of 69 N compared to 116 N when the suture vector was collinear with the anchor axis. This was thought to be secondary to increased friction experienced by the suture at the metal suture eyelet with this orientation. Even with the suture vector collinear with the anchor axis, the suture consistently failed at a lower force than the reported failure strength of the suture material. This is thought to be related to the sharp metal edges on the suture eyelet. Industry has responded to these

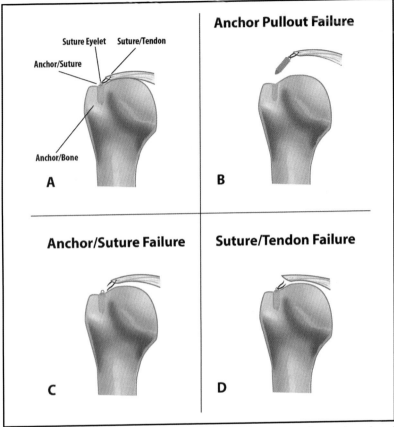

Figure 4-2. Illustration demonstrating suture–anchor implant interface and modes of failure.

findings with suture anchor eyelet design adaptations, and newer suture anchors now consist of a suture-based eyelet, eliminating the potential sharp edges of the metal or bioabsorbable polymer eyelets.

There is a case report in the literature detailing suture eyelet failure in a biocomposite anchor secondary to eyelet fracture with resultant loose body formation. Another case report details suture anchor eyelet loss of fixation to the anchor with resultant loose body formation and humeral head chondral damage as a result of the suture eyelet loose body.[6] These reports are exceedingly rare in the literature, and complications related to the suture–eyelet interface are reported to have an incidence of around 0.000167% based on information from US Food and Drug Administration medical device reporting database data.[7]

The 2 primary mechanisms of fixation between the anchor–bone interface are screw-in and impaction-type anchors. These anchors have been found to show similar pullout strengths in patients with normal bone density, but screw-in type anchors have been found to have superior pullout strength in low bone density. Screw threads allow for increased contact between the bone and the implant, and these anchors also displace less bone with placement.[8,9] It is important to understand the type of anchor in place when planning revision surgery in the setting of prominent or loose hardware to understand proper removal techniques.

Anchor Materials

With the evolution of arthroscopic surgical techniques have come several advances in arthroscopic anchor fixation mechanisms. The first arthroscopic anchors used were primarily metal composed of titanium and stainless steel. These anchors had initial problems with anchor loosening, formation of loose bodies, chondral injury, technical difficulty with revision surgeries, and issues with advanced imaging modalities such as magnetic resonance imaging (MRI) for postoperative evaluation of persistent pain and repair integrity. A benefit of these anchors is the ability to evaluate implant positioning postoperatively with plain-film radiographs.

Due to complications associated with metal anchor use, bioabsorbable suture anchors were developed. Potential advantages of bioabsorbable anchors included initial strong fixation of repair, which over time as soft tissue heals to bone slowly resorbs, loses strength, and is broken down to consumable metabolites. Different bioabsorbable polymers have been used in orthopedic surgery anchors within the shoulder, with differing crystalline structures that affect the rate of degradation. These include polyglycolic acid (PGA), poly-L-lactic acid (PLLA), and poly-L/D-lactic acid (PLDLA), which is composed of varying ratios of the L and D stereoisomers. Complications reported in the literature related to these bioabsorbable implants include inflammatory responses such as synovitis and osteolysis, premature degradation with loose body formation and failure of repair, and implant loosening with resultant prominent hardware and chondral injury. Studies have also shown that upon degradation, there is a lack of bone formation within the hardware tunnels.[10] These anchors are radiolucent and unable to be evaluated on plain-film radiographs but do not have artifact generation on MRI and thus do not interfere with postoperative imaging of surgical repairs. Despite the theoretical advantages of bony biointegration with absorbable suture anchors, the complications associated with these anchors, mainly inflammatory reactions and loosening at the bone–anchor interface, have resulted in these anchors falling out of favor.

More recently, biocomposite anchors have been developed to address the possible issues of lack of bony ingrowth into the suture anchor holes following resorption. These anchors are composed of bioabsorbable polymers such as poly(lactide-coglycolide) and osteoconductive bioceramics such as β-tricalcium phosphate. These anchors allow for strong initial fixation, with similar degradation profiles to some of the bioabsorbable implants and osteoconductive material promoting bony ingrowth following absorption.

Additional biostable polymers such as polyether ether ketone (PEEK) have been developed and show good results in orthopedic implants within other subspecialties. These anchors have advantages over bioabsorbable anchors in that they are inert and do not produce an inflammatory response, do not lose strength over time, and, like absorbable anchors, are MRI compatible and can be drilled through in revision scenarios. These advantages of PEEK suture anchors have the led the authors to adopt this material as the primary method for fixation of soft tissue rotator cuff and labral repairs.

Complications With Respective Anchor Materials

Metal

Several complications associated with metal anchors have been described in the literature, which have led to a transition away from metal anchor use in shoulder arthroscopy (Figure 4-3). Godinho et al[8] described 28 cases of complications from loose or prominent metal anchors in shoulder arthroscopy for SLAP repair, anterior/posterior instability, and rotator cuff repair. The majority of the cases involved traumatic anterior instability, and the most frequently symptomatic anchor position in this surgery was found to be the 5-o'clock position. They found that 47 out of 82 anchors (57.31%) among the 28 patients were determined to be inadequately positioned, and 43 of these required removal. Upon repeat arthroscopy, all patients had chondral damage, with 19 out of the 28 patients having grade 3 or 4 chondral injury based on the Outerbridge classification.

Kaar et al[9] described 8 cases of complications with metallic suture anchors in patients with anterior instability, SLAP tears, and rotator cuff tears. Patients presented an average of 12 months after the initial operation with persistent pain and underwent repeat arthroscopy. They found that all the patients who had more than 3 glenoid anchors placed had at least one anchor in an extraosseous position, leading them to conclude that there should be high concern for anchor misplacement if greater than 3 anchors were used in the initial repair. Three of the 8 patients were found to have severe articular damage at the time of repeat arthroscopy.

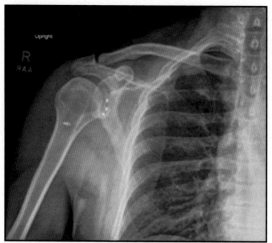

Figure 4-3. Right shoulder radiograph demonstrating pullout of a metal labral impaction suture anchor.

Another study looking at Bankart repairs found 5 cases with metallic anchor complications and proud screw heads in the 5- to 7-o'clock anchor position. Patients presented an average of 12 months postoperatively with sharp pain, catching symptoms, and decreased range of motion. All of their cases were found to have severe articular cartilage damage on repeat arthroscopy.[11]

Bioabsorbable

Bioabsorbable implants are degraded by hydrolysis, resulting in long polymer chain breakdown and eventual implant fragmentation with macrophage activation and phagocytosis, leading to cleavage of fragments into final lactic acid by-products. This absorption happens over a course of weeks to months to years depending on the crystalline structure of the implant, with PGA being the fastest absorbing, followed by PLDLA compositions and PLLA absorbing the slowest.[12] Research shows that this degradation process is associated with an inflammatory response, and it is hypothesized that the rate of degradation correlates with the intensity of the inflammatory response. The faster-absorbing polymers have shown greater rates of synovitis associated with their use.[12] With bioabsorbable implants, there is debate on the mechanism of chondral injury seen after failure, and both biologic and mechanical etiologies have been proposed. Biologic cartilage injury is postulated to be in response to hypertrophic synovitis and inflammatory response incited by the breakdown of the polymers seen in some patients. Mechanical injury has been shown to be related to loose body formation within the glenohumeral joint with implant breakdown.[12]

PGA was among the first bioabsorbable materials to be used in shoulder arthroscopy and was primarily used in tack implants. There were several issues associated with its use; most important was its quick degradation process, reported to undergo complete degradation from 4 to 6 weeks up to 6 months after insertion. This led to several issues with loss of fixation. Additionally, there have been several case reports of foreign body reactions and massive synovitis, as well as issues with loose body formation related to PGA use. One study found a 22% rate of synovial reaction to PGA implants. Burkhart et al[13] describe a foreign body reaction to PGA implants in the early postoperative period. They detail case reports of 4 patients who underwent treatment of SLAP and anterior instability with arthroscopic stabilization using PGA tack implants, 3 of which developed massive synovitis postoperatively. Three of the 4 patients were found to have broken tack devices with intra-articular loose body fragments.

PLLA was developed in response to early failures with PGA and thought to have a better and slower degradation profile with advertised degradation in the 10- to 30-month time frame, but some studies have shown the presence of PLLA implants up to 12 years after implantation. This polymer was initially used with tacks as well and was associated with complications including failure of tacks at the transition zone between the head and shaft. One study demonstrated 6 cases of transition zone failure with PLLA tack use for SLAP repairs at an average of 9.5 months postoperatively. Additionally, 3 patients had failure of the SLAP repairs, and 2 patients had chondral injury on repeat arthroscopy.[14]

Another study looked at 44 patients with complications who underwent rotator cuff repair or labral repair with either suture or tack PLLA implants. Patients were brought back to the operating room at an average of 18.8 months postoperatively and were found to have macroscopic debris within the joint in 55% of cases. Histologic samples taken at the time of surgery revealed papillary synovitis in 79% of patients and histologic giant cell reaction in 84% of patients. Seventy percent of patients were found to have grade 3 or 4 Outerbridge classification chondral damage, with increased damage correlated to increased time from initial surgery. Four patients required extensive synovectomy secondary to persistent PLLA breakdown products.[15]

In contrast to this study, other studies have shown low rates of suture anchor complications with PLLA suture anchors. One study evaluated 360 patients who underwent rotator cuff or labral repair with PLLA suture anchors and found 18 patients (5%) requiring repeat surgery, with anchor-specific adverse events accounting for only 2 of 18 cases, suggesting an incidence of 0.5% of anchor-associated complications with PLLA suture anchors. They did not find any inflammatory reactions secondary to the breakdown products in their study.[12]

Other studies evaluating PLLA anchors, specifically the BioKnotless suture anchor (Mitek), have shown complications in Bankart and SLAP repairs. Athwal et al[16] described 4 cases of osteolysis, loss of fixation, and severe glenohumeral arthropathy following the use of the above listed anchor. On repeat arthroscopy, they found sharply demarcated regions of cartilage loss adjacent to loose anchors suggestive of a mechanical etiology of chondral damage. They postulated that a large number of anchors used in the repairs (5 anchors per patient) may have caused convergence of the anchors, leading to poor fixation. Additionally, they mention that the knotless concept requires deeper bone fixation and thus may not achieve the same relative proportion of cortical fixation as traditional suture anchors. Additionally, they noted that the anchor design, which primarily resists pullout by frictional interference, was insufficient. All of these factors may have contributed to the initial loss of fixation that initiated a cascade of micromotion leading to osteolysis and further anchor loosening, creating a prominent anchor or intra-articular loose body that ultimately induced chondral damage.

Another study relating to BioKnotless anchor use demonstrated 3 patients with painful symptoms 11 to 15 months postoperatively. In this study, fewer anchors were used per patient (2 to 3 per case), and reactive synovitis, osteolysis, and arthritis were seen in all cases. The authors postulated that the time frame (11 to 15 months postoperatively) coincided with PLLA degradation, and they felt that exposed PLLA anchor components to the synovial fluid led to a synovial reaction in addition to the anchor-loosening cascade described previously. They endorsed the additional technique point of avoiding leaving any PLLA exposed to the synovial environment.[17]

PLDLA is composed of a combination of L and D stereoisomers of lactic acid in variable concentrations. Most common ratios include 70% L and 30% D or 96% L and 4% D. These have differing crystalline structures that result in a faster degradation profile than PLLA but slower than PGA. Complications associated with the use of PLDLA anchors are similar to other bioabsorbable polymers, and one recent study has shown significantly higher reoperation rates and rates of SLAP repair failure in patients with these anchors. This study looked at 348 patients over a 10-year period who underwent SLAP repair. The authors found an overall 6.3% reoperation rate and 4.3% revision repair rate. They had patients who underwent repair with titanium, PEEK, PLLA, and PLDLA 70/30 as well as PLDLA 96/4 anchors. All of their reoperations were within the PLDLA anchor group, including 7 of 169 PLDLA 70/30 anchor patients (4.1% revision rate) and 15 of 62 PLDLA 96/4 anchor patients (24.2% revision rate). Statistical analysis revealed a 12.7 times increased odds ratio of failure with PLDLA anchors. On repeat arthroscopy, anchors were found to have lost structural integrity and contained surrounding synovitis. The authors concluded that they would recommend avoiding the use of bioabsorbable materials in SLAP repairs.[18]

Biocomposite

Limited literature exists on biocomposite anchors within shoulder arthroscopy and associated complications; however, one study assessing pooled results of patients who have undergone knee and shoulder surgeries quotes complications of tunnel widening in 3% of patients, joint effusion in 5% of patients, and cyst formation in 4% of patients.[10] Biocomposite implants composed of poly(lactide-coglycolide) and β-tricalcium phosphate are reported to absorb at a faster rate than PLLA implants; however, complications with synovitis have not been reported in the literature, and this is thought to be related to buffering of the inflammatory response to the lactic acid generation associated with breakdown products by the bioceramic calcium–based material. Additionally, these implants have shown improved osteoconductive activity compared to their bioabsorbable counterparts. Postoperative imaging has shown partial or complete ossification of implant tracts in 63% of patients at an average of 27 months postoperatively, as well as implant volume loss of 88% at 30 months postoperatively.[10]

Biostable

PEEK anchors also have limited complications reported within the literature and, along with biocomposite anchors, are newer to the market, and thus complications may not have become apparent at this point. One study previously discussed in this review included 87 patients treated with PEEK anchors. There were no reoperations in this group, as well as no reported complications with these patients.[18] In the authors' experience, complications have been primarily limited to user error (Figure 4-4). PEEK appears to be a promising material for use in orthopedic implants with favorable outcomes to date.

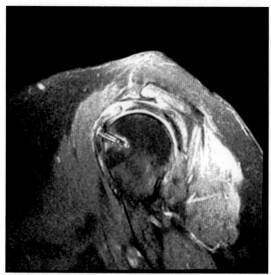

Figure 4-4. T2 parasagittal MRI demonstrating prominence of a PEEK suture anchor due to inadequate seating upon initial implant placement.

Appropriate Workup for Loose Anchors

Most patients with loose or prominent implants present in the postoperative period with persistent pain that does not improve with time and is often worsened once active range of motion exercises are progressed. Typical presentation includes persistent or worsening pain, crepitus or mechanical symptoms, and decreased range of motion. Appropriate workup depends slightly on the type of fixation used but generally should include laboratory tests to rule out infectious etiology, including white blood cell count, erythrocyte sedimentation rate, and C-reactive protein. The risks and benefits of joint aspiration may be weighed based on laboratory results. From an imaging standpoint, radiographs to assess for progressive arthropathy in the case of radiolucent implants and to assess for implant positioning in the case of metallic implants can be useful. Advanced imaging such as a computed tomography scan can be useful to assess for osteolysis surrounding anchors, and MRI is the modality of choice to evaluate the integrity of the soft tissue repair and anchor positioning (not applicable with metallic implants secondary to artifact generation).

Figure 4-5. Right shoulder ultrasound of a 54-year-old woman 6 weeks postoperatively from arthroscopic rotator cuff repair and biceps tenodesis demonstrating pullout of a PEEK suture anchor.

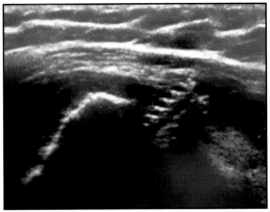

A study by Magee et al[19] validated the usefulness of MRI for evaluating rotator cuff repairs postoperatively in the setting of bioabsorbable implants. They found that among 30 patients with recurrent pain after isolated supraspinatus tendon rotator cuff repair who underwent MRI evaluation, imaging assessment correlated excellently with arthroscopy results. Nine patients were found to have anchor dislodgment and retear, 4 patients were found to have loose anchors with intact repair, 3 were found to have intact anchors and retear (all 16 cases were verified with repeat arthroscopy), and 14 were found to have intact anchors and repair (5 of which were verified by repeat arthroscopy). This study highlights the utility of MRI to accurately diagnose anchor loosening and displacement postoperatively and, in the correct clinical situation, assists in diagnosis and preoperative planning. Rarely, there are instances in which MRI is nondiagnostic of loose or dislodged implants, such as the scenario where failure occurs at the suture–eyelet interface. It should be noted that in the setting of appropriate soft tissue healing, MRI results would likely not show the small loose body associated with the suture eyelet failure, and repeat arthroscopy remains the gold standard for evaluation of repair and suture anchor integrity.[6]

While ultrasound has been used for decades in soft tissue imaging studies, it is highly user dependent, and its utility for evaluating musculoskeletal structures is evolving. While MRI yields images with greater definition, the use of MRI is limited by implant artifact and substantial cost. The utility of ultrasound for diagnoses of rotator cuff pathology as well as guidance of subacromial and intra-articular injections has been well established in the literature.[20] Ultrasound may become more helpful and mainstream in the workup of patients with concerning postoperative pain and stiffness from suspected early implant failure (Figure 4-5) during the early postoperative period.

Proper Surgical Techniques

Appropriate surgical techniques with rotator cuff repair and labral instability fixation must be adhered to in order to minimize complications of implant loosening or dislodgment. Appropriate use of implants as detailed by the manufacturer and adequate surgical training are imperative to avoid potentially disastrous complications of glenohumeral arthropathy. Specific points of emphasis regarding surgical techniques are discussed below.

General Anchor Insertion Concepts

As discussed previously, the role of eyelet orientation in anchors with solid eyelets (those not composed of suture) is important in order to minimize friction on the suture and decrease risk of suture failure at the suture-eyelet interface. Additionally, depth of anchor insertion is important, as leaving an anchor proud leads to devastating chondral damage, and burying an anchor too deep decreases cortical bone contact and pullout strength, as well as leads to suture abrasion on the cortical bone edges.[2] For these reasons, careful attention to detail with suture anchor insertion cannot be emphasized enough. Additionally, other variables such as loop and knot security as well as tissue quality play a large role in ensuring appropriate repair strength and facilitating tissue healing but are beyond the scope of this chapter.

Rotator Cuff Repair

Cadaveric studies have shown that along the rotator cuff footprint, the thicker cortex lies proximally between the articular surface and the greater tuberosity, and as one moves distally toward and past the tip of the tuberosity, the bone density decreases significantly. As a result of this, anchor placement should be positioned proximally at the edge of the articular surface to ensure optimal fixation strength with higher-density cortical bone. Additionally, care must be taken during preparation of the rotator cuff footprint to avoid excessive decortication.

In the setting of poor bone mineral density, screw-in suture anchors have been shown to be preferential to impaction suture anchors yielding higher pullout strengths. As such, proper assessment of bone and tissue quality is imperative at the time of repair.

Insertion angle of anchors has been discussed in the literature, and the "deadman's angle" (45 degrees) was coined by Dr. Stephen Burkhart[21] to provide the optimal anchor pullout strength and reduce suture tension. Biomechanical studies have since challenged this concept, and a study by Strauss et al[4] shows higher cyclic loads to failure in anchors inserted at a 90-degree angle (380 cycles) as opposed to the traditional 45-degree angle (297 cycles) proposed by Burkhart. They explain these results by highlighting the fact that most failures occur at the tissue–suture interface and not the implant–bone interface. They also found widening within the cancellous bone tunnels of the anchors implanted at a 45-degree angle and proposed that micromotion within the anchor at this angle leads to increased motion in the anchor-suture construct and allows the suture to saw through the tendon. Additionally, they state that the deadman's angle causes increased shear forces on the suture–tendon interface. For these reasons, some authors advocate for suture anchor placement perpendicular to the articular surface as opposed to the traditional deadman's angle.[4]

Labral Instability

In labral instability, studies have shown that the anterior inferior quadrant of the glenoid has the lowest bone mineral density and thus the lowest pullout strength for anchor fixation. Most loose anchors placed within the glenoid are found within this anterior inferior quadrant, which is difficult to access arthroscopically but also shown to be the most important fixation point for shoulder instability cases. Additionally, studies evaluating insertion angle of screws relative to the glenoid rim show that the highest pullout strength is found when anchors are placed orthogonal to the glenoid rim. Anchors placed at 20 and 40 degrees of deviation from the orthogonal have been evaluated and show statistically significant decreased pullout strength in all glenoid quadrants at 40 degrees of deviation from the orthogonal. Within the anterior-inferior quadrant, statistically significantly decreased pullout strength at only 20 degrees of deviation has been shown.[22] This highlights the importance of increased vigilance on the part of the surgeon to ensure appropriate placement of anchors within this difficult region of the glenoid to avoid potentially catastrophic damage to the joint with prominent or loose anchors, in addition to ensuring a successful clinical outcome in preventing recurrent instability.

Rhee et al[11] describe important technique points to avoid anchor complications. They state that placement of the anterior-inferior portal is important in Bankart repair and should be placed far lateral to the middle glenohumeral ligament to gain an appropriate angle for anchor insertion.

They also emphasized the importance of inserting the bone punch 1 to 2 mm from the glenoid rim at a 45-degree medial angle and ensuring that the anchor is fully seated within the glenoid to the point where it is below the subchondral bone and not just below the cartilage. Additionally, they emphasize avoiding excessive forceful handling of the screw, as this can lead to blunting of the tip, which both impairs insertion and increases difficulty of possible removal if needed.

STRATEGIES FOR ANCHOR REMOVAL

Once a dislodged, loose, or prominent anchor has been identified, arthroscopic evaluation and removal of the implant is the treatment of choice. Rarely does anchor removal require an open shoulder arthrotomy approach, but it may require larger than normal portal incisions to facilitate hardware removal. It is important for the treating surgeon to be aware of the tools available at the time of the case and understand the type of anchor they are dealing with. The appropriate equipment from the manufacturer of the anchor should be available if known to assist in retrieval. Careful assessment of preoperative imaging can assist in localization of dislodged anchors as well as evaluation for other loose or prominent anchors. Dislodged anchors are treated differently than loose or prominent anchors, and the latter may require additional tools not present in standard arthroscopic trays.

Dislodged Anchors

Dislodged implants are best evaluated with diagnostic arthroscopy and, much like other loose bodies within the shoulder, often settle in the subscapular or axillary recess. These spaces must be visualized on diagnostic arthroscopy to ensure that no fragments of anchor or suture material remain within the glenohumeral joint that could continue to cause damage. Removal may necessitate large-diameter cannulas, and standard arthroscopic tools such as graspers or pituitary rongeurs are often helpful in retrieval. If the anchor is composed of metal, it can be useful to have magnetic retrieval tools to assist in removal. Often times in the case of bioabsorbable anchors, the dislodged anchor is fragmented. Depending on the number of fragments and the size of these pieces, suction-shaver devices can be useful to remove these loose bodies.

Loose or Prominent Anchors

Arthroscopic retrieval of loose and proud anchors can be difficult as anchors are often covered with scar tissue. The first step in removal involves exposure of the anchor head. This can be achieved with radiofrequency ablators or shavers. Care should be taken to avoid damage to adjacent cartilage with the use of these devices. Once exposed, anchors can be evaluated for loosening or prominence and may be treated with either removal or impaction depending on the clinical circumstances. Often times, impaction-type anchors can be far more difficult to remove than screw anchors as the barbs prevent removal. Arthroscopic elevators and pituitary rongeur devices are particularly useful in freeing loose anchors from surrounding soft tissue and assisting in retrieval. Attention to bone loss with anchor removal is important especially when dealing with the glenoid to avoid fracture and preserve bone stock for revision fixation if needed. When prominent anchors without loosening are encountered and cannot be removed with the assistance of appropriate manufacturer insertion devices, this can present a challenging problem. Several strategies have been described for these scenarios in the literature.

Impaction

For anchors within the humeral head, impaction of the anchor below the subchondral bone is often the easiest treatment option, especially for impaction-type anchors for which the design resists removal. However, this is not recommended in the glenoid, as it can be associated with fracture due to the hard cortical bone surrounding the glenoid neck. The original insertion device can be helpful in impacting the anchor if available, and if not available, a narrow bone tamp can be used. Care should be taken to impact the device collinear to the axis of the anchor, and judgment should be used to avoid fracture or worsening of the clinical problem.

Drilling

For biodegradable and biostable anchors, if it is not possible to remove the implant, then the implant can be drilled out using a drill bit the same size as the anchor width. For this technique, it is recommended to use high-flow fluid settings to allow for appropriate removal of anchor debris from the joint.[23]

Loosening

Another method described in the literature involves attempting to dislodge the anchor from the surrounding bone to allow removal. This method was described in a case series of 6 patients with proud metallic suture anchors who presented after Bankart repair without subsequent complication. The authors recommend using a screwdriver with a diameter larger than that of the anchor and wedging the screw driver between the proud anchor and the bone to loosen the anchor. They report good results with this technique in their small case series, but this strategy should be attempted with care and has not been the treatment choice of the authors.[2]

Trephination

In situations where the aforementioned techniques are not available or unsuccessful, another strategy for implant removal is to pass a trephine over the anchor and remove the anchor with the column of bone it is attached to. Trephination is performed in a counterclockwise direction collinear to the anchor axis. This procedure can carry with it significant bone loss, and use of bone graft for the resulting defect may be considered. Burkhart et al[24] describe this technique with the use of an osteochondral allograft transplant harvester. When using this technique, it is important to be aware of the width and length of the tools available to you, as it is necessary for the trephine or allograft transplant harvester to be long enough and narrow enough to reach the anchor through the arthroscopic portal while minimizing excess bone loss.

CONCLUSION

Protruding or dislodged implants in shoulder arthroscopy are rare but potentially catastrophic complications of common shoulder procedures such as Bankart, SLAP, and rotator cuff repair. An appropriate knowledge of implant-specific potential complications and meticulous attention to proper implant placement are the fundamental means to avoid these complications. Patients presenting in the postoperative period with worsening pain, decreased range of motion, and mechanical symptoms should be assessed for implant-associated complications and appropriate workup obtained. Many strategies exist for removal of these implants, and it is imperative for the treating surgeon to have knowledge of the instrumentation available and have a preoperative plan for removal strategies.

REFERENCES

1. Weber SC, Abrams JS, Nottage WM. Complications associated with arthroscopic shoulder surgery. *Arthroscopy.* 2002;18(2)(suppl 1):88–95.
2. Jeong J-H, Shin S-J. Arthroscopic removal of proud metallic suture anchors after Bankart repair. *Arch Orthop Trauma Surg.* 2009;129(8):1109–1115.

3. Wilkerson JP, Zvijac JE, Uribe JW, Schürhoff MR, Green JB, Failure of polymerized lactic acid tacks in shoulder surgery. *J Shoulder Elbow Surg.* 2003;12(2):117–121.

4. Strauss E, Frank D, Kubiak E, Kummer F, Rokito A. The effect of the angle of suture anchor insertion on fixation failure at the tendon-suture interface after rotator cuff repair: deadman's angle revisited. *Arthroscopy.* 2009;25(6):597–602.

5. Meyer DC, Nyffeler RW, Fucentese SF, Gerber C. Failure of suture material at suture anchor eyelets. *Arthroscopy.* 2002;18(9):1013–1019.

6. Barber FA. Biodegradable shoulder anchors have unique modes of failure. *Arthroscopy.* 2007;23(3):316–320.

7. Cole BJ, Provencher MT. Safety profile of bioabsorbable shoulder anchors. *Arthroscopy.* 2007;23(8):912–913.

8. Godinho GG, França FO, Alves Freitas JM, Aguiar PN, de Carvalho Leite M. Complications resulting from the use of metal anchors in shoulder arthroscopy. *Rev Bras Ortop.* 2009;44(2):143–147.

9. Kaar TK, Schenck RC, Wirth MA, Rockwood CA. Complications of metallic suture anchors in shoulder surgery: a report of 8 cases. *Arthroscopy.* 2001;17(1):31–37.

10. Barber FA, Spenciner DB, Bhattacharyya S, Miller LE. Biocomposite implants composed of poly(lactide-co-glycolide)/β-tricalcium phosphate: systematic review of imaging, complication, and performance outcomes. *Arthroscopy.* 2017;33(3):683–689.

11. Rhee YG, Lee D-H, Chun IH, Bae SC. Glenohumeral arthropathy after arthroscopic anterior shoulder stabilization. *Arthroscopy.* 2004;20(4):402–406.

12. Cobaleda Aristizabal AF, Sanders EJ, Barber FA. Adverse events associated with biodegradable lactide-containing suture anchors. *Arthroscopy.* 2014;30(5):555–560.

13. Burkhart A, Imhoff AB, Roscher E. Foreign-body reaction to the bioabsorbable suretac device. *Arthroscopy.* 2000;16(1):91–95.

14. Sassmannshausen G, Sukay M, Mair SD. Broken or dislodged poly-L-lactic acid bioabsorbable tacks in patients after SLAP lesion surgery. *Arthroscopy.* 2006;22(6):615–619.

15. McCarty LP, Buss DD, Datta MW, Freehill MQ, Giveans MR. Complications observed following labral or rotator cuff repair with use of poly-L-lactic acid implants. *J Bone Joint Surg Am.* 2013;95(6):507–511.

16. Athwal GS, Shridharani SM, O'Driscoll SW. Osteolysis and arthropathy of the shoulder after use of bioabsorbable knotless suture anchors: a report of four cases. *J Bone Joint Surg Am.* 2006;88(8):1840–1845.

17. Boden RA, Burgess E, Enion D, Srinivasan MS. Use of bioabsorbable knotless suture anchors and associated accelerated shoulder arthropathy: report of 3 cases. *Am J Sports Med.* 2009;37(7):1429–1433.

18. Park MJ, Hsu JE, Harper C, Sennett BJ, Huffman GR. Poly-L/D-lactic acid anchors are associated with reoperation and failure of SLAP repairs. *Arthroscopy.* 2011;27(10):1335–1340.

19. Magee T, Shapiro M, Hewell G, Williams D. Complications of rotator cuff surgery in which bioabsorbable anchors are used. *AJR Am J Roentgenol.* 2003;181(5):1227–1231.

20. Strakowski JA, Visco CJ. Diagnostic and therapeutic musculoskeletal ultrasound applications of the shoulder. *Muscle Nerve.* 2019;60(1):1–6.

21. Burkhart SS. The deadman theory of suture anchors: observations along a south Texas fence line. *Arthroscopy.* 1995;11:119–123.

22. Ilahi OA, Al-Fahl T, Bahrani H, Luo Z-P. Glenoid suture anchor fixation strength: effect of insertion angle. *Arthroscopy.* 2004;20(6):609–613.

23. Grutter PW, McFarland EG, Zikria BA, Dai Z, Petersen SA. Techniques for suture anchor removal in shoulder surgery. *Am J Sports Med.* 2010;38(8):1706–1710.

24. Burkhart SS, Lo IKY, Brady PC. Tricks and tips. In: Burkhart SS, Lo IKY, Brady PC, eds. *Burkhart's View of the Shoulder: A Cowboy's Guide to Advanced Shoulder Arthroscopy.* Lippincott Williams & Wilkins; 2006:298.

5

Medical and Anesthetic Complications of Arthroscopic Shoulder Surgery

Emmanuel N. Osadebey, MD;
Christopher G. Salib, MD, MS;
and Terry L. Thompson, MD

Arthroscopic shoulder surgery is a valuable technique used by experienced surgeons to diagnose and treat a wide variety of musculoskeletal pathology involving the shoulder. The advantages of this surgical technique include the ability to visualize a majority of the shoulder anatomy through a limited approach. Improved techniques and optimization of equipment over the years continue to improve postoperative patient outcomes and function. However, arthroscopic shoulder surgery is not without perioperative complications. As such, the purpose of this chapter is to review the medical and anesthetic complications of arthroscopic shoulder surgery.

MEDICAL COMPLICATIONS

Deep Vein Thrombosis

Deep vein thrombosis (DVT) affecting the arm is rare, with an overall incidence of 4%.[1] Burkhart[2] was the first to report a case of shoulder arthroscopy complicated by thromboembolism in 1990. The reported prevalence

Thompson TL, ed.
*Arthroscopic Shoulder Surgery:
Complications and Management* (pp 63-82).
© 2022 Taylor & Francis Group.

of DVT is 0.31% after shoulder arthroscopy. The condition is found to affect the axillary vein, humeral veins, homolateral basilica vein, cephalic vein, and jugular vein.[1-5] Although shoulder arthroscopy does not impose a surgical insult to the lower extremities, DVT after shoulder arthroscopy has been found to stem from the popliteal vein and the tibiofibular branch.[4] Proposed etiologies support that patients' postoperative pain and desire to rest may contribute to the sedentary postoperative course, which increases the risk of developing a venous clot. There has been wide variation in reported timing of presentation of a thrombosis after shoulder arthroscopy, from the fourth postoperative day to 6 weeks postoperatively.[1,3,4] If there is a concern for a DVT, multiple imaging modalities have been used to find the source, including ultrasound Doppler, arteriovenous Doppler, and echo Doppler, all with variable success.[1,4]

Multiple anticoagulation therapies to treat DVT sustained after a shoulder arthroscopy have been used. Warfarin with and without anticoagulation bridging therapy has been used.[1] Low molecular weight heparin and acenocoumarol (a vitamin K antagonist) have also been successfully used to manage postoperative DVT.[3,4] Development of DVT has been shown to propagate further complications that negatively affect patient morbidity and mortality.[1] Full recovery after DVT, however, is possible with anticoagulation therapy. According to Kuremsky et al[1] and Moen et al,[6] following anticoagulation therapy, their patients' DVT resolved, and full shoulder range of motion without residual pain or apprehension was achieved. However, the systemic anticoagulation effects of therapy can be potentially problematic, ranging from additional clinical interventions to subsequent operative procedures or even fatality.[1] The development of adhesive capsulitis with and without evidence of hemarthrosis has also been documented in the literature. Kuremsky et al[1] reported a patient who developed adhesive capsulitis secondary to hemarthrosis requiring manipulation under anesthesia, capsular plication, bursectomy, and "filter" placement. This patient was thought to have had a good outcome despite the torturous postoperative course from the index procedure. There has also been a report of a patient with protein C deficiency forming a second clot while being anticoagulated for the initial clot. This subsequent complication resulted in the patient having a slow and incomplete shoulder recovery stemming from pain and lack of consistent rehabilitation.[1]

The etiology or contributing factors for the development of DVT have been said to be multifactorial, being the culmination of the simultaneous presence of multiple risk factors and the interaction with one another.[4] Controversy remains over the general risk factors for DVT and pulmonary embolism and their relationship to shoulder arthroscopy.[6] Smoking, hereditary thrombophilia, overweight/obesity, hormone therapy, and neoplasm have the potential to produce a systemic hypercoagulable state increasing the risk of thrombosis in shoulder arthroscopy.[4,5] An arthroscopic etiology for the generation of a clot has been postulated to be contributed by venous compression by the motorized shaver, an interscalene block, lateral decubitus position, arm traction, pacemakers with electrodes, and venous catheters.[1,3] Paget-Schroetter disease, an axillosubclavian thrombosis typically seen in physically active patients who perform vigorous activities of the upper extremities, has also been mentioned to be associated with thrombosis. It has been seen in shoulder arthroscopy in the setting of a history of vein catheters and electrodes for pacemakers.[3]

In 2007, National Institute for Health and Clinical Excellence in England and Wales produced guidelines recommending that all orthopedic inpatients, including those undergoing shoulder arthroscopy, be offered anticoagulation during their hospital stay in the form of low molecular weight heparin. The guidelines were later amended to affect only those who were thought to be high risk, which included age over 60 years, patients with obesity, patients with "significant" comorbidities, and operations in which the surgical and anesthesia time exceeded 90 minutes.[7] Jameson et al[8] found that there was no significant difference in venous thromboembolism event or mortality before or after the introduction of the guidelines in 2007. Upon analysis of the demographics of those who underwent shoulder arthroscopy, the authors noted that more than half of the patients were deemed "high risk." The study found that mortality and venous thromboembolism rates ranged from 0.03% to 0.47% and 0.01% to 0.2%, respectively, with the incidence of these events being similar to the nonsurgical population.

Moen et al[6] also reported that antithrombotic prophylaxis did not significantly decrease the risk of DVT after shoulder arthroscopy. At this time, international guidelines for thromboembolism do not exist for shoulder arthroscopy. Authors have proposed preoperative clotting cascade testing to screen patients for an occult hypercoagulable state that could increase their risk of postoperative thrombosis.[4]

Pulmonary Embolism

Pulmonary embolism is rare after shoulder arthroscopy, with the literature reporting a risk of 0.2% to 2% and a mortality rate of 1%.[9] Clinical manifestations of a pulmonary embolism after shoulder arthroscopy, such as DVT, have a wide range of date of presentation. Patients have been diagnosed as early as 2 days postoperatively and as late as 29 days from the procedure.[4,9] There is no evidence to support routine prophylaxis for pulmonary embolism for patients undergoing shoulder arthroscopy. Some surgeons who plan to perform or have performed shoulder arthroscopy have used preoperative hematology assessment and certoparin sodium in hopes of preventing a pulmonary embolism.[3,5] Edgar et al[9] described a patient on chronic warfarin therapy for a history of thrombophilia and 2 previous pulmonary embolisms who was referred to his hematologist for preoperative anticoagulation recommendations. His postoperative course was complicated by a pulmonary embolism, and it was noted after the procedure that the patient was noncompliant with starting enoxaparin after discontinuing warfarin in preparation for his operation. Polzhofer et al[5] reported a 48-year-old man who developed a pulmonary embolism while being anticoagulated with subcutaneous certoparin sodium for thromboprophylaxis.

The pulmonary site of embolism may be bilateral or unilateral, affecting the larger segmental and the smaller subsegmental branches.[4,9] Infarction may affect the perihilar and suprahilar regions of the lungs as well.[1,9] Various imaging techniques have been used to determine the location and source of thromboembolism, including duplex ultrasound, chest computed tomography (CT), and lung scintigraphy.[1,5,9] The etiology of a pulmonary embolism often stems from breakage of an initial DVT that has traveled to the lungs, but the source has not always been discovered. Edgar et al[9] reported a case of negative bilateral and upper and lower extremity duplex ultrasounds in a 26-year-old man after shoulder arthroscopy, exhibiting that the lack of appreciable thrombus or embolism does not preclude its existence.

Similar to patients who develop a DVT, the postoperative course is variable. There are documented cases of pulmonary embolism stemming from a known DVT with patients being able to attain satisfactory, uneventful recoveries with full function and strength after 6 months.[1,9] Conversely, Polzhofer et al[5] reported a patient who was given thromboprophylaxis who sustained a pulmonary embolism requiring multiple resuscitations, thrombus lysis therapy, and a tracheotomy for long-term ventilation.

There have been numerous postulated contributing factors for the development of a pulmonary embolism after shoulder arthroscopy. Modifiable operative factors have included lateral decubitus position, traction use, and subclavian vein compression by the motor-driven shaver.[1,5] The National Institute for Health and Clinical Excellence guidelines for prophylaxis against pulmonary embolism have not proven to have a significant impact on the development of either DVT or pulmonary embolism.[7]

The position of the patient during arthroscopic shoulder surgery has been a topic of controversy as to which position, lateral decubitus or beach chair, negatively influences or is protective against thromboembolism development. Moen et al[6] reported that the incidence of thromboembolic complications is equal when comparing lateral decubitus and beach chair positions. Pharmacologic prophylaxis against thromboembolic events after shoulder arthroscopy has had a minimal efficacy in combatting their manifestation, even if patients have factors that make them more susceptible to developing these complications. Currently, the optimal strategy to curtail the rare but profound risk of thromboembolism after shoulder arthroscopy is unknown.

Moen et al[6] recommended counseling the patient preoperatively that thromboembolism is a risk that may affect surgical outcomes. In the acute setting, medical consultation or vascular consultation should be acquired for anticoagulation management with intensive care unit admissions and thrombolysis possibly being necessary for hemodynamically unstable patients.

Cerebrovascular Desaturation and Ischemia

Cerebrovascular complications after shoulder arthroscopy may be due to a general lack of perfusion or a decrease in oxygenation. The literature on this topic appears to focus on the upright beach chair position being a contributing factor to the development of intraoperative ischemia and desaturation, with approximately two-thirds of shoulder surgeries being performed in the beach chair position.[10] The beach chair position, in comparison to the lateral decubitus position, offers a more anatomic position, less traction and risk of injury on the brachial plexus, improved better airway access, and easier conversion to an open approach if needed.[10,11] Although the beach chair position offers numerous advantages over the lateral decubitus position, the disadvantage of the beach chair position can be catastrophic even in relatively healthy individuals with no known risk factors, including risk of cerebral hypoperfusion and hypoxia, neurologic injury, severe brain damage, and death.[10]

Studies have shown that cerebral desaturation during shoulder arthroscopy has an incidence of 18%.[10] Salazar et al[10] reported 1.89 cerebral desaturation events in patients during shoulder arthroscopy, ranging from 21% to 62% from their preoperative baseline oxygen levels.

Anesthesia and seated position angle influence the body's ability to perfuse the brain. The sympathetic nervous system is stimulated upon assuming a seated position in the normal physiologic state. The sympathetic nervous system subsequently raises the heart rate and systemic vascular resistance to maintain mean arterial pressure and cardiac output. However, anesthesia diminishes the effects of the sympathetic nervous system due to its vasodilatory effects. As well, the transition from the supine to the seated position in anesthetized and awake patients substantially changes the body's hemodynamics in regards to decreased cardiac index, arterial pressure, and stroke volume.[12]

Monitoring the body's hemodynamics in the form of blood pressure takes careful consideration. Cerebral blood pressure may be overestimated by blood pressure cuff measurements taken at the brachial artery. A hydrostatic column of blood is created from the heart to the brain when a patient is placed in the seated beach chair position. This decreases arterial pressure as blood flows vertically directly linked to the fluid column's weight.[12] This is called the "waterfall" effect.[10] Numerous studies have been performed to understand how the beach chair position affects oxygenation to the brain. The studies use near-infrared spectroscopy (NIRS) to evaluate cerebral desaturation. NIRS has been used in procedures that are high risk for adverse neurologic outcomes such as transplant, cardiac, vascular, and major abdominal surgery. This noninvasive technique has been shown to accurately recognize desaturation events with continuous monitoring of cerebral oxygenation, which would be unnoticed with typical intraoperative monitoring.[12]

The thresholds for a clinically relevant decrease in oxygenation include desaturation of or over 20% from baseline determined by the regional oxygen saturation index mean value over the first minute after induction or a decrease in oxygen saturation below 55% for 15 seconds. A 20% reduction in the oxygenation in the frontal lobe is associated with clinical manifestations of cerebral hypoperfusion in conscious patients, such as syncope.[12] A decrease in oxygenation of 20% from baseline has been used as a predictor of neurologic compromise in patients monitored by NIRS during shoulder arthroscopy. This drop in 20% from baseline has been termed an *cerebral desaturation event*.[13]

Cerebral desaturation at increasing beach chair position angles has shown to be statistically significant, with a decline in oxygenation as beach chair position angles increase, but the oxygenation levels have been shown to remain within the accepted range to prevent neurologic compromise. The cerebral desaturation magnitude appears to be linear with Songy et al[13] showing the largest decrease in cerebral oxygenation occurring from supine to 30 degrees. Interestingly, the regional oxygen saturation index levels fluctuate throughout the procedure during shoulder arthroscopy performed in the beach chair position. This makes it difficult to understand the clinical relevance of cerebral oxygenation given its dynamic behavior.

The duration and magnitude of cerebral ischemia necessary to result in neurocognitive dysfunction are unclear. Furthermore, the clinical relevance of intraoperative cerebral desaturation events is not well understood.[12] Salazar et al[12] performed a prospective cohort study using serial cognitive examinations to better understand intraoperative desaturation via NIRS during shoulder arthroscopy. The Repeatable Battery for the Assessment of Neuropsychological Status was analyzed after being administered preoperatively and postoperatively on day 3. No statistically significant association between postoperative cognitive dysfunction and intraoperative cerebral desaturation events was found. Measurable cognitive decline was also not demonstrated in the Repeatable Battery for the Assessment of Neuropsychological Status analysis. The authors attributed their findings to prompt reversal of transient cerebral desaturation made possible by continuous cerebral monitoring.

There is a paucity of literature regarding guidelines to deter cerebrovascular desaturation and ischemia during shoulder arthroscopy. Songy et al[13] excluded length of surgery as a risk factor for cerebrovascular desaturation events, finding no statistical difference in patients who had cerebral deoxygenating events and those who did not. Furthermore, they recommended a beach chair position angle of 30 to 45 degrees for shoulder arthroscopy. Interscalene block has been shown to decrease the incidence of cerebral desaturation events, and it can be an effective anesthetic for operative shoulder procedures.[13] Moen et al[6] found that the rate of cerebral desaturation can be substantially lowered by use of regional anesthesia.

Stroke

Neurocognitive complications after shoulder arthroscopy have been shown to have an incidence that ranges for 0.004% to 0.0067% while in the beach chair position.[12,13] Although the clinical manifestations are rare, there can be catastrophic complications, including ophthalmoplegia, vision loss, optic neuropathy, and cerebral stroke.[11,12] The perioperative period during which a clinically apparent ischemic event such as a stroke is considered to be in relation to the operation is 30 days.[11] Zeidan et al[11] reported on a 52-year-old man who underwent right shoulder arthroscopy and, on postoperative day 5, presented to the hospital with Broca's aphasia, memory disturbance, and mild dysarthria. There were no motor or sensory deficits noted. Imaging thereafter included CT scan of the brain, echocardiogram, and carotid Doppler, which were all negative. The patient was diagnosed with a cerebral stroke affecting the anterior region of the brain, including the left inferior frontal gyrus. He was able to make a significant recovery after 1 month. Review of his records revealed a mean blood pressure drop of 37% that exceeded the recommended value and may have been the cause of his neurologic deficits. Salazar et al[12] discovered an anomalous circle of Willis as the possible etiology of a postoperative right-sided hemiplegia that went unresolved in a 50-year-old man after arthroscopic subacromial decompression and open rotator cuff repair. Diminished perfusion to the left middle and anterior cerebral artery distributions may have caused the clinically significant pathology.

Bijker and Gelb[14] found that intraoperative hypotension itself increased the risk of stroke by 1.3% per minute of hypotension, with a 30% decrease in mean blood pressure from baseline defined as a safe intraoperative hypotension. The pathophysiology of intraoperative hypotension and the subsequent development of a stroke has not been definitively determined. There is an assumption that as perfusion decreases, the ability to clear micro-emboli within blood vessels reduces, extending the area of hypoperfusion. The authors further postulate that the duration of intraoperative hypotension potentially may have a direct causation with stroke postoperatively.

Although there is an incomplete understanding regarding the association of stroke and beach chair positioning, authors have advised use of the lateral decubitus position as the easiest way to decrease the risk of a catastrophic neurologic incident given the exclusivity or near exclusivity of these incidents using beach chair positioning.[6,11] However, if the beach chair position is the position of choice, the risk of stroke can be managed by a number of modalities. The placement of the blood pressure cuff at the level of the patient's heart and using an arterial line can both optimize accurate assessments of the blood pressure. Attentively monitoring and maintaining intraoperative and perioperative blood pressure may deter dangerous decreases in the perfusion of the central nervous system. Situating the cervical spine at a neutral position while using the beach chair position is paramount due to a potential predisposition to stroke caused by excessive cervical spine extension.[6]

Although a decrease in oxygenation of 20% from baseline has been used as a predictor of neurologic compromise, the clinical relevance of intraoperative cerebrovascular ischemia and desaturation requires further study.[12,13] Nonetheless, the absolute values of cerebral perfusion appear to pale in comparison to changes in baseline perfusion with regard to the importance of predicting ischemia. Furthermore, oxygen saturation trends are believed to be the more clinically pertinent measurement for neurologic complications and should be a focal point of investigation in future research.

Cardiovascular Compromise

The literature on perioperative cardiovascular complications during shoulder arthroscopy is sparse, with contribution from case reports and retrospective studies. However, the information from these studies is remarkable given the manageable insulting cardiovascular etiologies and variation in hemodynamic compromise that have be reported. A key contributor to these uncommon complications appears to be the composition of the irrigation fluid used during shoulder arthroscopy, which has shown to destabilize the cardiovascular system intraoperatively.

Epinephrine-infused irrigation fluid is often used in shoulder arthroscopy to aid in visualization and reduce bleeding. Often the use is benign, but there have been a handful of reports detailing their grave effects on the cardiovascular system. Abrons and Ellis[15] reported severe refractory hypertension in a 52-year-old man undergoing an arthroscopic rotator cuff repair. Abruptly after initiation of the surgical irrigation, the patient's systolic blood pressure rose to 220 to 230 mm Hg, with minimal change after being medicated with a benzodiazepine and 2 administrations of both a β-blocker and an anesthetic sedative. Upon recounting the addition of epinephrine in the surgical irrigation, the irrigation was discontinued and replaced with epinephrine-free irrigation with a return of appropriate blood pressure measurements shortly thereafter. The case was completed devoid of any further hemodynamic instability.[15]

Irrigation fluid–induced cardiac arrest, with and without epinephrine infusion, has been reported in the literature. Manual expression of the irrigation fluid at the conclusion of shoulder arthroscopy is a common occurrence by many surgeons to decrease the volume in the shoulder. This expression of fluid is not benign. Chung et al[16] reported a case of coronary artery spasm while compressing the shoulder, causing the patient to go into ventricular fibrillation requiring cardiopulmonary resuscitation and defibrillation. An echocardiogram was obtained immediately after return of spontaneous circulation, which was devoid of regional wall motion abnormalities and showed normal ventricular contractions. The patient remained intubated and was transferred to the intensive care unit to manage his hemodynamic instability. Coronary angiography was performed, showing no considerable stenosis, but rapid contraction and obstruction were observed in the right coronary artery upon injection of ergonovine with return to normal size after administration of nitroglycerin. The patient was diagnosed with variant angina. The authors postulated that due to fluid accumulation in the shoulder with subsequent gravity and position-dependent spread of the fluid into the neck, the carotid sinus was aroused by fluid stimulation.[16]

Intraoperative cardiac arrest was reported in a 19-year-old man and a 49-year-old woman by Cho et al,[17] which the authors concluded was caused by an improper mixture of the epinephrine in the surgical irrigation. The male patient was undergoing shoulder stabilization surgery, and 5 minutes after infusion of the epinephrine-saline irrigation, the patient's electrocardiogram was notable for paroxysmal supraventricular tachycardia, which progressed to ventricular fibrillation. The irrigation was discontinued and cardiopulmonary resuscitation was immediately performed. During the resuscitation, pink frothy secretion was appreciated from the endotracheal tube, which was considered an indicator of pulmonary edema. An emergent bedside echocardiogram was obtained notable for global hypokinesia devoid of bubbles and diminished ejection fraction. Electrocardiogram showed no ST segment or T-wave abnormalities, but abnormal elevation of creatine kinase, myoglobin, and troponin I was noted. A repeat echocardiogram was performed on postoperative day 5 that showed no abnormal findings, and the patient was discharged home on postoperative day 8.[17]

The 49-year-old woman in the report by Cho et al[17] followed a similar pattern, undergoing paroxysmal supraventricular tachycardia that deteriorated into ventricular tachycardia 5 minutes after epinephrine-infused irrigation was used.[17] The patient was cardioverted 5 times and administered lidocaine before a normal cardiac rhythm was obtained. She was then admitted to the intensive care unit, where an echocardiogram was performed showing global hypokinesia devoid of air bubbles within the circulation and diminished ejection fraction of 30%. On postoperative day 12, a second echocardiogram was obtained that showed no abnormalities. The patient was later discharged home.

A retrospective study by Rubenstein et al[18] using the National Surgical Quality Improvement Program database was aimed at better understating postoperative complications within 30 days of shoulder arthroscopy in patients 60 years and older. They reported an adverse event percentage of 1.6%, with myocardial infarction comprising 0.1% of the adverse events and 3 total reports of cardiac arrest.[18] A recent retrospective study by Rubenstein et al[19] using the National Surgical Quality Improvement Program database noted a correlation of cardiovascular complications of shoulder arthroscopy with body mass index.[19] Patients with a body mass index over 40 kg/m^2 had an odds ratio of 1.8 in regard to major complications after shoulder arthroscopy, which included cardiac arrest. The risk factors for cardiovascular complications in shoulder arthroscopy are an area of research longing for more understanding, but given the infrequent occurrence, it may be difficult to establish pertinent influential characteristics.[19] Cho et al[17] reported on 2 shoulder arthroscopy patients who developed ventricular tachycardia. The authors describe the experimental results of improper mixing of gentacin with a dye-infused saline solution designed to mimic epinephrine. The authors found that the dye, which was intended to represent epinephrine, would localize to the irrigation outlet and be more rapidly infused through the outlet if the bag was poorly mixed. They believed inadequate mixing caused high concentrations of epinephrine to be infused rapidly, resulting in cardiac arrest in their patients. This was newly appreciated due to a recent change in volume of saline used, switching from a 3-L bag of saline to a 1-L bag of saline.[17]

Although cardiovascular destabilization is a rare occurrence, it is life threatening and may be combated by proper handling of the irrigation fluid. The surgeon should be vigilant about obtaining an adequate homogeneous mixture of epinephrine if it is to be used in shoulder arthroscopy as to safeguard the cardiovascular system.

Obesity

A national database study by Sing et al[20] found that 43% of all shoulder arthroscopies from 2011 to 2013 were performed on patients with obesity, with body mass index ranging from 30 to 39 kg/m^2. Complications of shoulder arthroscopy in relation to obesity have included DVT and pulmonary embolism. However, the overall risk of any complications after shoulder arthroscopy does not appear to be statistically significant when compared to nonobese patients. Infection of the surgical site has shown to be statistically significant in patients with obesity, but it may not be clinically significant given the difference in rate between the 2 groups was only 0.3%. Furthermore, surgical site infection in patients with obesity was not found to be an independent predictor of overall 30-day postoperative complications, diminishing its clinical relevance.[20]

ANESTHETIC COMPLICATIONS

Shoulder arthroscopy can be performed under general or regional anesthesia (interscalene block). The main advantage of general anesthesia is that the airway is secured, and induced hypotension can be used to decrease the irrigating fluid requirements. Merits of regional anesthesia are that it avoids polypharmacy, provides for postoperative analgesia, and promotes early ambulation.

Subcutaneous Emphysema, Pneumothorax, and Pneumomediastinum

Arthroscopic shoulder surgery has demonstrated a 5.8% to 9.5% cumulative risk of developing perioperative complications.[20] Documented respiratory complications are rare but have been implicated in relation to anesthesia and to surgical technique or the surgical equipment used. Spontaneous pneumothorax is a serious complication following arthroscopic surgery with endotracheal intubation that has been reported in patients with a history of asthma or heavy smoking[21] (Figure 5-1).

Calvisi et al[21] reported the case of a 52-year-old woman who underwent arthroscopic surgery for subacromial impingement. The patient underwent a scalene brachial plexus block with a long-acting local anesthetic and was positioned upright in the beach chair position. Surgery was uncomplicated except for a single 15-minute episode of dry coughing with spontaneous resolution. On postoperative day 1, emphysema was noted in the supraclavicular fossa extending up the left side of the neck. A chest

Figure 5-1. This computed tomography scan of a 31-year-old woman shows a small pneumothorax (see arrows).

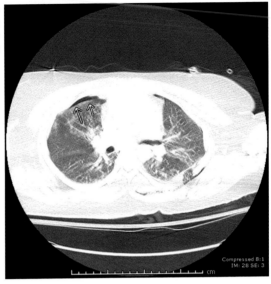

radiograph revealed pneumomediastinum and subcutaneous emphysema in the left thoracic and neck region. A CT scan confirmed the findings and increased clinical suspicion of a full-thickness linear tear extending through the left posterolateral tracheal wall at the level of T4. An emergent thoracic surgery consult was performed, and the patient underwent fiber-optic tracheobronchoscopy that ruled out the suspected injury to the airway and pharynx.[21] Monitoring for these complications is paramount, as unrecognized symptoms can lead to potential adverse events.

Respiratory complications following arthroscopic shoulder surgery can potentially be devastating. Lee et al[22] reported on 3 patients who developed subcutaneous emphysema, pneumomediastinum, and tension pneumothorax following arthroscopic subacromial decompression. The authors did not report on the patients' smoking history or on the presence or absence of preexisting pleuropulmonary comorbidities. Patients were operated on in the upright position under general anesthesia with endotracheal intubation and positive pressure ventilation. The authors hypothesized that negative pressure in the subacromial space may result from transient pressure drops when the motorized shaver coupled to high suction is used during the decompression technique. Air can be sucked internally through the working portal and forced by the infusion pressure into the axillary sheath. Pneumomediastinum develops if air penetrates the visceral space of the neck. In addition, a rise in mediastinal pressure during expiration or because of positive pressure ventilation could tear the parietal pleura, causing pneumothorax.

Similarly, Lau[23] reported on one patient having subcutaneous emphysema and pneumomediastinum after arthroscopic debridement for a glenoid labral tear under general anesthesia by endotracheal intubation. The author postulated that faulty or suboptimal surgical equipment setup may be the culprit for this complication and suspected that a loose junction between the saline solution bag and the valve of the inflow tube could have potentially injected air into the joint. Portal-related capsular openings would allow water and air extravasation into the surrounding soft tissues and ultimately cause pneumomediastinum.[23]

These studies underline the importance of noting patient risk factors but also the meticulous attention to the proper functioning of surgical equipment. It is unclear from the previous studies whether arthroscopic cannulas equipped with a sealing dam were used. Sealing dams have been associated with a reduced risk of air entrance. The pathogenetic mechanisms postulated by the above authors imply that air leakage from the airway system should be definitely ruled out. However, a chest CT scan was used in only 1 of the 3 patients reported by Lee et al,[22] and none underwent fiber-optic bronchoscopy to exclude injury during intubation. Since tears of the tracheal membranous portion have been associated with endotracheal intubation, their reported complication could potentially be dependent upon anesthetic factors. The literature review would thus suggest that both anesthesia- and surgery-related variables may be implied in the onset of subcutaneous emphysema and pneumomediastinum. Furthermore, heavy smoking and pulmonary comorbidities could represent predisposing conditions to spontaneous pneumothorax when shoulder surgery is performed under endotracheal intubation. Last, prompt physical and imaging evaluation is recommended if the patient demonstrates respiratory symptoms during or after surgery.

Interscalene Block

Interscalene block regional anesthesia offers many advantages over general anesthesia for both arthroscopic and open surgeries of the shoulder. It provides excellent intraoperative anesthesia and muscle relaxation as well as analgesia that continues into the postoperative period[24] (Figure 5-2).

Bishop et al[24] performed a retrospective chart review of 568 consecutive patients undergoing shoulder surgery with interscalene regional block. Ninety-seven percent of patients with an interscalene block alone had a successful block, and the remaining 3% had block failure requiring the conversion to general anesthesia. Comparatively, the complication rate was 1.4% for those receiving an interscalene regional block for arthroscopy vs 3.2% for those who had open shoulder surgery.[24] There were no complications

Figure 5-2. Anesthesiologist performing an interscalene block.

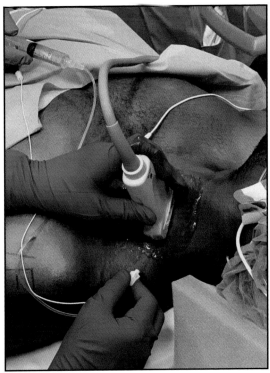

of general anesthesia. As demonstrated by this study, surgeons must understand the anatomic limitations of the block and the necessity to supplement blocks, and they should not consider this cooperative effort to be a sign of block failure.

It could be hypothesized that inadvertent puncture of the prevertebral fascia during interscalene block might draw in air and produce the clinical picture of subcutaneous and mediastinal emphysema. This phenomenon is thought to be propagated by a Bernoulli effect, which may create conditions favoring air entrance into the subacromial space. Since the centrifugal fluid pump maintains a constant flow rate, the change of cross-sectional area and resistance between the subacromial space and the outflow cannula would increase the outflow velocity and consequently cause a pressure drop according to Bernoulli's law. Hence, transient pressure drops in the subacromial space could suck in air when, for example, the threaded cannula is switched from one portal to another or a portal is not engaged by the cannula. A high-suction pressure would add to the Bernoulli effect, as advocated by Lee et al.[22]

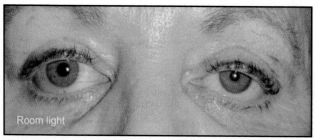

Figure 5-3. This 65-year-old patient with Horner syndrome has ptosis and miosis on the left. (Reproduced with permission from Martin TJ. Horner syndrome: a clinical review. *ACS Chem Neurosci.* 2018;9[2]:177–186. © 2018 American Chemical Society.)

Horner Syndrome Associated With Interscalene Block

Horner syndrome is not an uncommon finding immediately after performance of an interscalene block, and its clinical manifestations are generally transient. Transient Horner syndrome is a well-known side effect of stellate ganglion block, interscalene block of the brachial plexus, and occasionally of epidural analgesia. However, prolonged Horner syndrome occurring after interscalene block is rare and a matter of significant concern because it may represent traumatic interruption of the sympathetic cervical chain (Figure 5-3).

Ekatrodramis et al[25] described prolonged Horner syndrome in 2 patients in whom the formation of a lateral neck hematoma after interscalene block was believed to be the cause of this complication. The authors presented the case of a 48-year-old woman undergoing treatment of persistent complex regional pain syndrome type I of the right hand. Treatment was performed under continuous interscalene analgesia. The catheter was tunneled subcutaneously by an 18-gauge intravenous cannula without complication. On the third day after interscalene catheter placement, the patient reported blurred vision and painful swelling on the right lateral aspect of her neck. Inspection revealed a swelling around catheter site insertion and concomitant Horner syndrome on the ipsilateral side: myosis, ptosis, enophthalmia, anhydrosis on the whole ipsilateral side of the face, and conjunctival hyperemia, which was not present at the time of the initial block. Eight hours after removing the catheter, sensory block of the right arm resolved, but Horner syndrome remained. Residual ptosis was the only remaining symptom for approximately 1 year, after which the Horner syndrome resolved completely.

Spontaneous Pneumothorax

Dietzel and Ciullo[26] reported on 4 patients developing spontaneous pneumothorax after arthroscopic shoulder surgery. All patients were smokers, and 2 had asthma. Surgery was performed in the lateral decubitus position under general anesthesia. The authors hypothesized that the onset of pneumothorax would have been caused by rupture of a bullae. The increase of the negative pleural pressure on the operated side in the lateral decubitus could have added to the potential of bullae rupture.[26] These authors recommend that patients with respiratory comorbidities with preoperatively identified bullae undergo interscalene block to reduce the risk of spontaneous pneumothorax. Unfortunately, bullae can be detected only in 20% of patients by means of routine examination.[26] There are very little other documented data on this devastating complication.

Tracheal Compression Caused by Fluid Extravasation

Shoulder arthroscopy requires visualization of 2 main areas: the encapsulated glenohumeral joint and the unencapsulated subacromial space. Proper visualization of the glenohumeral joint requires expansion of the joint space by irrigating fluid from a normal capacity of 3 to 4 mL to approximately 60 mL. Alternatively, the subacromial space is an unencapsulated anatomic area that communicates well via various anatomic planes to the soft tissues of the neck and chest. This space requires higher pressures for proper visualization and poses risk of fluid escape into the neck and chest, leading to airway swelling and further to respiratory compromise. Amount of fluid extravasation will depend on the amount and pressure of the irrigating fluid used and duration of surgery. Lateral position and obesity also predispose to fluid accumulation. Fluid extravasation not only complicates surgical field visualization with large amounts of fluid escaping into the neck and chest but also can accumulate and cause external compression on and swelling of the laryngeal and tracheal tissue structures, leading to life-threatening airway obstruction. Thus, measures that decrease fluid extravasation play a very important role in shoulder arthroscopy.[27]

Ozhan et al[28] reported on a 33-year-old man who underwent arthroscopic acromioplasty and repair of the rotator cuff for impingement syndrome of the right shoulder. The patient underwent general anesthesia with interscalene brachial plexus block for postoperative pain management. According to anesthetic monitoring, the capnographic curve showed a sloped shape indicating an obstructive pattern with a decreasing oxygen saturation and intraoperative physical examination revealing a tense and swollen neck, right chest, and shoulder on palpation. A portable chest radiograph examination showed soft tissue swelling in the right shoulder and neck, and pneumothorax and hemothorax were excluded. A fiber-optic bronchoscopic evaluation through the endotracheal tube revealed that the trachea was compressed but not completely obstructed. It was determined that the irrigation fluid had leaked subcutaneously from the shoulder joint to the neck. The operation was resumed and completed without further complication, and the patient was extubated without complication.[28]

Berjano et al[29] performed a retrospective series comparing the complication rates of arthroscopic shoulder surgery vs arthroscopic plus open procedures performed by the same surgeon. The complication rate was 10%, with one case of respiratory distress requiring reintubation and intensive care for 24 hours, with no subsequent complications. The underlying mechanism of this complication is the leakage of excessive amounts of irrigation fluid into extracapsular tissues and then accumulation in the soft tissues near the neck and in the mucous membranes of the upper airway. The predisposing factors established in the literature are prolonged surgery, subacromial procedures, using a high-pressure irrigation pump, and surgeon proficiency. Procedures performed in the lateral decubitus position tend to accumulate fluid due to gravity. The beach chair position, however, is a special concern for anesthesiologists because it has unique risks for air embolism, hypotensive and bradycardic events, and brain and spinal cord ischemia.[29]

Association Between Sleep Apnea and Perioperative Outcomes

An increasing percentage of orthopedic surgeries is performed in ambulatory surgery centers. Whether or not patients with obstructive sleep apnea (OSA) are suitable candidates for operative procedures in this type of setting is controversial given their presumed increased risk of adverse events.

Masaracchia et al[30] examined the extent to which OSA is associated with decrements in perioperative outcomes using data from a large population-based patient cohort. They identified 128,932 patients who underwent shoulder arthroscopy at 583 hospitals between 2010 and 2015, with approximately 6% of patients having a sleep apnea diagnosis. Patients with OSA were more likely to be of older age, White (non-Hispanic), and male. The preexisting comorbidity data revealed a higher comorbid burden in patients with OSA, especially regarding uncomplicated diabetes and chronic obstructive pulmonary disease. An increase in complication rates was identified for the OSA group, as were the increased odds of patients with OSA experiencing any complication (2.23 times higher) and pulmonary complications (4.92 times higher). Patients with OSA were also found to have higher rates of hospital resource utilization, including substantially greater odds of receiving blood transfusions, intensive care unit transfers, and the need for a hospital admission. This may be related to the overall health status of patients with OSA requiring greater medical intervention for health maintenance.

Negative Pressure Pulmonary Edema

Negative pressure pulmonary edema has been increasingly reported in the surgical literature since the 1970s, yet there are limited references to this complication in the orthopedic literature. A case by Gogia et al[31] reports on negative pressure pulmonary edema occurring during an elective shoulder arthroscopy for recurrent shoulder dislocation in an 18-year-old man. The procedure was uneventful, but after extubation, the patient exhibited obstructed breathing that progressed to complete airway obstruction, with massive swelling extending to the neck and chest. Considering the threat of airway obstruction, the trachea was immediately reintubated after direct laryngoscopy. On further examination, auscultation of the chest revealed bilateral crepitus, and neck circumference was measured as 52 cm. A diagnosis of postobstructive noncardiogenic pulmonary edema was made. The patient was monitored in the intensive care unit and extubated following chest x-ray confirmation of resolution after 24 hours. The patient was discharged home without any further complication.

Arthroscopic shoulder surgery has several advantages over open procedures, including reduced postoperative pain, reduced hospital stay, and early mobilization. It is considered a fairly safe procedure with limited complications, but anesthesia-related complications are indeed very serious and must be preemptively recognized by an astute surgeon in collaboration with the anesthesia team, addressed promptly, and monitored closely in the immediate postoperative period to ensure successful patient outcomes.

REFERENCES

1. Kuremsky MA, Cain EL Jr, Fleischli JE. Thromboembolic phenomena after arthroscopic shoulder surgery. *Arthroscopy.* 2011;27(12):1614–1619.
2. Burkhart SS. Deep venous thrombosis after shoulder arthroscopy. *Arthroscopy.* 1990;6(1):61–63.
3. Delos D, Rodeo SA. Venous thrombosis after arthroscopic shoulder surgery: pacemaker leads as a possible cause: pacemaker leads as a possible cause. *HSS J.* 2011;7(3):282–285.
4. Garofalo R, Notarnicola A, Moretti L, Moretti B, Marini S, Castagna A. Deep vein thromboembolism after arthroscopy of the shoulder: two case reports and a review of the literature. *BMC Musculoskelet Disord.* 2010;11:65.
5. Polzhofer GK, Petersen W, Hassenpflug J. Thromboembolic complication after arthroscopic shoulder surgery. *Arthroscopy.* 2003;19(9):E129–E132.
6. Moen TC, Rudolph GH, Caswell K, Espinoza C, Burkhead WZ Jr, Krishnan SG. Complications of shoulder arthroscopy. *J Am Acad Orthop Surg.* 2014;22:410–419.
7. National Institute for Health and Clinical Excellence. Venous thromboembolism in over 16s: reducing the risk of hospital-acquired deep vein thrombosis or pulmonary embolism. 2018. http://www.nice.org.uk/NG89. Accessed October 15, 2020.
8. Jameson SS, James P, Howcroft DWJ, et al. Venous thromboembolic events are rare after shoulder surgery: analysis of a national database. *J Shoulder Elbow Surg.* 2011;20:764–770.
9. Edgar R, Nagda S, Huffman R, Namdari S. Pulmonary embolism after shoulder arthroscopy. *Orthopedics.* 2012;35(11):e1673–e1676.
10. Salazar D, Sears BW, Aghdasi B, et al. Cerebral desaturation events during shoulder arthroscopy in the beach chair position: patient risk factors and neurocognitive effects. *J Shoulder Elbow Surg.* 2013;22(9):1228–1235.
11. Zeidan A, Bluwi M, Elshamaa K. Postoperative brain stroke after shoulder arthroscopy in the lateral position. *J Stroke Cerebrovasc Dis.* 2014;23:384–386.
12. Salazar D, Hazel A, Tauchen AJ, Sears BW, Marra G. Neurocognitive deficits and cerebral desaturation during shoulder arthroscopy with patient in beach-chair position: a review of the current literature. *Am J Orthop (Belle Mead NJ).* 2016;45:E63–E68.
13. Songy CE, Siegel ER, Stevens M, Wilkinson JT, Ahmadi S. The effect of the beach-chair position angle on cerebral oxygenation during shoulder surgery. *J Shoulder Elbow Surg.* 2017;26:1670–1675.
14. Bijker JB, Gelb AW. Review article: the role of hypotension in perioperative stroke. *Can J Anaesth.* 2013;60(2):159–167.
15. Abrons RO, Ellis SE. Severe refractory hypertension during shoulder arthroscopy. *Saudi J Anaesth.* 2016;10(2):236–237.
16. Chung J, Gong HY, Park J, et al. Coronary artery spasm induced by carotid sinus stimulation during arthroscopic shoulder surgery: a case report. *Medicine (Baltimore).* 2019;98(5):e143–e152.
17. Cho SH, Yi JW, Kwack YH, Park SW, Kim MK, Rhee YG. Ventricular tachycardia during arthroscopic shoulder surgery: a report of two cases. *Arthrosc Sports Med.* 2010;130:353–356.
18. Rubenstein WJ, Pean CA, Colvin AC. Shoulder arthroscopy in adults 60 or older: risk factors that correlate with postoperative complications in the first 30 days. *Arthroscopy.* 2017;33:49–54.

19. Rubenstein WJ, Lansdown DA, Feeley BT, Ma CB, Zhang AL. The impact of body mass index on complications after shoulder arthroscopy: should surgery eligibility be determined by body mass index cutoffs? *Arthroscopy.* 2016;84(1):27–33.

20. Sing DC, Ding DY, Aguilar TU, et al. The effects of patient obesity on early postoperative complications after shoulder arthroscopy. *Arthroscopy.* 2016;32(11):2212–2217.

21. Calvisi V, Lupparelli S, Rossetti S. Subcutaneous emphysema and pneumomediastinum following shoulder arthroscopy with brachial plexus block: a case report and review of the literature. *Arch Orthop Trauma Surg.* 2009;129(3):349–352.

22. Lee HC, Dewan N, Crosby L. Subcutaneous emphysema, pneumomediastinum, and potentially life-threatening tension pneumothorax: pulmonary complications from arthroscopic shoulder decompression. *Chest.* 1992;101(5):1265–1267.

23. Lau KY. Pneumomediastinum caused by subcutaneous emphysema in the shoulder: a rare complication of arthroscopy. *Chest.* 1993;103:1606–1607.

24. Bishop JY, Sprague M, Gelber J. Interscalene regional anesthesia for shoulder surgery. *J Bone Joint Surg Am.* 2005;87:974–979.

25. Ekatrodramis G, Macaire P, Borgeat A. Prolonged Horner syndrome due to neck hematoma after continuous interscalene block. *Anesthesiology.* 2001;95(3):801–803.

26. Dietzel DP, Ciullo JV. Spontaneous pneumothorax after shoulder arthroscopy: a report of four cases. *Arthroscopy.* 1996;12(1):99–102.

27. Borgeat A, Bird P, Ekatodramis G, Dumont C. Tracheal compression caused by periarticular fluid accumulation: a rare complication of shoulder surgery. *J Shoulder Elb Surg.* 2000;9(5):443–445.

28. Ozhan MO, Suzer MA, Cekmen N, Caparlar CO, Eskin MB. Tracheal compression during shoulder arthroscopy in the beach-chair position. *Curr Ther Res Clin Exp.* 2010;71(6):408–415.

29. Berjano P, González BG, Olmedo JF, et al. Complications in arthroscopic shoulder surgery. *Arthroscopy.* 1998;14:785–788.

30. Masaracchia MM, Sites BD, Herrick MD, Liu H, Davis M. Association between sleep apnea and perioperative outcomes among patients undergoing shoulder arthroscopy. *Can J Anaesth.* 2018;65:1314–1323.

31. Gogia AR, Bajaj J, Sahni A, Saigal D. Negative-pressure pulmonary oedema in a patient undergoing shoulder arthroscopy. *Indian J Anaesth.* 2012;56(1):62–65.

6

Nerve and Vascular Injury

Filippo Familiari, MD; Jorge Rojas, MD;
Prashant Meshram, MS, DNB; Gazi Huri, MD;
and Edward G. McFarland, MD

INTRODUCTION

Shoulder surgery has undergone a paradigm shift over the past 20 to 30 years. The introduction, development, and refinement of arthroscopic instrumentation and surgical techniques have prompted many surgeons to transition away from open procedures in favor of arthroscopic techniques. As the popularity of arthroscopic surgery has increased, proponents of these techniques have cited its numerous advantages over open surgery, including lower complication rates.[1] However, complications are ubiquitous in surgery of any kind, and this is true of arthroscopic shoulder surgery as well.

It might be more appropriate to suggest that complications of arthroscopic surgery are similar to those seen in open surgery, albeit at a different rate and type. For example, infections after some open shoulder surgical procedures may be more frequent than with arthroscopic shoulder surgery,[2] but this should not lull the surgeon into not taking adequate precautions to avoid them intraoperatively and to be aware of them postoperatively. Among the most distressing complications after shoulder surgery

Thompson TL, ed.
Arthroscopic Shoulder Surgery:
Complications and Management (pp 83-97).
© 2022 Taylor & Francis Group.

are neurologic or vascular injuries, which can occur with either open or arthroscopic procedures. These complications can result in permanent disability of the shoulder and have the potential to be life and limb threatening.

The Brachial Plexus and Pertinent Shoulder Anatomy in Arthroscopy

For the safe performance of arthroscopic shoulder procedures, knowledge of the specific anatomy of nerves and vessels, their location relative to standard portal placement, and their proximity during specific procedures is critical. The distance of neurovascular structures from easily identifiable bony landmarks has been reported in the literature, and identifying the borders of these structures is important to safe and accurate portal placement during arthroscopic shoulder surgery.

Direct injury to nerves and blood vessels during arthroscopic surgery fortunately is uncommon. Knowledge of the location of these structures around the shoulder is just as important as when performing an open surgery. While axillary nerve, cephalic vein, and suprascapular artery and nerve are the structures at most risk during shoulder arthroscopy,[3-5] information of the location of the brachial plexus and major vessels is also important. Knowledge of their locations and courses is critical to avoid traumatic injury during portal placement.

The brachial plexus is medial and inferior to the shoulder joint and, for most arthroscopic procedures, is not at risk. However, the plexus can be at risk during acromioclavicular joint stabilizations, subscapularis tendon repairs, and anterior instability operations. The brachial plexus is reported to be within 2 cm from the anterior glenoid rim (Figure 6-1A).[5] If the subscapularis tendon and muscle is torn or atrophied, the plexus may be closer to the glenoid rim (Figure 6-1B). The anterior arthroscopic portal has a safe zone which was defined by Matthews et al.[6] This portal should be placed lateral to the coracoid. When placed and viewed from inside the joint, the safe zone is between the upper border of subscapularis tendon and the biceps tendon.

One of the nerves that is commonly at risk of injury during arthroscopic shoulder surgery is the axillary nerve. The axillary nerve travels posterior to the coracoid and inferior to the lateral border of the subscapularis medial to the musculotendinous junction (see Figure 6-1B). The nerve can be as close as 3.1 cm from the leading edge of the acromion with arm abduction.[7] Typically, the axillary nerve then gives off 2 branches that supply the inferior capsule. In a cadaver study, Uno et al[8] found that the axillary nerve is connected to the capsule with loose tissue between the 5- and 7-o'clock

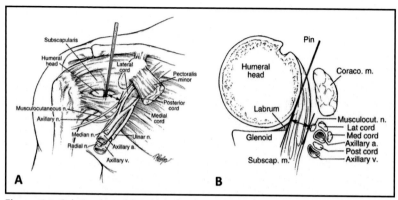

Figure 6-1. Relationship of brachial plexus with the glenoid rim. (A) Anterior view of shoulder demonstrating the relationship of the anterior glenoid rim with the brachial plexus. (B) A cross-sectional diagram of the shoulder joint viewed from below demonstrates the relationship of the brachial plexus to the subscapularis muscle. a., artery; Coraco. m., coracobrachialis muscle; Lat cord, lateral cord; Med cord, medial cord; Musculocut. n., musculocutaneous nerve; Post cord, posterior cord; subscap. m., subscapularis muscle; v., vein. (Illustrations: Tim Phelps © 2001 JHU AAM, Department of Art as Applied to Medicine, The Johns Hopkins University School of Medicine. Reproduced with permission.)

positions and lies close to the glenoid in the neutral position, extension, and internal rotation. Abduction, external rotation, and traction cause the capsule to distend and, thus, move the nerve away from the anteroinferior portion of joint, possibly making this position safer during arthroscopic surgery. After passing the capsule, the axillary nerve travels posteriorly through the quadrilateral space and gives off a posterior and an anterior trunk. The posterior trunk has 3 terminations: the superolateral cutaneous branch, the posterior branch to the deltoid muscle, and the nerve to the teres minor.[9] The anterior trunk travels around the humerus and supplies the 3 heads of the deltoid muscle.[7] Traditionally, this anterior branch of the axillary nerve was thought to be an average of 5 to 7 cm distal to the lateral tip of the acromion.[10] While the nerve has also been described as 3.5 cm distal to the superior prominence of the greater tuberosity,[11] another cadaveric study revealed that this section of the axillary nerve can be much closer, especially in short women.[7] Overall, the nerve has been reported to be from 3 to 7 cm from the lateral acromion depending on patient size and arm length.[7,12] Abducting the arm brings the axillary nerve branch even closer to the acromion; at 90 degrees, this distance is decreased by 30%.[7]

In the upper arm, the cephalic vein travels in the superficial fascia of the deltopectoral interval and extends downward through the coracoclavicular fascia to the axillary vein beneath the clavicle. It is at this deltopectoral interval that the vein is most at risk for injury during portal placement, typically resulting in a superficial hematoma. A cadaveric study reported the cephalic vein to be located less than 1 cm from the anterior portal in 25% of the specimens.[3] While the cephalic vein may be at risk of injury during arthroscopic portal placement, damage to this vessel has not been reported to cause deep venous thrombosis (DVT) or other complications.

The suprascapular nerve arises from the upper trunk of the brachial plexus, traveling then through the posterior triangle of neck. The suprascapular artery runs with the nerve until it reaches the suprascapular notch. The nerve lies 3 cm (range, 2.5 to 3.9 cm) medial to the supraglenoid tubercle at the suprascapular notch.[13] At this point, while the nerve travels underneath the transverse scapular ligament, the artery passes above this ligament and outside the notch. Within 1 cm of exiting the notch, the nerve gives its motor branch to the supraspinatus. Then the nerve then follows an oblique course laterally toward the base of scapular spine. The nerve lies at an average of 1.8 cm (range, 1.4 to 2.5 cm) from the midline of the posterior glenoid at the base of scapular spine. The nerve then curves medially to innervate the infraspinatus.[13]

Adverse Neurologic Events

Patient Positioning

While neurologic complications associated with shoulder arthroscopy are uncommon, a wide variety of injuries have been reported after shoulder arthroscopy. Adverse events such as neurapraxia of the great auricular nerve or cranial nerve,[14] injury to the cervical plexus,[15] ophthalmoplegia,[16,17] and fatal venous air embolism[18] have been reported. However, the most severe and well-studied complications are ischemic events caused by cerebral hypoperfusion such as stroke,[19,20] central nervous system infarct,[21] and vision loss.[16] These events are reported, almost exclusively, when shoulder arthroscopy was performed with the patient in the beach chair position. While the patient is awake, the autonomic nervous system regulates systemic blood pressure to maintain cerebral perfusion, particularly when moving from a supine to an upright position.[22,23] General anesthesia impairs the autonomic nervous system's ability to maintain blood pressure with change in the position. Thus, cerebral circulation is at risk of hypoperfusion during arthroscopic shoulder surgery performed using the beach chair position, placing the patient at risk for an ischemic event. Friedman et al[19] surveyed American shoulder surgeons who had performed more than 200,000 shoulder procedures in the beach chair position, mostly arthroscopic. They reported 8 cerebrovascular events with an overall incidence of 0.003%. Despite this very low incidence, the neurologic sequelae can be devastating for the patient and the providers. Pohl and Cullen[21] reported 4 cases of ischemic brain injury after shoulder surgery in the beach chair position that resulted in the death of 1 patient and severe brain damage in 3 patients. Drummond et al[24] reported one case of stroke and right hemiparesis after shoulder surgery in the beach chair position in a patient with congenital variation of circle of Willis anatomy.

Cogan et al[14] and Boisseau et al[25] reported 2 cases of neurapraxia of the 9th, 10th, and 12th cranial nerve pairs after arthroscopic rotator cuff repair in the beach chair position. Although cerebral hypoperfusion was considered a possible cause, the most likely cause for nerve palsy proposed by those authors was an extracranial mechanical compression. Isolated cranial nerve injuries after beach chair positioning have also been reported. There have been 5 cases of isolated hypoglossal nerve neurapraxia reported in the literature in patients undergoing shoulder surgery in the beach chair position.[26-30] While the exact mechanism is not exactly known, either compression or distraction of the nerve due to positioning has been speculated. Eight cases of neurapraxia of the greater auricular nerve have been reported in the literature after shoulder surgery in the beach chair position, and direct nerve compression by the headrest was considered the etiology.[15,31-33]

Other neurologic injuries reported in the literature with the beach chair position are direct external nerve compressions, which are probably related to patient positioning. Lateral femoral cutaneous nerve palsy after shoulder surgery in the beach chair position is an uncommon complication, with a reported incidence of 1.3%.[34] Patient body mass index and body weight were found to be the risk factors for its development. Other potential factors contributing to the development of lateral femoral cutaneous nerve palsy include the positioning and tightness of the restraining belt.

The easiest way to minimize the risk of a catastrophic neurologic event is to perform shoulder arthroscopy using the lateral decubitus position. This position has been associated with substantially fewer cerebral hypoperfusion events than has the beach chair position.[35-37] However, if arthroscopy must be performed using the beach chair position, the surgeon and anesthesiologist can take measures to maintain an accurate assessment of the patient's blood pressure, including positioning the blood pressure cuff at the level of the patient's heart and inserting an arterial line. They also can vigilantly monitor and maintain the intraoperative and perioperative blood pressure to avoid a severe decrease in perfusion pressure of the central nervous system.[38] Additionally, recent research has shown that shoulder arthroscopy performed with regional anesthetic and intravenous sedation has a substantially lower rate of cerebral desaturation events.[39]

The most commonly reported cause of neurologic injury when shoulder arthroscopy is performed in the lateral decubitus position is either excessive strain on the brachial plexus due to intraoperative traction, direct external nerve compression, or iatrogenic injury during the arthroscopic procedure. The reported incidence of transient paresthesia or nerve palsies after arthroscopic surgery in the lateral decubitus position has been reported to be 0.2% to 10%.[40-45] Despite this relatively high incidence of nerve injuries, in almost all cases reported, the injuries were neurapraxias, which recovered with no sequelae. Andrews et al,[40] in a series of 120 patients who underwent shoulder arthroscopy in the lateral decubitus position, reported 3 cases of clinically detectable neurapraxia. The musculocutaneous nerve was involved in 1 patient and ulnar nerve in 2 patients. Ogilvie-Harris and Wiley[41] studied 439 patients who underwent arthroscopic surgical procedures in the lateral decubitus position and reported one case of musculocutaneous nerve palsy. This injury resolved in about 6 weeks without any long-term sequelae. Berjano et al[43] reported 3 ulnar nerve neurapraxias attributed to the use of a traction device in a series of 156 patients who underwent shoulder arthroscopy in the lateral decubitus position. Similarly, Paulos and Franklin,[45] in a series of 76 patients, reported one case of axillary nerve neurapraxia with deltoid muscle dysfunction that resolved after 2 months.

Pitman et al[42] used somatosensory evoked potentials (SEPs) to evaluate the onset of neurapraxia during shoulder arthroscopy performed in the lateral decubitus position in 20 patients. They found a 100% incidence of abnormal SEP of the musculocutaneous nerve. Fifty percent of patients also had varying combinations of involvement of the median, ulnar, and radial nerves. Fortunately, injury was subclinical in all but 2 patients (10%) who had a neurapraxia that recovered fully. Abnormal SEPs were related to the amount of weight used in the traction system. No abnormal SEP was found in any of the nerves of the brachial plexus with a weight lower than 12 pounds used for long-axis traction and with a weight lower than 7 pounds used for perpendicular midhumerus traction.

Traction during shoulder arthroscopy with the patient in the lateral decubitus position can cause a partial or complete tourniquet effect, which could potentially impair the perfusion of the operative extremity. Hennrikus et al[46] studied the effect of 3 methods of shoulder traction during arthroscopy on arterial oxygen saturation (SaO$_2$) measured by a pulse oximeter applied to the fingertip of the arm in traction of 30 patients. They found that simple longitudinal traction was the safest method in terms of limb perfusion. Only 1 of 30 patients had decrease of SaO$_2$ with this method of traction. On the other hand, when perpendicular traction was applied with a narrow 2-inch sling, compression of the brachial artery by the sling caused a decrease of SaO$_2$ in 25 of 30 limbs. The wider 4-inch sling used for perpendicular traction resulted in a decrease of limb perfusion in only 7 of 30 patients and was found safer than the narrow sling. Despite this concern, vascular lesions associated with traction have not been reported. For the lateral decubitus position, many traction devices involve a stocking or a device to hold the hand, on which the traction is applied. As a result, compression of the digital nerves in the hand with subsequent neurapraxias has been reported. Ellman[44] reported 3 cases of transient dysesthesia of the dorsal digital nerve of the thumb believed to be due to poor padding of the extremity at the wrist.

In the lateral decubitus position, brachial plexus palsy has also been reported in the nonoperative extremity, which is in contact with the bed.[47] There has been only one report of a patient with a cervical rib who developed a transient C7-T1 contralateral neurapraxia after a shoulder arthroscopy in the lateral decubitus position. Although the presence of the cervical rib was suggested as the possible cause, use of a gel type of axillary roll between the chest and the bed is recommended to prevent these types of injuries to the nonoperative extremity.

Neurovascular injuries seen in patients in the lateral decubitus position may also be related to difficulty in the arthroscopic portal placement as a virtue of lateral patient position. Only one cadaveric study[48] has compared the risk of neurovascular injuries as they relate to the patient positioning. In that study, compared to the beach chair position, the lateral decubitus position had an increased risk of injury to the musculocutaneous and axillary nerves when a 5-o'clock trans-subscapular or anteroinferior portal was used.

Portal Placement

A significant portion of the nerve injuries during shoulder arthroscopy is believed to occur during placement of the portals. Segmüller and colleagues,[49] for example, reported a 7% rate of cutaneous nerve neuropathies after shoulder arthroscopy, with nearly half of these lesions remaining symptomatic at 8 months after surgery. They noted that most of the nerve injuries' locations were close to the portal sites and attributed them to blunt trauma during introduction of the trocar.

The axillary, suprascapular, and musculocutaneous nerves are most vulnerable to direct injury during portal placement. The normal and variant anatomy of the axillary nerve has been well described.[5,8,9,50,51] The axillary nerve is at risk of injury during the placement of standard arthroscopic portals, most notably, the anterior and inferior portals. In a study of cadaver specimens and clinical data, placement of a standard anterior portal lateral to the coracoid and through the rotator interval has been shown to be safe.[52]

However, given the proximity of the axillary nerve to the inferior glenoid and joint capsule, the margin of safety diminishes as the portal is placed in progressively inferior positions.[3,53] Posterior portals are typically safe in terms of the risk of neurovascular injury. Classic posterior portal placement, 2 cm medial and 2 cm inferior to the posterolateral corner of the acromion, is typically a minimum of 2 to 3 cm away from the axillary nerve.[3,53] When placed properly, an accessory portal created at the 7-o'clock position has also been described as safe, because it is 3.9 cm from the axillary nerve.[54] Proper placement of lateral portals also can prevent injury to the axillary nerve. Burkhead et al[7] described a "safe zone" located within 3 cm of the lateral border of the acromion; lateral working portals placed within this zone avoid the axillary nerve injury. Placement of the Port of Wilmington (located approximately 1 cm lateral and 1 cm anterior to the posterolateral corner of the acromion) and antero-supero-lateral portals is also safe given the distance from the portal to the adjacent neurovascular structures.[3,53]

Specific surgical procedures, particularly glenohumeral capsular release, thermal capsulorrhaphy, and arthroscopic stabilization, have been shown to have an increased risk of axillary nerve injury. Arthroscopic capsular release through the anteroinferior and posteroinferior axillary pouch and recess places the axillary nerve at risk of injury because of its proximity to the inferior capsule.[50] Capsulolabral sutures used during arthroscopic stabilization have been implicated in injury to the axillary nerve, especially when they are used in a capsular shift of the anteroinferior band of the inferior glenohumeral ligament.[1] However, sutures placed within the glenohumeral capsule no further lateral than 1 cm from the glenoid rim are at a relatively safe distance from the axillary nerve.[55] During more advanced arthroscopic techniques, such as the arthroscopic Latarjet and arthroscopic axillary nerve release, surgical instruments are in close proximity to the axillary nerve; therefore, these procedures should be performed with caution.[56-58]

The unique anatomy of the suprascapular nerve makes it vulnerable to injury during shoulder arthroscopy, although the incidence of nerve injury is low.[13,59] Historically, the suprascapular nerve was considered vulnerable to injury during "blind" transglenoid drilling while performing surgery for glenohumeral instability. The use of suture anchors has become more prevalent, helping to diminish the risk of injury to the suprascapular nerve.[60] This injury is not unique to arthroscopic shoulder surgery; it has also been documented with overly aggressive lateral mobilization of a retracted rotator cuff tear.[59] A safe zone of no more than 2 cm medial to the superior glenoid rim must be respected during juxtaglenoid capsulotomy and cuff mobilization. Arthroscopic surgical decompression at the suprascapular and spinoglenoid notch also puts the nerve at risk of injury and requires a thorough knowledge of suprascapular nerve anatomy.[61,62]

The musculocutaneous nerve is also at risk of injury during arthroscopic shoulder surgery. The studies on procedures such as arthroscopic Latarjet have focused on determining the relationship of the musculocutaneous nerve to the specific portals.[57,63] Standard placement of an anterior working portal is typically midway between the coracoid and the anterolateral corner of the acromion. Inferior or medial placement of this portal can place the musculocutaneous nerve at risk of injury. This risk can be diminished with the insertion of a spinal needle through the rotator interval under direct visualization or by creation of an inside-out portal. In a systematic review, Griesser et al[64] reported a 1.4% rate of neurovascular injury across open and arthroscopic techniques. There were 11 musculocutaneous nerve injuries, of which 2 were either partial or temporary and 9 were either partial permanent or complete injuries, resulting in nerve deficit. Dauzère et al[65] noted one case (1.5%) of axillary nerve palsy that resolved by 3 months. Kany et al[66] also found only one transient axillary nerve palsy (0.9%), while Castricini et al[67] did not encounter any neurologic injuries. No injuries to the suprascapular nerve have been described in the arthroscopic Latarjet technique, but the risk is present if fixation is made more than 2 cm medial to the posterior glenoid rim.[68]

Vascular Injuries

Arterial Injures

While injuries to the blood vessels of the shoulder region during arthroscopic shoulder surgery are uncommon, they can be catastrophic depending upon the extent of the injury to the vessels and to the success of the arterial repair.[69-73] Knowledge of the location of vessels is important when placing portals or performing complex arthroscopic procedures.

Cameron[74] first reported the formation of a venous pseudoaneurysm in a 39-year-old patient on renal dialysis after arthroscopic irrigation of a septic shoulder. There are also several cases of pseudoaneurysm formation from branches of the thoracoacromial artery following arthroscopic procedures.[70] All of these injuries were associated with the anterior portal site. Three of these cases underwent embolization, while the fourth patient had an open ligation and hematoma evacuation. All of them were reported to have uneventful recoveries after the treatment of pseudoaneurysm.

Historically, the management of arterial injuries has primarily relied upon an open surgical intervention. As technology advanced, ultrasound-guided compression became a commonly used treatment for postcatheterization-associated pseudoaneurysms. Success rates were initially very promising, ranging from 90% to 100%. However, as experience with ultrasound-guided compression grew, relatively lower success rates have been consistently reported between 62% and 88%.[75] Percutaneous thrombin injection has also proven to be a very effective means of sealing pseudoaneurysms. Existing literature suggests that thrombin injection is successful in 93% to 100% of cases, with most pseudoaneurysms successfully thrombosed with the first treatment.[75]

Venous Injuries

While DVT can occur after arthroscopic shoulder surgery, it is not known to be related with direct injury to the veins during the procedure. Traction on the vascular structures during arthroscopic surgery may be a contributing factor for the development of DVT in the upper extremity. However, in many cases, the pulmonary emboli (PE) may come from the legs and not the upper extremities. Fortunately, the risk of DVT and PE after shoulder arthroscopic surgery remains very low, and in-hospital anticoagulation treatment of patients having DVT or PE is usually effective. In a study from the United Kingdom, the rates of DVT and PE were reported to be below 0.01% after arthroscopic shoulder surgery, which were similar to the nonsurgical population.[76] In comparison, the reported rate for DVT after fracture surgery and total shoulder replacement was around 0.2% to 0.4%. Chemoprophylaxis for DVT and PE was not reported to affect the number of events. Kuremsky et al[77] reported 6 cases on 1900 shoulder arthroscopies over a period of 4 years, resulting in an incidence of 0.3%. All of these patients required in-hospital treatment. Randelli et al[78] reported 0.6 per 1000 events with no influence of chemoprophylaxis, but they were aware of a possible bias of the study due to their surgeon-reported survey design. Ojike et al,[79] in a systematic review, studied 8 articles with a total of 40,000 shoulder surgeries, including 16,000 arthroplasties, and found an overall incidence of 0.24% for DVT and 0.11% for PE.

CONCLUSION

Shoulder surgery has undergone a paradigm shift over the past 20 to 30 years. The introduction, development, and refinement of arthroscopic instrumentation and surgical techniques have prompted many surgeons to transition away from open procedures in favor of arthroscopic techniques. As the popularity of arthroscopic surgery has increased, proponents of these techniques have cited numerous advantages over open surgery, including lower complication rates.

However, complications are ubiquitous in surgery of any kind, and this is true of arthroscopic shoulder surgery as well. Among the most distressing complications after shoulder surgery are neurologic or vascular injuries, which can occur with either open or arthroscopic procedures. These complications have the potential to be life and limb threatening, as well as result in permanent disability of the shoulder. Knowledge of the specific anatomy of nerves and vessels, their location relative to standard portal placement, and their proximity during specific procedures is critical for the safe performance of arthroscopic shoulder procedures.

REFERENCES

1. Weber SC, Abrams JS, Nottage WM. Complications associated with arthroscopic shoulder surgery. *Arthroscopy.* 2002;18(2)(suppl 1):88–95.
2. Hughes JD, Hughes JL, Bartley JH, Hamilton WP, Brennan KL. Infection rates in arthroscopic versus open rotator cuff repair. *Orthop J Sports Med.* 2017;5(7):2325967117715416.
3. Meyer M, Graveleau N, Hardy P, Landreau P. Anatomic risks of shoulder arthroscopy portals: anatomic cadaveric study of 12 portals. *Arthroscopy.* 2007;23(5):529–536.
4. Paxton ES, Backus J, Keener J, Brophy RH. Shoulder arthroscopy: basic principles of positioning, anesthesia, and portal anatomy. *J Am Acad Orthop Surg.* 2013;21(6):332–342.
5. McFarland EG, Caicedo JC, Guitterez MI, Sherbondy PS, Kim TK. The anatomic relationship of the brachial plexus and axillary artery to the glenoid. Implications for anterior shoulder surgery. *Am J Sports Med.* 2001;29(6):729–733.
6. Matthews LS, Zarins B, Michael RH, Helfet DL. Anterior portal selection for shoulder arthroscopy. *Arthroscopy.* 1985;1(1):33–9.
7. Burkhead WZ Jr, Scheinberg RR, Box G. Surgical anatomy of the axillary nerve. *J Shoulder Elbow Surg.* 1992;1(1):31–36.
8. Uno A, Bain GI, Mehta JA. Arthroscopic relationship of the axillary nerve to the shoulder joint capsule: an anatomic study. *J Shoulder Elbow Surg.* 1999;8(3):226–230.
9. Ball CM, Steger T, Galatz LM, Yamaguchi K. The posterior branch of the axillary nerve: an anatomic study. *J Bone Joint Surg Am.* 2003;85(8):1497–1501.
10. Hoppenfeld S, DeBoer P, Buckley R. *Surgical Exposures in Orthopaedics: The Anatomic Approach.* 4th ed. Lippincott Williams & Wilkins; 2009.
11. Gardner MJ, Boraiah S, Helfet DL, Lorich DG. The anterolateral acromial approach for fractures of the proximal humerus. *J Orthop Trauma.* 2008;22(2):132–137.
12. Cetik O, Uslu M, Acar HI, Comert A, Tekdemir I, Cift H. Is there a safe area for the axillary nerve in the deltoid muscle? A cadaveric study. *J Bone Joint Surg Am.* 2006;88(11):2395–2399.
13. Bigliani LU, Dalsey RM, McCann PD, April EW. An anatomical study of the suprascapular nerve. *Arthroscopy.* 1990;6(4):301–305.
14. Cogan A, Boyer P, Soubeyrand M, Hamida FB, Vannier JL, Massin P. Cranial nerves neuropraxia after shoulder arthroscopy in beach chair position. *Orthop Traumatol Surg Res.* 2011;97(3):345–348.
15. Park TS, Kim YS. Neuropraxia of the cutaneous nerve of the cervical plexus after shoulder arthroscopy. *Arthroscopy.* 2005;21(5):631.

16. Bhatti MT, Enneking FK. Visual loss and ophthalmoplegia after shoulder surgery. *Anesth Analg.* 2003;96(3):899–902.

17. Mumith A, Scadden J. Postoperative vision loss after reverse shoulder arthroplasty. *Case Rep Orthop.* 2014;2014:850950.

18. Zmistowski B, Austin L, Ciccotti M, Ricchetti E, Williams G Jr. Fatal venous air embolism during shoulder arthroscopy: a case report. *J Bone Joint Surg Am.* 2010;92(11):2125–2127.

19. Friedman DJ, Parnes NZ, Zimmer Z, Higgins LD, Warner JJ. Prevalence of cerebrovascular events during shoulder surgery and association with patient position. *Orthopedics.* 2009;32(4):orthosupersite.com/view.asp?rID=38058.

20. Dippmann C, Winge S, Nielsen HB. Severe cerebral desaturation during shoulder arthroscopy in the beach-chair position. *Arthroscopy.* 2010;26(9)(suppl):S148–S150.

21. Pohl A, Cullen DJ. Cerebral ischemia during shoulder surgery in the upright position: a case series. *J Clin Anesth.* 2005;17(6):463–469.

22. Frey MA, Tomaselli CM, Hoffler WG. Cardiovascular responses to postural changes: differences with age for women and men. *J Clin Pharmacol.* 1994;34(5):394–402.

23. Van Lieshout JJ, Wieling W, Karemaker JM, Secher NH. Syncope, cerebral perfusion, and oxygenation. *J Appl Physiol (1985).* 2003;94(3):833–848.

24. Drummond JC, Lee RR, Howell JP Jr. Focal cerebral ischemia after surgery in the "beach chair" position: the role of a congenital variation of circle of Willis anatomy. *Anesth Analg.* 2012;114(6):1301–1303.

25. Boisseau N, Rabarijaona H, Grimaud D, Raucoules-Aimé M. Tapia's syndrome following shoulder surgery. *Br J Anaesth.* 2002;88(6):869–870.

26. Mullins RC, Drez D Jr, Cooper J. Hypoglossal nerve palsy after arthroscopy of the shoulder and open operation with the patient in the beach-chair position: a case report. *J Bone Joint Surg Am.* 1992;74(1):137–139.

27. Choi WJ, Shin HK, Kim DO, Park SW, Lee DI, Kim DS. Transient hypoglossal nerve palsy after general anesthesia in beach chair position for shoulder arthroscopic Bankart repair: a case report. *Korean J Anesthesiol.* 2004;47(2):277–280.

28. Hung NK, Lee CH, Chan SM, et al. Transient unilateral hypoglossal nerve palsy after orotracheal intubation for general anesthesia. *Acta Anaesthesiol Taiwan.* 2009;47(1):48–50.

29. Rhee YG, Cho NS. Isolated unilateral hypoglossal nerve palsy after shoulder surgery in beach-chair position. *J Shoulder Elbow Surg.* 2008;17(4):e28–e30.

30. Kim C, Oh H, Park J-j, Chung M. Cranial nerve XII (hypoglossal nerve) palsy after arthroscopic shoulder surgery under general anesthesia combined with sono-guided interscalene brachial plexus block: a case report. *Anesth Pain Med.* 2016;11:322–325.

31. Joshi M, Cheng R, Kamath H, Yarmush J. Great auricular neuropraxia with beach chair position. *Local Reg Anesth.* 2017;10:75–77.

32. Ng AK, Page RS. Greater auricular nerve neuropraxia with beach chair positioning during shoulder surgery. *Int J Shoulder Surg.* 2010;4(2):48–50.

33. LaPrade CM, Foad A. Greater auricular nerve palsy after arthroscopic anterior-inferior and posterior-inferior labral tear repair using beach-chair positioning and a standard universal headrest. *Am J Orthop (Belle Mead NJ).* 2015;44(4):188–191.

34. Holtzman AJ, Glezos CD, Feit EJ, Gruson KI. Prevalence and risk factors for lateral femoral cutaneous nerve palsy in the beach chair position. *Arthroscopy.* 2017;33(11):1958–1962.

35. Murphy GS, Szokol JW, Marymont JH, et al. Cerebral oxygen desaturation events assessed by near-infrared spectroscopy during shoulder arthroscopy in the beach chair and lateral decubitus positions. *Anesth Analg.* 2010;111(2):496–505.

36. Jeong H, Jeong S, Lim HJ, Lee J, Yoo KY. Cerebral oxygen saturation measured by near-infrared spectroscopy and jugular venous bulb oxygen saturation during arthroscopic shoulder surgery in beach chair position under sevoflurane-nitrous oxide or propofol-remifentanil anesthesia. *Anesthesiology.* 2012;116(5):1047–1056.
37. Lee JH, Min KT, Chun YM, Kim EJ, Choi SH. Effects of beach-chair position and induced hypotension on cerebral oxygen saturation in patients undergoing arthroscopic shoulder surgery. *Arthroscopy.* 2011;27(7):889–894.
38. Papadonikolakis A, Wiesler ER, Olympio MA, Poehling GG. Avoiding catastrophic complications of stroke and death related to shoulder surgery in the sitting position. *Arthroscopy.* 2008;24(4):481–482.
39. Koh JL, Levin SD, Chehab EL, Murphy GS. Neer Award 2012: cerebral oxygenation in the beach chair position: a prospective study on the effect of general anesthesia compared with regional anesthesia and sedation. *J Shoulder Elbow Surg.* 2013;22(10):1325–1331.
40. Andrews JR, Carson WG Jr, Ortega K. Arthroscopy of the shoulder: technique and normal anatomy. *Am J Sports Med.* 1984;12(1):1–7.
41. Ogilvie-Harris DJ, Wiley AM. Arthroscopic surgery of the shoulder: a general appraisal. *J Bone Joint Surg Br.* 1986;68(2):201–207.
42. Pitman MI, Nainzadeh N, Ergas E, Springer S. The use of somatosensory evoked potentials for detection of neuropraxia during shoulder arthroscopy. *Arthroscopy.* 1988;4(4):250–255.
43. Berjano P, González BG, Olmedo JF, Perez-España LA, Munilla MG. Complications in arthroscopic shoulder surgery. *Arthroscopy.* 1998;14(8):785–788.
44. Ellman H. Arthroscopic subacromial decompression: analysis of one- to three-year results. *Arthroscopy.* 1987;3(3):173–181.
45. Paulos LE, Franklin JL. Arthroscopic shoulder decompression development and application: a five year experience. *Am J Sports Med.* 1990;18(3):235–244.
46. Hennrikus WL, Mapes RC, Bratton MW, Lapoint JM. Lateral traction during shoulder arthroscopy: its effect on tissue perfusion measured by pulse oximetry. *Am J Sports Med.* 1995;23(4):444–446.
47. Pavlik A, Ang KC, Bell SN. Contralateral brachial plexus neuropathy after arthroscopic shoulder surgery. *Arthroscopy.* 2002;18(6):658–659.
48. Gelber PE, Reina F, Caceres E, Monllau JC. A comparison of risk between the lateral decubitus and the beach-chair position when establishing an anteroinferior shoulder portal: a cadaveric study. *Arthroscopy.* 2007;23(5):522–528.
49. Segmüller HE, Alfred SP, Zilio G, Saies AD, Hayes MG. Cutaneous nerve lesions of the shoulder and arm after arthroscopic shoulder surgery. *J Shoulder Elbow Surg.* 1995;4(4):254–258.
50. Jerosch J, Filler TJ, Peuker ET. Which joint position puts the axillary nerve at lowest risk when performing arthroscopic capsular release in patients with adhesive capsulitis of the shoulder? *Knee Surg Sports Traumatol Arthrosc.* 2002;10(2):126–129.
51. Yoo JC, Kim JH, Ahn JH, Lee SH. Arthroscopic perspective of the axillary nerve in relation to the glenoid and arm position: a cadaveric study. *Arthroscopy.* 2007;23(12):1271–1277.
52. Matthews LS, Zarins B, Michael RH, Helfet DL. Anterior portal selection for shoulder arthroscopy. *Arthroscopy.* 1985;1(1):33–39.
53. Lo IK, Lind CC, Burkhart SS. Glenohumeral arthroscopy portals established using an outside-in technique: neurovascular anatomy at risk. *Arthroscopy.* 2004;20(6):596–602.
54. Davidson PA, Rivenburgh DW. The 7-o'clock posteroinferior portal for shoulder arthroscopy. *Am J Sports Med.* 2002;30(5):693–696.

55. Eakin CL, Dvirnak P, Miller CM, Hawkins RJ. The relationship of the axillary nerve to arthroscopically placed capsulolabral sutures: an anatomic study. *Am J Sports Med.* 1998;26(4):505-509.

56. Boileau P, Mercier N, Old J. Arthroscopic Bankart-Bristow-Latarjet (2B3) procedure: how to do it and tricks to make it easier and safe. *Orthop Clin North Am.* 2010;41(3):381-392.

57. Lo IK, Burkhart SS, Parten PM. Surgery about the coracoid: neurovascular structures at risk. *Arthroscopy.* 2004;20(6):591-595.

58. Millett PJ, Gaskill TR. Arthroscopic trans-capsular axillary nerve decompression: indication and surgical technique. *Arthroscopy.* 2011;27(10):1444-1448.

59. Warner JP, Krushell RJ, Masquelet A, Gerber C. Anatomy and relationships of the suprascapular nerve: anatomical constraints to mobilization of the supraspinatus and infraspinatus muscles in the management of massive rotator-cuff tears. *J Bone Joint Surg Am.* 1992;74(1):36-45.

60. Chan H, Beaupre LA, Bouliane MJ. Injury of the suprascapular nerve during arthroscopic repair of superior labral tears: an anatomic study. *J Shoulder Elbow Surg.* 2010;19(5):709-715.

61. Lafosse L, Piper K, Lanz U. Arthroscopic suprascapular nerve release: indications and technique. *J Shoulder Elbow Surg.* 2011;20(2)(suppl):S9-S13.

62. Romeo AA, Ghodadra NS, Salata MJ, Provencher MT. Arthroscopic suprascapular nerve decompression: indications and surgical technique. *J Shoulder Elbow Surg.* 2010;19(2)(suppl):118-123.

63. Flatow EL, Bigliani LU, April EW. An anatomic study of the musculocutaneous nerve and its relationship to the coracoid process. *Clin Orthop Relat Res.* 1989;(244):166-171.

64. Griesser MJ, Harris JD, McCoy BW, et al. Complications and re-operations after Bristow-Latarjet shoulder stabilization: a systematic review. *J Shoulder Elbow Surg.* 2013;22(2):286-292.

65. Dauzère F, Faraud A, Lebon J, Faruch M, Mansat P, Bonnevialle N. Is the Latarjet procedure risky? Analysis of complications and learning curve. *Knee Surg Sports Traumatol Arthrosc.* 2016;24(2):557-563.

66. Kany J, Flamand O, Grimberg J, et al. Arthroscopic Latarjet procedure: is optimal positioning of the bone block and screws possible? A prospective computed tomography scan analysis. *J Shoulder Elbow Surg.* 2016;25(1):69-77.

67. Castricini R, De Benedetto M, Orlando N, Rocchi M, Zini R, Pirani P. Arthroscopic Latarjet procedure: analysis of the learning curve. *Musculoskelet Surg.* 2013;97(suppl 1):93-98.

68. Hawi N, Reinhold A, Suero EM, et al. The anatomic basis for the arthroscopic Latarjet procedure: a cadaveric study. *Am J Sports Med.* 2016;44(2):497-503.

69. Yang AE, Hall JM, Vincent GS, Chambers L. Deep brachial artery pseudoaneurysm following arthroscopic shoulder debridement. *Vasc Endovascular Surg.* 2018;52(5):378-381.

70. Ishida Y, Chosa E, Taniguchi N. Pseudoaneurysm as a complication of shoulder arthroscopy. *Knee Surg Sports Traumatol Arthrosc.* 2015;23(5):1549-1551.

71. Webb BG, Elliott MP. Pseudoaneurysm after arthroscopic subacromial decompression and distal clavicle excision. *Orthopedics.* 2014;37(6):e596-e599.

72. Choo HJ, Kim JH, Kim DG. Arterial pseudoaneurysm at the arthroscopic portal site as a complication after arthroscopic rotator cuff surgery: a case report. *J Shoulder Elbow Surg.* 2013;22(12):e15-e19.

73. Godin JA, Mayer SW, Garrigues GE, Mather RC III. Pseudoaneurysm after shoulder arthroscopy. *J Shoulder Elbow Surg.* 2013;22(10):e12-e17.

74. Cameron SE. Venous pseudoaneurysm as a complication of shoulder arthroscopy. *J Shoulder Elbow Surg.* 1996;5(5):404–406.

75. Morgan R, Belli A-M. Current treatment methods for postcatheterization pseudoaneurysms. *J Vasc Intervent Radiol.* 2003;14(6):697–710.

76. Jameson SS, James P, Howcroft DW, et al. Venous thromboembolic events are rare after shoulder surgery: analysis of a national database. *J Shoulder Elbow Surg.* 2011;20(5):764–770.

77. Kuremsky MA, Cain EL Jr, Fleischli JE. Thromboembolic phenomena after arthroscopic shoulder surgery. *Arthroscopy.* 2011;27(12):1614–1619.

78. Randelli P, Castagna A, Cabitza F, Cabitza P, Arrigoni P, Denti M. Infectious and thromboembolic complications of arthroscopic shoulder surgery. *J Shoulder Elbow Surg.* 2010;19(1):97–101.

79. Ojike NI, Bhadra AK, Giannoudis PV, Roberts CS. Venous thromboembolism in shoulder surgery: a systematic review. *Acta Orthop Belg.* 2011;77(3):281–289.

7

Postoperative Septic Arthritis

Rajeev Pandarinath, MD; Seth Stake, MD; and Taylor Swansen, MD, MS

INTRODUCTION

Septic arthritis is a rare but feared complication of shoulder arthroscopy. These surgeries are at an intrinsically low risk for infection given the minimally invasive nature and constant irrigation. Most arthroscopic shoulder cases are brief, with minimal blood loss.[1] However, the rare cases of septic arthritis that do occur after arthroscopy have historically poor outcomes with great cost to the health care system.[2] This chapter will explore risk factors, epidemiology, microbiology, diagnosis, and management of postarthroscopy septic arthritis. Long-term outcomes and salvage procedures will be described.

EPIDEMIOLOGY

Postoperative septic arthritis of the shoulder is a serious complication that is typically treated with surgery. The rate of infection after shoulder surgery has been significantly reduced by the advent of arthroscopic

Thompson TL, ed.
*Arthroscopic Shoulder Surgery:
Complications and Management* (pp 99-113).

techniques.[3] The incidence of deep infection after arthroscopic shoulder surgery is between 0.16% and 1.9%.[4] D'Angelo and Ogilvie-Harris[5] performed a large series of 4000 arthroscopic procedures and noted 9 (0.23%) cases of septic arthritis. This study was done without preoperative antibiotic prophylaxis and led the authors to recommend routine prophylaxis to possibly reduce hospital cost and patient morbidity associated with this complication.[6] These recommendations were implemented by Randelli et al[7] in a series of 9385 patients undergoing shoulder arthroscopies performed over a 1-year period. The authors of this study noted 15 infections (0.16%) with a significant difference in infection rate between patients who received antibiotics prophylaxis and those who did not (0.095% vs 0.58%, $P = .01$).[7] More recent studies have continued to show low rates of postarthroscopic septic arthritis. Noud and Esch[6] published a recent study on 263 patients with only one infection (0.38%).

Rates of postoperative septic arthritis differ based on both intrinsic and extrinsic factors. Among different arthroscopic surgeries, rotator cuff repair has shown the highest infection rate, while Bankart repair has shown the lowest.[3] Revision arthroscopic surgeries are typically more complex and carry a higher infection rate of 2.1%.[3] Infection rates are increased when arthroscopic cases are converted to open procedures. Moen et al[2] performed a study of 360 patients treated with mini–open rotator cuff repair following arthroscopic subacromial decompression and reported an infection rate of 1.9%. The authors of this study noted a significant reduction in this rate when the surgical site is prepared with a Betadine (povidone iodine) paint between arthroscopic and open portions of the procedure.[2] Patient-specific factors that increase risk of postarthroscopic septic arthritis include age older than 60 years, previous ipsilateral shoulder surgery, chronic lymphedema, venous stasis, vascular compromise, and radiation fibrosis.[2] Werner et al[8] employed a national database to evaluate the relationship between preoperative corticosteroid injections and postarthroscopic infection. The authors found a significantly greater incidence of infection in patients who underwent infection within 3 months compared to controls.[8] A study by Yeranosian et al[9] suggested the incidence of septic arthritis varies significantly across regions, with the highest incidence in the southern United States (0.37%) and the lowest incidence in the Midwest (0.11%).

With a rate 10 times lower than the frequency of neurologic complications, septic arthritis is a rare complication.[10] However, this incidence is likely underestimated. *Cutibacterium acnes* is the most frequently isolated causative organism and tends to cause very slowly developing infections. In addition, *C acnes* infection is difficult to diagnose using standard culture media.[10] Horneff et al[11] conducted a prospective study on the rate of

C acnes infections in arthroscopy patients with postoperative pain. In this study, intraoperative cultures were positive for *C acnes* in 23.5% of cases.[11] The authors concluded that the rate of *C acnes* is greater than previously published in patients requiring revision procedures.[11]

MICROBIOLOGY

The most commonly isolated bacteria associated with shoulder infections after arthroscopy are *C acnes* and *Staphylococcus*.[3] These pathogens are most commonly isolated around the shoulder and account for nearly all infectious cases.[3] Hair follicles and sebaceous glands provide a suitable habitat for these pathogens.[3]

C acnes is a non–spore-forming, commensal, gram-positive rod that has drawn great interest in recent years.[3] It is part of the normal superficial skin flora and lives deep to hair follicles and sebaceous pores.[11] In addition to being isolated from the axilla, these bacteria are found in the face, scalp, chest, and back. Its high concentration in the face and shoulders has made it a commonly isolated organism in acne.[12] *C acnes* is implicated as the chief causative pathogen in postoperative infections in shoulder infections due to its high concentration about the shoulder.[12] In addition to its role in orthopedic and dermatologic conditions, these bacteria are implicated in systemic conditions affecting the cardiac, urologic, ophthalmologic, and neurologic systems.[11] Chuang et al[12] documented the skin colonization and deep tissue inoculation rates of *C acnes* index arthroscopic procedures in a prospective trial of 51 patients. These patients received antibiotic prophylaxis and a standard surgical preparation prior to having their skin and portal sites swabbed intraoperatively and portal site swabbed at the end of the procedure.[12] Superficial and deep cultures grown on a *Brucella* medium were positive in 72.5% and 19.6% of samples, respectively.[12] A higher incidence of positive superficial cultures was associated with male sex (81.6% vs 46.1%, $P = .027$).[12] Other studies have found a range of *C acnes* superficial skin colonization at arthroscopic portal sites between 47.7% and 72.5%.[3]

Patients infected with *C acnes* typically do not present with typical inflammatory symptoms such as drainage, fever, and erythema. Inflammatory markers are routinely normal and aspirate cultures are oftentimes negative. Symptoms typically include shoulder stiffness and pain following shoulder arthroscopy. This subacute presentation includes minimal fever and only mild local tissue inflammation. In rare cases, acute presentations may occur with purulent drainage and elevated inflammatory markers, as evidenced by Dodson et al.[13] Multiple studies have shown that confirmation of *C acnes* may take up to 3 weeks on culture-based methods.[11]

Adding to the fastidious nature of the organism, *C acnes* typically requires a chocolate agar medium and anaerobic environment for identification.[12] Prior failure to recognize the specialized conditions needed to isolate this agent have led to historic underreporting of *C acnes* infection.[12] Outcomes after treatment of *C acnes* infections are extremely poor according to current literature.[12] *C acnes* infection has been correlated to the pathogenesis of glenohumeral osteoarthritis, even in subacute cases.[12] In addition, up to 38% of patients report unsatisfactory results following completion of treatment for *C acnes* septic arthritis.[12]

Staphylococcal species are the other frequently isolated skin contaminant causing septic arthritis following arthroscopic shoulder surgery.[2] These bacteria are less investigated in current literature as they cause more typical inflammatory symptoms and are easily isolated on basic culture media.[2] The ability of these bacteria to cause suppurative infection depends in part on bacterial adherence. With the ability to form a biofilm, these bacteria have an enhanced ability to bind orthopedic implants and evade host immune mechanisms.[2] More rarely, isolated pathogens have been reported in case studies, including *Pseudomonas aeruginosa*, *Mycobacterium tuberculosis*, and *Actinomyces* species. In 2009, a case study by Tosh et al[14] described an outbreak of *P aeruginosa* following arthroscopic surgeries in Texas. Seven deep surgical site infections occurred during a 2-week window.[14] This was thought to be secondary to surgical instrument contamination with the pathogen during instrument reprocessing.[14] Thus, outbreak of infection with unlikely organisms should prompt the investigation of decontamination processes, especially of orthopedic cannulae and shaver handpieces. This theory was tested by Armstrong and Bolding,[1] who investigated a 2% infection rate in a series of 352 arthroscopic procedures performed over a 9-month period at a single institution. The authors found inadequate use of a disinfectant solution and decreased the infection rate by a factor of 10 following correction of the sterilization process.[1] Two of these infections were *P aeruginosa* attributed to contaminated electrocardiogram cables.[1]

RISK FACTORS AND PREVENTION

Modifications can be made in the preoperative, intraoperative, and postoperative setting to attempt to reduce the risk of postarthroscopic septic shoulder arthritis.

Patient-specific risk factors for complications have been identified in the literature to limit readmission for prolonged antibiotic treatment and increased cost. In the preoperative setting, patient demographic information and medical history can be used to stratify patient risk for septic arthritis. Cancienne et al[15] performed a Medicare database study of 530,754 patients who underwent arthroscopic shoulder surgery with 1409 infections within a 90-day postoperative window. The study was well powered and represented the largest study group to date on this topic.[15] The authors isolated chronic anemia, malnutrition, male sex, morbid obesity, and chronic depression as independent risk factors for acute infection postoperatively.[15] Cancienne et al[15] also linked obesity to postarthroscopic septic arthritis, but the study lacked a true regression analysis to isolate it as an independent risk factor. Various other studies have also linked male sex to increased risk for infection.[15] The exact reasoning for difference between sexes has not yet been fully established, but it has been hypothesized that there are differences in skin microbiology, particularly in the concentration of C acnes.[15] Yeranosian et al[9] looked at demographic factors in a study of 165,000 patients and isolated age as an independent risk factor. The authors of this study showed that patients older than 60 years were twice as likely to become infected compared to patients younger than 40 years.[9] The authors linked this to age-related comorbidities and immunocompromised status but suggested that future studies that stratified by age should be conducted to infer causality.[9]

Different arthroscopic surgeries carry different risks of infection postoperatively. Yeranosian et al[9] found an increased risk during rotator cuff surgery (0.29%), as compared to capsulorrhaphy (0.16%) or distal claviculectomy (0.21%). Other studies have found increased risk with preoperative steroid injection or prior arthroscopic surgery. Werner et al[8] performed a large Medicare database study examining the effect of timing of elective shoulder surgery after shoulder injection on infection risk. The authors reported that performing shoulder injections in the 3-month window prior to surgery increases the risk of infection by 2.2 times.[8] They added that performing even one injection in the 6-month window increases risk by 1.6 times.[8] Cancienne et al[15] found prior arthroscopic shoulder surgery to be the greatest independent risk factor for septic arthritis following arthroscopic shoulder surgery. Other studies have found revision arthroscopic shoulder surgery to be an independent risk factor. Cancienne et al[15] evaluated 94 patients undergoing revision arthroscopic rotator cuff repair and found an infection rate of 2.1%.

In the perioperative and intraoperative period, risk factors have been identified in the literature leading to alterations in management of patients undergoing arthroscopic shoulder surgery. In a landmark review in 1988, D'Angelo and Ogilvie-Harris[5] noted 9 cases of septic arthritis confirmed with cultures of joint aspirate after 4000 arthroscopic procedures (0.23%). The increased morbidity and hospital cost associated with the postoperative care of these patients prompted the authors to investigate the use of antibiotic prophylaxis.[5] Randelli et al[7] followed this study by noting a decreased risk of postarthroscopic infection for patients who received antibiotic prophylaxis vs those who did not in a study of 9385 cases (0.095% vs 0.58%). Other studies have found a similarly decreased risk of infection with the use of antibiotic prophylaxis (1.54% to 0.28%).[3] Surgical duration has a large impact on the risk of postoperative infection. The risk of surgery lasting more than 45 minutes increases 3.63 times, and in cases lasting more than 90 minutes, the risk of infection increases to 4.4 times.[3] Steroid injection at the time of surgery has been frequently cited as an independent risk factor for infection.[15] This may be performed for frozen shoulder, symptomatic rotator cuff, or degenerative conditions at the time of surgery. The notion of increased risk of infection with intraoperative steroid injection is validated by studies showing similar effects of intraoperative injection in other joints, such as the knee and elbow.[15] Armstrong and Bolding[1] cited intraoperative corticosteroids as having a major potentiating effect on the occurrence of postoperative infection. The authors of this study found a greater than 20 times risk of infection with intra-articular steroids delivered at the time of surgery. It is important for the operating surgeon to recognize the increased risk of surgical site infection with injection and weigh this against the possible short-term benefits of improved motion and pain control postoperatively.[15] Specific surgical site preparations can diminish the risk of infection by lowering loads of bacterial skin flora. Saltzman et al[16] investigated the use of three different solutions with skin preparation by taking intraoperative cultures after preparation with each of them. The authors found the lowest rate of positive culture with Chloraprep (chlorhexidine gluconate and isopropyl alcohol; 7%) compared to Duraprep (iodine povacrylex and isopropyl alcohol) and povidone-iodine (19% and 31%, respectively).

While the use of antibiotic prophylaxis and skin preparation has decreased the overall incidence of infection following shoulder arthroscopy, it has shifted the most common pathogen from staphylococci species to C acnes species. C acnes has been shown to be scarcely influenced by standard antibiotic prophylaxis and semiresistant to current standard skin preparation techniques.[16] While early studies supported the notion that skin preparation decreases the risk of postoperative infection with C acnes, recent studies have shown that there may be no difference in terms of C acnes colonization following disinfection with chlorhexidine compared with controls.[3] Chuang et al[12] took intraoperative cultures from 51 patients undergoing shoulder arthroscopy following standard skin preparation and tested them for C acnes. Even following standard skin preparation, 72.5% of patients had a superficial colonization rate with a 19.6% incidence in deep cultures.[12] This rate was found to be especially high in men, likely due to increased bacterial load deep within hair follicles and sebaceous pores.[12] Furthermore, clipping of the axilla has been shown to increase, rather than decrease, the rate of infection.[3] Some recent studies have found encouraging results with the use of clindamycin phosphate and benzoyl peroxide, with colonization rates as low as 3.1%.[3] Postoperative use of antibiotics has not been shown to decrease rates of infection in the literature. Encouraging results have also been cited with use of an axillary sterile drape, with decreased colonization rates from 33% down to 9.3%.[3] Sircana et al[3] provided patients with a 7-day course of doxycycline following outpatient arthroscopic procedures and found no difference in *C acnes* culturing outcomes when compared to controls.

DIAGNOSIS

Diagnosis of a deep infection following shoulder arthroscopy is often delayed due to relatively nonspecific patient complaints. Delayed diagnosis can cause chronic pain, implant failure, or even sepsis; therefore, a timely diagnosis is imperative.[17] Workup of possible infection following shoulder arthroscopy is most often initiated by physical examination findings. Cellulitis or fibrinous exudate from arthroscopic portal wounds may be an early indicator. Deeper infections may have a delayed presentation and are characterized by stiffness and increased pain. Patients may describe a feeling of fullness and endorse warmth and night pain. In a review performed in 2011 of 14 studies involving 6242 patients, joint pain was found to be 85% sensitive, while fever and joint effusion were found to have sensitivities of 57% and 78%, respectively.[18] When compared to staphylococcal species, *C acnes* is even harder to diagnose as a causative organism due to more insidious onset and nonspecific symptoms. A retrospective study by Horneff et al[11] found that of 10 patients who were later diagnosed with deep *C acnes* shoulder infections, the only complaint for 9 of these patients was shoulder pain for an average of 3 months.

Conventional radiographs are usually the first imaging modality used in patients with shoulder pain, but they are insensitive to early infection. They may be used to evaluate the joint if the infection progresses and show joint space narrowing and marginal erosions from cartilage destruction.[19] Radiographs also evaluate late septic arthritis and can demonstrate joint destruction, calcifications of periarticular tissues, subchondral bone loss, and sclerosis.[19]

Magnetic resonance imaging is infrequently used in the setting of septic arthritis but may be used in ambiguous cases or to determine the extent of infection in the setting of known septic arthritis. In early infections, T2-weighted images display distention of the joint capsule with high-intensity fluid. Progression of septic arthritis demonstrates joint effusion with articular cartilage destruction and cellulitis around the joint. T2-weighted images at that stage show nonhomogeneous fluid with intermediate signal intensity, indicating infected fluid and blood. Cellulitis is indicated by signal hyperintensity around the joint.[19] A study completed by Bremell et al[20] using an animal model demonstrated that cartilage destruction and erosion of the subchondral bone may occur within several days of infection. Later stages of infection will show extension of the infectious process from the joint and into the surrounding bone.[21] Ultrasound has also been used to evaluate for effusions or loculations within an effusion.[22]

Scintigraphy is a useful adjunct for determining the extent and severity of infection, although it has several pitfalls. Tagged white blood cell (WBC) scintigraphy can be considered when the diagnosis of infection is questionable, but studies have shown that it varies in sensitivity and specificity, making interpretation difficult.[16] Both gallium and WBC scintigraphy show increased periarticular uptake and are sensitive to joint inflammation but cannot differentiate between septic or inflammatory arthritis.[23] This imaging modality is useful to rule out adjacent osteomyelitis but may be difficult to identify in cases of severe septic arthritis with high periarticular uptake.[23]

Laboratory studies may be used to confirm a suspicion for infection. A peripheral leukocyte count may be normal in a more indolent infection or may be elevated with a left shift. Erythrocyte sedimentation rate (ESR) or C-reactive protein (CRP) will likely be elevated but is confounded by the fact that such markers are elevated after a surgical procedure or any other inflammatory state. A review by Dodson et al[17] in 2011 found that no patient with deep *C acnes* infections had an elevated WBC, while 46% had an elevated ESR and 72% had an elevated CRP. A retrospective study by Margaretten et al[18] found that absence of a fever or a normal serum leukocyte count, ESR, or CRP could not reliably exclude a diagnosis of septic arthritis irrespective of causative organism, however. Procalcitonin has been investigated as a laboratory marker indicating septic arthritis. A study by Hügle et al[24] found that serum procalcitonin has a sensitivity of 93% and specificity of 75% for septic arthritis, compared with CRP levels, which had a sensitivity of 79% and a sensitivity of 68%. The same study found no significant difference between serum WBC in septic arthritis when compared to nonseptic arthritis.

While imaging and serum laboratory values are useful to indicate the presence of infection, joint aspiration and culture for aerobic, anaerobic, acid-fast, and fungal organisms is the gold standard to diagnose septic arthritis. Slower-growing, indolent bacterial strains such as *C acnes* may require cultures to be incubated for an average of 9 days, with a range of 4 to 21 days.[17,25] Fungal or mycobacterial cultures may need to be incubated for up to 8 weeks.[16] The joint fluid should also be analyzed for crystals to evaluate for inflammatory arthropathy. A cell count should be sent for analysis as well. A synovial WBC of greater than 50,000 with more than 75% polymorphonuclear cells is strongly suggestive of infection. WBC counts of fewer than 25,000, 25,000 to 50,000, 50,000 to 100,000, and more than 100,000 were found to have likelihood ratios of septic arthritis of 0.32, 2.9, 7.7, and 28, respectively.[18] Synovial fluid glucose may also be used and will be low in patients with bacterial septic arthritis when compared with serum glucose level. This finding can be confounded in the setting of diabetes or rheumatoid arthritis, however.[26] Polymerase chain reaction of joint fluid has also been evaluated for improved diagnosis of the causative organism. While it has not been shown to offer an advantage for staphylococcal or streptococcal infections, it can be useful for organisms that are difficult to culture, such as *Borrelia*.[27]

Arthroscopic tissue culture has been investigated as an alternative method of diagnosis of deep infection and is especially useful with organisms that are more difficult to diagnose or culture by typical means. A retrospective review of 19 patients who underwent arthroscopic tissue biopsy due to concern for a chronic periprosthetic shoulder infection was performed by Dilisio et al[28] in 2014. The results of the tissue biopsies were compared with fluoroscopically guided glenohumeral aspiration, as well as open tissue biopsies when the patients underwent revision surgery. At the time of revision surgery, 41% of those patients had positive culture results, and each positive culture included *C acnes*. All arthroscopic tissue cultures were consistent with cultures obtained during the revision surgery, with a 100% sensitivity, specificity, negative predictive value, and positive predictive value. In comparison, glenohumeral aspirations had a 16.7% sensitivity, 100% specificity, 58.3% negative predictive value, and 100% positive predictive value.[28]

MANAGEMENT

Management of septic arthritis is dependent on identifying the causative organism and appropriate debridement along with antibiotic therapy. Surgical debridement of an infected joint and irrigation is the mainstay of treatment. The aim of this is to remove any purulent material, removing bacteria and mediators of destruction of the soft tissues in the shoulder. Sutures and anchors from the prior surgery should ideally be removed due to concern for a residual nidus of infection but should be removed on a patient-by-patient basis. Implant removal should be strongly considered in the setting of a *C acnes* infection, in which there is a high likelihood for biofilm formation.[29] Rerepair may be performed with nonbraided, absorbable suture if original implants are removed.[16] Conservative treatment with joint aspiration rather than surgical debridement is an alternative treatment option, although few studies have been done to demonstrate its efficacy.[27]

Antibiotic choice is based on the most likely causative organism until the organism is identified by culture or polymerase chain reaction. Broad-spectrum antibiotics are implemented initially and should be tailored to the identified or most likely causative organism. Consultation with an infectious disease specialist for treatment recommendations is useful in the setting of increasing antibiotic resistance. Intravenous antibiotic therapy for 4 to 6 weeks is commonly used to treat for the risk of osteomyelitis.[16] Standard broad-spectrum antibiotic regimens should be implemented based on patient risk factors, although the efficacy of different regimens has not been studied in comparison with one another. For patients with no risk factors for atypical organisms, flucloxacillin 2 g 4 times a day or gentamycin should be chosen. Clindamycin 450 to 600 mg 4 times a day or a second- or third-generation cephalosporin may be chosen for a penicillin allergic patient. In patients at high risk of gram-negative sepsis, including older patients, those with recurrent urinary tract infections, or patients who have had recent abdominal surgery, a second- or third-generation cephalosporin such as cefuroxime 1.5 g 3 times a day should be chosen. Flucloxacillin may be added depending on hospital policy. For patients with a methicillin-resistant *Staphylococcus aureus* (MRSA) risk, including intravenous drug users, a known MRSA history, or recent inpatients, vancomycin along with a second- or third-generation cephalosporin should be initiated. For patients with suspected gonococcal or meningococcal infections, ceftriaxone should be initiated.[27] Antibiotic choice for *C acnes* is variable and depends on the strains of resistance present. Up to 65% of *C acnes* strains have been found to be resistant to at least one antibiotic, likely due to increasing use of antibiotic regimens for dermatologic cases of acne vulgaris. Common regimens include penicillin, tetracyclines, vancomycin, and erythromycin.[29]

Supplementing antibiotic therapy with nonsteroidal anti-inflammatory medications has been shown to decrease the destruction of articular cartilage in animal models and may be beneficial.[30]

CASE PRESENTATION

A 56-year-old man presented with full-thickness supraspinatus and upper subscapularis tears. His medical comorbidities included coronary artery disease with a history of a coronary artery bypass graft, hypertension, obesity with a body mass index of 35 kg/m^2, type 2 diabetes, and sleep apnea. He underwent an outpatient arthroscopic rotator cuff repair with biceps tenotomy and acromioplasty (Figure 7-1). A single anchor was

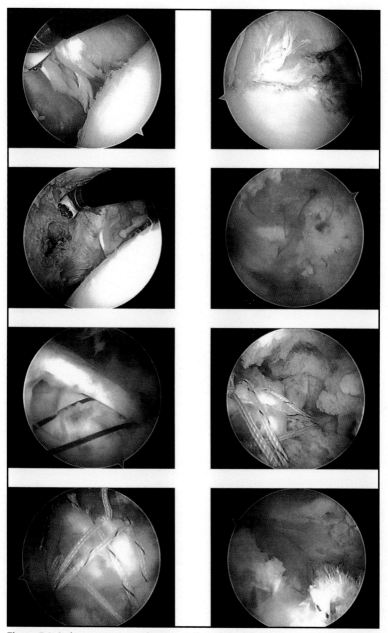

Figure 7-1. Arthroscopic views of rotator cuff repair for full-thickness supraspinatus and upper subscapularis tears in a 56-year-old man. The subscapularis was repaired via a single anchor and the supraspinatus was repaired with a double row. Biceps tenotomy and acromioplasty were also performed.

Figure 7-2. Cutaneous manifestations of a *C acnes* postarthroscopic infection 18 days following rotator cuff repair, biceps tenodesis, and acromioplasty in a 56-year-old man.

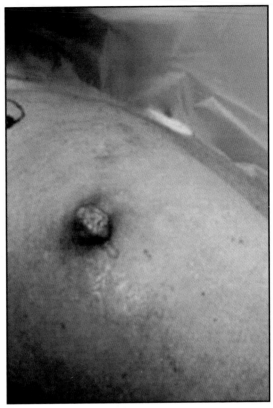

placed in the subscapularis, and a double-row repair was performed for the supraspinatus tear, which measured 3 by 2 cm. The procedure was well tolerated with no complications. He received cefazolin preoperatively per standard protocol at the institution.

On his second postoperative day, he had no concerns, although at his 9-day follow-up, he had mild erythema at his lateral portal site and reported elbow pain. At his 18-day follow-up, he was noted to have a tender and swollen lateral portal site, with subjective shoulder stiffness and pain (Figure 7-2). On examination, he was found to have pain throughout a normal arc of motion. He was prescribed cephalexin and was counseled on appropriate wound care. At 21 days postoperatively, he still had not improved. His serum WBC was 7200, ESR was 30 (normal value, 0 to 15), and CRP was 2.1 (normal, 0 to 0.6).

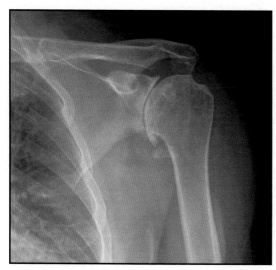

Figure 7-3. Left shoulder AP 6 years following irrigation and debridement for postarthroscopic infection with *C acnes* depicts severe glenohumeral osteoarthritis.

He was taken to the operating room for an irrigation and debridement of his portal wound and an arthroscopic debridement of his glenohumeral joint. The infection was found to have spread to the subacromial and glenohumeral space. His subscapularis anchor was loose and was removed, but the remaining anchors remained intact and were left in place. A Jackson-Pratt drain was placed and removed on postoperative day 2. His Gram stain was negative, and he was started on vancomycin, with ceftriaxone added by the infectious disease consult. Cultures grew *C acnes*, and the ceftriaxone was discontinued by the infection disease consult. He continued on intravenous vancomycin for 3 weeks. His ESR after he completed his antibiotic course was 7, and his CRP was 0.2. An ultrasound at 3 months postoperatively showed partial tearing of the subscapularis, with an intact supraspinatus. He was not experiencing pain, stiffness, or systemic signs of infection at that time. Long-term follow-up was significant for fairly rapid development of osteoarthritis (Figure 7-3). The patient was offered a shoulder arthroplasty, as he is now age 69, but after being counseled on the risks of prosthetic joint infection, he decided to pursue nonoperative treatment.

CONCLUSION

Due to historically poor outcomes, septic arthritis is a serious complication of shoulder surgery. The advent of arthroscopic techniques has helped to greatly reduce the incidence of postoperative shoulder septic arthritis.[1] Preoperative antibiotic prophylaxis has also been proven to be effective in reducing risk for postarthroscopic infection. *C acnes* is a particularly fastidious bacterium found deep in the sebaceous pores of the shoulder.[5,7] This organism requires that cultures with specialized mediums be held for up to 21 days for speciation. Preoperative surgical site preparation is less effective in reducing colonization with *C acnes*, and preoperative shaving and hair removal has actually been shown to increase the risk of postoperative infection in recent studies.[3,12]

Joint aspiration and bacterial culture remain the gold standard for diagnosis of septic arthritis. Cell count may also aid in evaluation, and intraoperative tissue culture can confirm the diagnosis of postarthroscopic shoulder septic arthritis, with sensitivity and specificity as high as 100%.[28] Management of postoperative septic arthritis consists of formal irrigation and debridement along with antibiotic therapy. Empiric antibiotic coverage should be initiated immediately following surgery and then narrowed based on identified or most likely bacteria.[16] Inflammatory markers should be checked periodically, and examinations should be trended to monitor progress.[30]

REFERENCES

1. Armstrong RW, Bolding F. Septic arthritis after arthroscopy: the contributing roles of intraarticular steroids and environmental factors. *Am J Infect Control.* 1994;22(1):16–18.
2. Moen TC, Rudolph GH, Caswell K, Espinoza C, Burkhead WZ Jr, Krishnan SG. Complications of shoulder arthroscopy. *J Am Acad Orthop Surg.* 2014;22:410–419.
3. Sircana G, Passiatore M, Capasso L, Saccomanno MF, Maccauro G. Infections in arthroscopy. *Eur Rev Med Pharmacol Sci.* 2019;23(2)(suppl):279–287.
4. Marecek GS, Saltzman MD. Complications in shoulder arthroscopy. *Orthopedics.* 2010;33(7):492–497.
5. D'Angelo GL, Ogilvie-Harris DJ. Septic arthritis following arthroscopy, with cost/benefit analysis of antibiotic prophylaxis. *Arthroscopy.* 1988;4(1):10–14.
6. Noud PH, Esch J. Complications of arthroscopic shoulder surgery. *Sports Med Arthroscopy Rev.* 2013;21(2):89–96.
7. Randelli P, Castagna A, Cabitza F, Cabitza P, Arrigoni P, Denti M. Infectious and thromboembolic complications of arthroscopic shoulder surgery. *J Shoulder Elbow Surg.* 2010;19(1):97–101.e.
8. Werner BC, Cancienne JM, Burrus MT, Griffin JW, Gwathmey FW, Brockmeier SF. The timing of elective shoulder surgery after shoulder injection affects postoperative infection risk in Medicare patients. *J Shoulder Elb Surg.* 2016;25(3):390–397.

9. Yeranosian MG, Arshi A, Terrell RD, Wang JC, McAllister DR, Petrigliano FA. Incidence of acute postoperative infections requiring reoperation after arthroscopic shoulder surgery. *Am J Sports Med.* 2014;42(2):437–441.

10. Bauer T, Boisrenoult P, Jenny JY. Post-arthroscopy septic arthritis: current data and practical recommendations. *Orthop Traumatol Surg Res.* 2015;101(8):S347–S350.

11. Horneff JG, Hsu JE, Voleti PB, O'Donnell J, Huffman GR. Propionibacterium acnes infection in shoulder arthroscopy patients with postoperative pain. *J Shoulder Elb Surg.* 2015;24(6):838–843.

12. Chuang MJ, Jancosko JJ, Mendoza V, Nottage WM. The incidence of Propionibacterium acnes in shoulder arthroscopy. *Arthroscopy.* 2015;31(9):1702–1707.

13. Dodson CC, Craig EV, Cordasco FA, et al. Propionibacterium acnes infection after shoulder arthroplasty: a diagnostic challenge. *J Shoulder Elbow Surg.* 2010;19(2):303–307.

14. Tosh PK, Disbot M, Duffy JM, et al. Outbreak of Pseudomonas aeruginosa surgical site infections after arthroscopic procedures: Texas, 2009. *Infect Control Hosp Epidemiol.* 2011;32(12):1179–1186.

15. Cancienne JM, Brockmeier SF, Carson EW, Werner BC. Risk factors for infection after shoulder arthroscopy in a large Medicare population. *Am J Sports Med.* 2018;46(4):809–814.

16. Saltzman MD, Marecek GS, Edwards SL, Kalainov DM. Infection after shoulder surgery. *J Am Acad Orthop Surg.* 2011;19(4):208–218.

17. Dodson CC, Craig EV, Cordasco FA, et al. Propionibacterium acnes infection after shoulder arthroplasty: a diagnostic challenge. *J Shoulder Elbow Surg.* 2010;19(2):303–307.

18. Margaretten ME, Kohlwes J, Moore D, Bent S. Does this adult patient have septic arthritis? Clinical scenario of septic arthritis. *JAMA.* 2007;297(13):1478–1488.

19. Weishaupt D, Schweitzer ME. MR imaging of septic arthritis and rheumatoid arthritis of the shoulder. *Magn Reson Imaging Clin N Am.* 2004;12(1):111–124.

20. Bremell T, Abdelnour A, Tarkowski A. Histopathological and serological progression of experimental *Staphylococcus aureus* arthritis. *Infect Immun.* 1992;60(7):2976–2985.

21. Chevalley P, Garcia J. Imaging of infectious sacroiliitis. *J Radiol.* 1991;72(2):1–10.

22. Diaz JD, Kumetz CA, Duran-Gehring P. Septic shoulder joint diagnosed via point of care ultrasound. *Vis J Emerg Med.* 2019;14:35–36.

23. Turpin S, Lambert R. Role of scintigraphy in musculoskeletal and spinal infections. *Radiol Clin North Am.* 2001;39(2):169–189.

24. Hügle T, Schuetz P, Mueller B, et al. Serum procalcitonin for discrimination between septic and non-septic arthritis. *Clin Exp Rheumatol.* 2008;26(3):453–456.

25. Seitz WH. Shoulder-joint infection: diagnosis and management. *Semin Arthroplasty.* 2011;22(1):42–47.

26. Parvizi J. Joint infection aspirate papers—comments. *JBJS.* 2010;15:1106–1107.

27. Mathews CJ, Kingsley G, Field M, et al. Management of septic arthritis: a systematic review. *Postgrad Med J.* 2008;84(991):265–270.

28. Dilisio MF, Warner JJP, Miller L, Higgins LD. Arthroscopic tissue biopsy for the evaluation of prosthetic shoulder infection. *J Shoulder Elbow Surg.* 2015;24(4):e117–e118.

29. Horneff JG, Hsu JE, Huffman GR. Propionibacterium acnes infections in shoulder surgery. *Orthop Clin North Am.* 2014;45(4):515–521.

30. Smith RL, Kajiyama G, Schurman DJ. Staphylococcal septic arthritis: antibiotic and nonsteroidal anti-inflammatory drug treatment in a rabbit model. *J Orthop Res.* 1997;15(6):919–926.

8

Postarthroscopic Arthrofibrosis

Craig Bennett, MD
and Jerome Colin Murray, BS

INTRODUCTION

Arthrofibrosis (frozen shoulder or adhesive capsulitis) is characterized by shoulder pain and limitation of shoulder joint movement. It is a cause of marked disability and can have a profound effect on a patient's quality of life. Arthrofibrosis arising as a complication following arthroscopic shoulder surgery is of concern to both patients and surgeons. Postoperative deficit of movement is a known complication of arthroscopic surgery of the shoulder. Most cases resolve within 6 months, with symptoms steadily improving during this time. Occasionally, patients deteriorate, and there is an establishment of arthrofibrosis. The limited glenohumeral joint range of motion results from fibrotic tissue, which can develop both deep and superficial to the glenohumeral joint. The fibrosis can present as a solitary contracture or in conjunction with adhesions and tendon contracture. Risk factors for developing postarthroscopic arthrofibrosis include diabetes, low patient motivation, lack of preoperative motion, decreased pain tolerance, and poor adherence with the postoperative rehabilitation protocol.[1,2]

107

Thompson TL, ed.
Arthroscopic Shoulder Surgery: Complications and Management (pp 115-130).
© 2022 Taylor & Francis Group.

Localization of the pathologic tissue is often difficult to identify. Following arthroscopic shoulder procedures, patients must be thoroughly evaluated for both passive and active motion loss. Additionally, certain arthroscopic procedures are associated with higher incidences of arthrofibrosis and in particular locations. Diagnostic imaging can also be useful to help localize and further delineate the pathologic tissue. Physical therapy is usually the initial treatment for arthrofibrosis. Additional options for management of this condition include intra-articular injections, manipulation under anesthesia, arthroscopic surgery, and finally open surgery. In this chapter, each of these treatment options will be discussed in detail.

ETIOLOGY AND DIAGNOSIS

Arthrofibrosis is a complex clinical condition with no uniform definition in literature. Shoulder stiffness can be subclassified broadly into idiopathic and acquired stiffness. Redler and Dennis[3] categorized (idiopathic) arthrofibrotic changes into 4 stages. Stage 1, termed the *preadhesive stage*, involves the proliferation of fibroblasts without the formation of adhesions. Patients may report painful movement, particularly at night, without the loss of range of motion. Stage 2, the *acute adhesive synovitis stage*, is described as the hypertrophy of synovial tissue and the initial formation of adhesions. This stage usually presents with a mild range of motion loss and with associated pain. The *maturation stage*, stage 3, comprises the transition of synovitis to fibrosis. Range of motion during this stage is noticeably limited. Patients are usually in less pain than in the previous stages. Stage 4, the *chronic stage*, is delineated by severe loss of range of motion and minimal pain, with the exception being when patients are forcibly moved past their fibrotic limitation.

Additionally, the British and the American Shoulder and Elbow Societies and the Orthopaedic Section of the American Physical Therapy Association have presented consensus definitions of frozen shoulder: first, an initially successful postoperative rehabilitation process after shoulder surgery followed by worsening pain in the shoulder with gradual loss of both active and passive range of motion; second, symptoms of true deltoid insertion shoulder pain and night pain of insidious onset; and third, painful restriction of active and passive movement, with passive movement limited to greater than 100 degrees elevation, greater than 30 degrees external rotation, and internal rotation limited to L5 or less. While these definitions were not designed to diagnose postoperative secondary frozen shoulder, the descriptions provide an appropriate framework for discussing the changes secondary to an arthroscopic surgical procedure. Typical arthrofibrosis involves intra-articular adhesions, but it can be associated with extra-articular scar accumulation within the subacromial, subcoracoid, and subdeltoid planes as well as along the humeroscapular motion interface. Capsular contracture that accumulates between these tissues can contribute to the stiffness that patients with arthrofibrosis experience.

INCIDENCE

The overall incidence of arthrofibrosis following arthroscopic shoulder surgery is relatively low. One study by Müller and Lundsiedl[4] found that among 846 patients who underwent an arthroscopic shoulder procedure, the incidence of postoperative arthrofibrosis was only 1%. Another retrospective analysis, by Evans et al,[5] evaluated 200 patients who underwent arthroscopic subacromial decompressions with or without distal clavicle excision. They found an incidence of arthofibrosis at 5.21% and 5.71%, respectively. In this study, the prognostic risk factors for the development of secondary frozen shoulder after arthroscopic shoulder procedures were age (between 46 and 60 years) and a previous idiopathic contralateral frozen shoulder.[5] Koorevaar et al[6] evaluated 505 patients who underwent elective shoulder surgery with a 6-month follow-up, and 368 of these patients had arthroscopic shoulder surgery. Eleven percent of the total number of patients who underwent surgery experienced arthrofibrosis (15% in women and 8% in men). Four prognostic factors identified for postoperative arthrofibrosis were: diabetes, arthroscopic shoulder surgery, specialized shoulder physiotherapy, and Disabilities of the Arm, Shoulder and Hand (DASH) score. Of note, this study found higher incidence rates of arthrofibrosis in patients who underwent arthroscopic procedures compared to patients who underwent open procedures. Arthroscopic surgery might violate the capsule during the arthroscopic procedure. The capsule, especially the rotator cuff interval, may be at greater risk of being traumatized during arthroscopic surgery compared to open surgery. Further research should analyze if different arthroscopic procedures and techniques will reduce the incidence of postoperative frozen shoulder.[6]

SPECIFIC ARTHROSCOPIC
SHOULDER PROCEDURES

Arthroscopic rotator cuff repair is a common orthopedic surgical procedure, and postprocedure stiffness is frequently a concern. Physical therapy is often recommended prior to surgery to improve range of motion before the repair. Stiffness following the procedure is typically associated with prolonged immobilization, poor adherence to the rehabilitation protocol, or limited shoulder motion secondary to excessive tensioning of the repair. Complete recovery from the repair typically takes up to a year, but some patients experience prolonged postrepair difficulty reclaiming full range of motion. Post–rotator cuff repair arthrofibrosis can be categorized into 4 groups: stiffness without repeat cuff tear, stiffness with repeat tear, stiffness in association with untreated glenohumeral osteoarthritis, and stiffness in combination with a deltoid and/or nerve injury without repeat tear.[7] Incidence rates of arthrofibrosis following arthroscopic rotator cuff repair are not clearly elucidated in the current literature. Huberty et al[8] reviewed of 489 patients who underwent arthroscopic rotator cuff repairs over a 3-year period. They found 4.9% of patients (24) experienced postoperative stiffness. When analyzed in the context of rotator cuff repair specifically, risk factors included calcific tendinitis, previous adhesive capsulitis, single-tendon cuff repair, and being under 50 years of age. The patients who developed postoperative arthrofibrosis underwent arthroscopic capsular release and lysis of adhesions, with all patients ultimately satisfied with their results. Factors associated with a lower incidence rate of developing postoperative stiffness included concomitant coracoplasty (acromioplasty) and rotator cuff tears involving more tendons and/or larger in size.

Selective anterior and posterior capsulorrhaphy are common procedures used to address shoulder instability. Arthroscopic shoulder instability procedures are also associated with an increased risk of postoperative arthrofibrosis. *Postcapsulorrhaphy arthropathy*, a term credited to Warner et al,[9] results in a loss of external rotation increasing the risk for posterior subluxation of the humoral head and osteoarthritis. Labral repair and capsulorrhaphy are sometimes associated with postoperative arthrofibrosis, usually due to prolonged immobilization and/or excessive tightening of the capsule. Loss of internal rotation, associated with posterior capsulorrhaphy, is a less common yet documented form of stiffness. Soft tissue lengthening procedures can often be used to treat these causes of arthrofibrosis. Incidence rates following labral and/or capsular repair are not clearly outlined in literature. When instability surgery leads to arthrofibrosis, conservative intervention to treat the arthrofibrosis is largely unsuccessful, with better outcomes observed with surgical intervention.[10]

TREATMENT INDICATIONS

The primary symptoms of arthrofibrosis are most often pain and limitation motion. Although radiographic imaging is typically normal in patients with arthrofibrosis, imaging can be used to rule out other potential causes of symptoms.[11,12] The indications for formal treatment are restricted motion as previously defined, pain associated with movement of the shoulder in any plane, and deltoid insertion pain. The principal goals of physical therapy are to improve passive and active range of motion and to produce sufficient strength to perform basic functional activities and to limit patients' pain. As previously discussed, a guideline for a shoulder arthrofibrosis in need of formal treatment demonstrates painful restriction of active and passive movement, passive movement limited to less than 100 degrees elevation, less than 30 degrees external rotation, and internal rotation limited to L5 or less. For idiopathic shoulder stiffness, the primary intervention is almost always physiotherapy, focused on passive stretching and techniques to reduce pain. Arthrofibrosis secondary to arthroscopic surgery, however, is usually less responsive to conservative therapy. For patients who do not respond to physical therapy, surgical intervention, such as arthroscopic or open release, is indicated. Surgical management begins with a presurgical consultation. All benefits and risks should be thoroughly explained to the patient preoperatively. Manipulation under anesthesia can help increase range of motion, yet this method is contraindicated in patients with a history of malnutrition, osteopenia, previous instability surgery, or nonunion. Contraindications to surgical intervention include any notable medical conditions that would increase risk and factors that would affect patient compliance with a postoperative therapeutic regimen.[13] Patients with reflex sympathetic dystrophy or cervical radiculopathy require special consideration as there is potential exacerbation of their condition due to postoperative pain. The decision between nonoperative and surgical treatment is multifactorial and reliant on the surgeons' discretion.

SURGICAL TREATMENT

Indications

Surgical intervention is generally indicated if nonsteroidal anti-inflammatory drugs (NSAIDs), physical therapy, and injections provide inadequate relief of symptoms by 6 to 9 months. Redler and Dennis[3] found, in a retrospective review of 105 patients, that 85% resolved arthrofibrotic symptoms with nonoperative intervention. These patients averaged treatment lengths of 3.8 months, while patients who received surgical intervention averaged treatment lengths of 12.4 months.

Presurgical Considerations

Prior to surgical intervention, patients must be thoroughly evaluated, and a detailed account of history of arthrofibrosis, physical therapy protocol, and any issues with compliance to the rehabilitation protocol must be noted. In addition, goals and outcomes for the procedure must be clearly summarized for the patient. Anesthesia will perform an interscalene nerve block to anesthetize the shoulder and upper arm. The option of an indwelling scalene catheter will also be discussed with the patient and anesthesia team.

Arthroscopic Release

The patient is positioned in either the lateral or beach chair position, once under general anesthesia, and the scalene block is performed. In the event an open anterior surgery is anticipated, the preference is the beach chair position, particularly if external rotation and anterior capsular tightness are markedly limited. If modest posterior capsular tightness and internal rotation are the primary preoperative concerns, the lateral position is an option, presuming an open release is not anticipated. Under anesthesia, evaluation of both shoulders is completed. The involved shoulder is sterilized, draped, and positioned in moderate distraction. The joint space is insufflated with saline to increase visualization and decrease the risk of iatrogenic chondral damage from arthroscopic tools. A diagnostic arthroscopy through an initial posterior portal is performed. An anterior portal placement is established between the biceps tendon and the superior border of the subscapularis tendon. In the relatively rare occurrence when it is not possible to insert the arthroscopic sheath via an anterior or posterior portal, the anterior rotator interval is identified and opened using a direct approach. Once opened, the arthroscope is inserted anteriorly, the posterior portal placement is visualized, and the capsular release begins from the anterior aspect of the shoulder (Figure 8-1).[13]

An anterior release from the inferior biceps to the inferior glenoid is often performed to increase external rotation in both adduction and abduction. The subscapularis must be identified prior to anterior release; otherwise, an open approach is indicated. A bipolar radiofrequency ablation probe is used to successfully release the capsulolabral junction posterior to the subscapularis. The rotator interval capsule is released first due to its relative thickness in these settings. The release is initiated beneath the biceps tendon and continued up to the superior border of the subscapularis. Performing a release at the base of the coracoid process is often necessary and can be done without additional risk to the neurovascular adjacent structures. Caution must be taken when performing a release inferiorly between

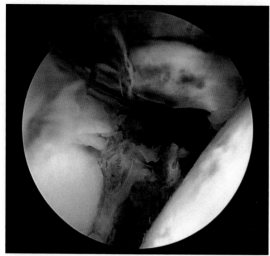

Figure 8-1. Arthroscopic image from a posterior portal in the beach chair position showing synovitis and fibrosis in a patient with adhesive capsulitis also typically seen in postarthroscopic arthrofibrosis.

the 5-o'clock and 7-o'clock positions due to the location of the axillary nerve. The nerve is often adherent to the inferior pouch after surgery, increasing the likelihood of injury. Dissection and release anterior to the subscapularis places neurovascular structures at risk and, as a result, is usually not necessary. Anterosuperior and anteroinferior release can restore external rotation with the arm at the side and in abduction, respectively.[13]

Posterior capsular release is performed under visualization via the anterior portal. The arthroscope is inserted through the anterior cannula, and the inflow is also changed to the anterior cannula. An arthroscopic cannula is placed posteriorly over a switching stick once the arthroscopic sheath is removed.[13] The release begins directly posterior to the biceps tendon and continues along the posterior labrum. Visibility of the infraspinatus muscle marks the completion of the release. Lateral deviation from the labrum increases risk of iatrogenic injury to the rotator cuff tendons as they become confluent with the posterior capsule near its insertion onto the humoral head. The suggested release location is from the 11-o'clock to 8-o'clock positions.

Some patients experience continued stiffness after surgical intervention. In these cases, repeated manipulation under anesthesia has been shown to be very effective. In a group of 730 patients, 141 patients underwent a second manipulation procedure. All of these patients experienced improvement from the first procedure.[13] Following arthroscopic debridement and capsulotomy, a postprocedure manipulation is performed as well with the patient in the beach chair or lateral position used to perform the arthroscopy (Figures 8-2 and 8-3).

Figure   8-2. Shoulder manipulation status post arthroscopic debridement and capsular release show-ing passive external rotation.

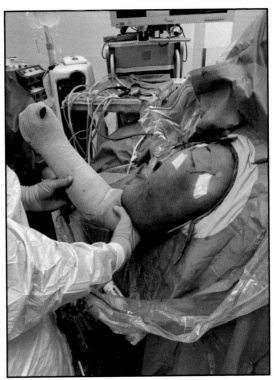

Open Surgical Release

Patients who fail to benefit from arthroscopic release or closed manipulation or have primarily extra-articular adhesions often benefit from open surgical release. This method is associated with extensive dis-tention and increased postoperative pain. Intraoperative soft tissue injec-tion with extended release bupivacaine can be used to mediate the pain associated with this procedure. Anatomic orientation is pivotal for success neurovascular safety during an open procedure. The preferred approach for an open release is a deltopectoral incision via a layer-by-layer dissection. The deltopectoral interval is opened, and release of subdeltoid adhesions is facili-tated by abduction and internally rotation of the arm with retraction on the deltoid.[13] The axillary nerve lies 3 to 5 cm distal to the lateral edge of the acromion on the deep surface of the deltoid, and its location must be con-sidered as adhesions are sharply released between the muscle and humerus. The surgeon should palpate the axillary nerve as it exits the posterior quad-rilateral space and keep all dissection above this. The subpectoral plane is

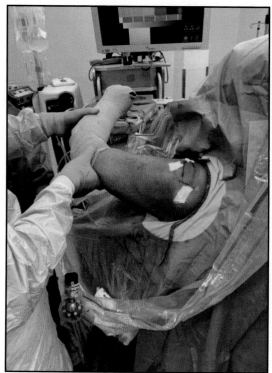

Figure 8-3. Shoulder manipulation status post arthroscopic debridement and capsular release showing passive internal rotation.

then released. The subacromial space is also released sharply. The interval between the conjoined tendon and the subscapularis is then released with careful attention to identify the axillary nerve anteriorly on the external surface of the subscapularis. A retractor is placed underneath the nerve proximally to protect it. Formal release of the rotator interval begins with transection of the coracohumeral ligament at the base of the coracoid process. This can be palpated as a thick band running from the coracoid to the upper portion of the subscapularis. Next the rotator interval is opened by dividing the tissue just above the subscapularis from lateral to medial to the base of the subscapularis.[14,15] Subsequent mobilization and repair of the subscapularis are indicated to preserve anterior stability.[16-18]

Fibrosis or contracture of the subscapularis may limit external rotation. If external rotation is significantly limited, the subscapularis can be lengthened with a Z-plasty, in which the tendon is cut in the coronal plane, leaving the deeper half attached to the lesser tuberosity and separating the superficial half. The deeper half is divided vertically at the glenoid level through the contracted capsule. The lateral edge of the superficial limb is then sutured to the medial edge of the deeper limb with the arm in external rotation after all releases have been completed. Often the subscapularis is scarred to the subscapular fossa and surrounding tissues. A global release should be performed to fully mobilize the muscle-tendon unit. This requires releases on the superior, inferior, anterior, and posterior surfaces. The axillary nerve should be identified during subscapularis mobilization. This can be performed by forward flexion and slight external rotation of the arm with some tension on the subscapularis. Once the axillary nerve is identified at the inferior edge of the subscapularis, a vessel loop can be passed for clear identification of the nerve. Abduction and internal rotation can also be improved through the deltopectoral incision. A retractor is used to displace the humeral head posteriorly, and a complete pericapsulotomy can be performed. The release is performed just lateral to the labral tissue and proceeds from posterosuperior to posteroinferior. Knowledge of the location of the axillary nerve during inferior dissection is critical. Once the releases are complete, the surgeon assesses the range of motion and determines the limitations for safe motion, especially external rotation in the setting of subscapularis lengthening.[13]

Postsurgical Considerations

Documentation of patients' passive range of motion is recorded preoperatively, while under anesthesia, and following the surgical release. The active range of motion preoperatively and postoperatively is documented as well. Analgesia is provided via an interscalene block, allowing for immediate postoperative movement. Patients are instructed to begin a physical therapy regimen once a day for a few weeks, beginning 24 hours after surgery. The number of weeks needed for daily and then biweekly physical therapy is very case dependent. Additionally, opioids are generally used for only a few days, as the interscalene blocks allow for significant pain relief. Oral NSAIDs are the mainstays of pain control postoperatively and surrounding therapy. Postoperative physical therapy is focused on maintaining adequate range of motion with slow, passive stretching. Patients are encouraged to stretch in the shower because the heat allows for some additional relief.[3] Dynamic bracing and continuous passive motion devices are also being used with increasing frequency. Continued passive range of motion with increasing active-assisted and active range of motion is moderated for months.

NONSURGICAL TREATMENT

Research surrounding some of the nonsurgical options is variable, and primarily, evaluations have been made relative to idiopathic arthrofibrosis management. Including the data in this chapter is important for completeness, as these treatments may be viable options for patients with arthrofibrosis secondary to arthroscopic surgery.

Oral Medication

NSAIDs are treatment options for analgesic effect. Oral corticosteroids have also been indicated for use in arthrofibrosis. A systematic review of the use of oral corticosteroids concluded that they provide notable short-term improvement for up to 6 weeks.[19]

Corticosteroid Injections

Intra-articular corticosteroid injections are commonly used to decrease inflammation and pain for patients with mild symptoms consistent with arthrofibrosis. A double-blind, placebo-controlled randomized study evaluating ultrasound-guided intra-articular and rotator interval corticosteroid injections in 122 patients with arthrofibrosis demonstrated a marked decrease in pain at a 6- and 12-week follow-up. These results were diminished at a 26-week follow-up, and there was no difference between patients who received an isolated intra-articular injection and patients who received a concomitant rotator interval injection.[20] In a separate study, the outcomes of patients who completed physical therapy were compared with outcomes of patients who received a corticosteroid injection, and no additional functional benefits were found. Patients who received a steroid injection did experience an increase in passive external movement. Additionally, other techniques offer an alternative to corticosteroid injections. These alternatives are particularly beneficial for patients with diabetes, for whom the effect corticosteroids have on blood glucose levels is a concern.[21]

Extracorporeal Shock Wave Therapy

Extracorporeal shock wave therapy has been shown to offer some benefit for patients with joint stiffness. Chen et al[22] observed significant short-term improvements in the range of motion of patients with shoulder adhesive capsulitis who underwent treatments with extracorporeal shock wave therapy.

Calcitonin

Calcitonin is a polypeptide hormone that acts to inhibit osteoclast activity and has been occasionally shown to increase bone density.[3] Rouhani et al[23] performed a double-blind randomized controlled trial comparing patients who underwent intranasal calcitonin treatment with patients who underwent physical therapy and NSAIDs. At a 6-week follow-up, improvements in pain, range of motion, and functional scores were all greater in the calcitonin group. While the calcitonin in this study was administered intranasally, intramuscular injections are available with potentially fewer associated adverse side effects. Chronic use of calcitonin has been proven to be a useful treatment option, without critical adverse effects. Of note, the calcitonin used clinically is derived from salmon and is contraindicated in patients with allergies to salmon.

Hyaluronic Acid Injections

Hyaluronic acid is an essential component of synovial fluid and is vital for protection of chondral surfaces and lubrication. Injection of hyaluronic acid into the joint space inhibits cytokine release, thus reducing pain and increasing joint function.[24,25] Well-established benefits of its use as a viscosupplement injection have been proven only for the treatment of osteoarthritis of the knee.[26,27] Use of hyaluronic acid to treat arthrofibrosis is largely experimental, and its use is currently off-label. A study completed by Rovetta and Monteforte[28] compared a combination of physical therapy and intra-articular hyaluronic acid/corticosteroid injection with intra-articular corticosteroid injection and physical therapy. Both groups showed improvements of pain and range of motion at 6-month follow-up. The group that received the hyaluronic acid experienced a greater degree of improvement in internal rotation than the group that received the combination injection.

Hydrodilation

Hydrodilation, or distention arthrograph, is the distention of the capsular space by injection of air or fluid.[29] This technique is done under fluoroscopic guidance using local anesthetic, with the goal being to stretch the capsular contracture and increase intracapsular volume. A mixture of long-acting analgesics, steroids, or saline can be used with this procedure. In a level 2 randomized controlled trial, reported by Le et al,[12] improved pain scores were seen in the group that received hydrodilation compared to the group that underwent manipulation under anesthesia alone. No difference in range of motion was observed between the 2 groups. The current research supports hydrodilation as a successful treatment option when done in conjunction with steroids and saline. The findings are unclear if hydrodilation offers better outcomes than isolated steroid injection treatments.[30] Lee et al[31] concluded that intra-articular hyaluronic acid injections as an isolated treatment option are not preferred over other conservative therapy options.

Whole-Body Cryotherapy

Whole-body cryotherapy is thought to provide both analgesic and anti-inflammatory effects. This procedure is done by exposing the shoulder in a chamber that circulates air within the temperatures range of −110°C and −140°C for 2 to 3 minutes. In a study comparing patients who completed physical therapy alone with those who received whole-body cryotherapy with physical therapy, patients who received whole-body cryotherapy had greater improvements in active range of motion and self-assessed functional scores.

Enzymatic Capsulotomy

Collagenase, isolated from the bacterium *Clostridium histylyticum*, is an enzyme that breaks down the peptide bonds in collagen. Its current approved use by the US Food and Drug Administration is for the treatment of other fibrotic pathologies, such as Dupuytren disease and Peyronie disease. A phase 2 placebo-controlled double-blind randomized trial found improvements in functional scores, range of motion, and pain scores in patients who received the enzymatic capsulotomy via extra-articular collagenase injection as compared to the placebo group (0.9% saline/2 mM $CaCl_2$). Improvements were still seen in patients at the 1.8-year follow-up. Noted side effects were injection site tenderness and ecchymosis that lasted up to 2 weeks.[32] There was no evidence on magnetic resonance imaging of damage to surrounding tissues (ie, rotator cuff) as a result of this treatment.[33]

Manipulation Under Anesthesia

Manipulation under anesthesia is typically performed under short general anesthesia with a brachial plexus block. The patient is placed in the supine position, and the preprocedure range of motion can be measured at this time. It is important during the procedure to stabilize both the scapula and humerus to prevent iatrogenic fracture. Pressure is then applied to the shoulder joint to break up the fibrotic tissue. The method used to manipulate often differs between surgeons to maximize the potential postprocedural range of motion and decrease the associated risks (Figure 8-4).

Figure 8-4. Manipulation under anesthesia showing passive abduction.

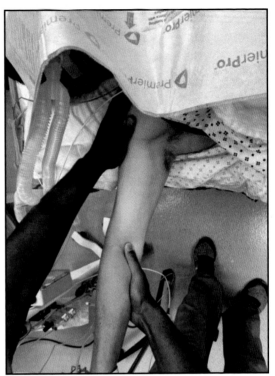

REFERENCES

1. Janda DH, Loubert P. Basic science and clinical application in the athlete's shoulder: a preventative program focusing on the glenohumeral joint. *Clin Sports Med.* 1991;10:955–971.
2. Allen AA, Warner JJP. Management of the stiff shoulder. *Oper Techn Orthop.* 1995;5:238–247.
3. Redler L, Dennis E. Treatment of adhesive capsulitis of the shoulder. *J Am Acad Orthop Surg.* 2019;27(12):e554.
4. Müller D, Lundsiedl F. Arthroscopy of the shoulder joint: a minimal invasive and harmless procedure? *Arthroscopy.* 2000;16:425.
5. Evans JP, Guyver PM, Smith CD. Frozen shoulder after simple arthroscopic shoulder procedures: what is the risk? *Bone Joint J.* 2015;97B:963–966.
6. Koorevaar RCT, van't Riet E, Ipskamp M, Bulstra SK. Incidence and prognostic factors for postoperative frozen shoulder after shoulder surgery: a prospective cohort study. *Arch Orthop Trauma Surg.* 2017;137(3):293–301.
7. Warner JJ, Greis PE. The treatment of stiffness of the shoulder after repair of the rotator cuff. *Instr Course Lect.* 1998;47:67–75.
8. Huberty DP, Schoolfield JD, Brady PC, et al. Incidence and treatment of postoperative stiffness following arthroscopic rotator cuff repair. *Arthroscopy.* 2009;25:880–890.

9. Warner JJ, Allen AA, Marks PH, et al. Arthroscopic release of postoperative capsular contracture of the shoulder. *J Bone Joint Surg Am.* 1997;79:1151–1158.

10. Katz LM, Hsu S, Miller SL, et al. Poor outcomes after SLAP repair: descriptive analysis and prognosis. *Arthroscopy.* 2009;25:849–855.

11. Warner JJ, Allen A, Marks PH, et al. Arthroscopic release for chronic, refractory adhesive capsulitis of the shoulder. *J Bone Joint Surg Am.* 1996;78:1808–1816.

12. Le HV, Lee SJ, Nazarian A, Rodriguez EK. Adhesive capsulitis of the shoulder: review of pathophysiology and current clinical treatments. *Shoulder Elbow.* 2017;9(2):75–84.

13. Vezeridis PS, Goel DP, Shah AA, Sung S, Warner JJP. Postarthroscopic arthrofibrosis of the shoulder. *Sports Med Arthrosc Rev.* 2010;18(3):198–206.

14. Neer CS II, Satterlee CC, Dalsey RM, et al. The anatomy and potential effects of contracture of the coracohumeral ligament. *Clin Orthop Relat Res.* 1992;280:182–185.

15. Neer CS II. Frozen shoulder. In: Neer CS II, ed. *Shoulder Reconstruction.* WB Saunders; 1990:422.

16. Kieras DM, Matsen FA III. Open release in the management of refractory frozen shoulder. *Orthop Trans.* 1991;15:801–802.

17. Ozaki J, Nakagawa Y, Sakurai G, et al. Recalcitrant chronic adhesive capsulitis of the shoulder: role of contracture of the coracohumeral ligament and rotator interval in pathogenesis and treatment. *J Bone Joint Surg Am.* 1989;71:1511–1515.

18. Leffert RD. The frozen shoulder. *Instr Course Lect.* 1985;34:199–203.

19. Buchbinder R, Green S, Youd JM, Johnston RV, Cumpston M. Arthrographic distension for adhesive capsulitis (frozen shoulder). *Cochrane Database Syst Rev.* 2008;1(1):CD007005.

20. Prestgaard T, Wormgoor MEA, Haugen S, Harstad H, Mowinckel P, Brox JI. Ultrasound-guided intra-articular and rotator interval corticosteroid injections in adhesive capsulitis of the shoulder. *Pain.* 2015;156:1683–1691.

21. Santoboni F, Balducci S, D'Errico V, et al. Extracorporeal shockwave therapy improves functional outcomes of adhesive capsulitis of the shoulder in patients with diabetes. *Diabetes Care.* 2017;40:e12–e13.

22. Chen CY, Hu CC, Weng PW, et al. Extracorporeal shockwave therapy improves short-term functional outcomes of shoulder adhesive capsulitis. *J Shoulder Elbow Surg.* 2014;23:1843–1851.

23. Rouhani A, Mardani-Kivi M, Bazavar M, et al. Calcitonin effects on shoulder adhesive capsulitis. *Eur J Orthop Surg Traumatol.* 2016;26:575–580.

24. Iwata H. Pharmacologic and clinical aspects of intraarticular injection of hyaluronate. *Clin Orthop Relat Res.* 1993;289:285–291.

25. Waddell DD, Kolomytkin OV, Dunn S, Marino AA. Hyaluronan suppresses IL-1β-induced metalloproteinase activity from synovial tissue. *Clin Orthop Relat Res.* 2007;465:241–248.

26. Bannuru RR, Natov NS, Dasi UR, Schmid CH, McAlindon TE. Therapeutic trajectory following intra-articular hyaluronic acid injection in knee osteoarthritis—meta-analysis. *Osteoarthritis Cartilage.* 2011;19(6):611–619.

27. Bellamy N, Campbell J, Robinson V, Gee T, Bourne R, Wells G. Viscosupplementation for the treatment of osteoarthritis of the knee. *Cochrane Database Syst Rev.* 2006;2:CD005321.

28. Rovetta G, Monteforte P. Intraarticular injection of sodium hyaluronate plus steroid versus steroid in adhesive capsulitis of the shoulder. *Int J Tissue Reactions.* 1998;20(4):125–130.

29. Georgiannos D, Devetzi E, Bisbinas I. Adhesive capsulitis of the shoulder: is there a consensus regarding the treatment? A comprehensive review. *Open Orthop J.* 2017;11:65–76.

30. Buchbinder R, Green S, Youd JM, et al. Arthrographic distension for adhesive capsulitis (frozen shoulder). *Cochrane Database Syst Rev.* 2008;1:CD007005.
31. Lee L-C, Lieu F-K, Lee H-L, Tung T-H. Effectiveness of hyaluronic acid administration in treating adhesive capsulitis of the shoulder: a systematic review of randomized controlled trials. *BioMed Res Int.* 2015;2015:314120.
32. Badalamente MA, Wang E. Enzymatic capsulotomy for adhesive capsulitis of the shoulder. Paper presented at American Academy of Orthopaedic Surgeons Annual Meeting; March 17–26, 2006; Chicago, IL.
33. Wang ED, Badalamente MA, Mackenzie S, et al. Phase 2a study of safety/efficacy of collagenase (CCH) in patients with adhesive capsulitis: level 2 evidence. Paper presented at American Society for Surgery of the Hand Annual Meeting; September 10–12, 2015; Seattle, WA.

9

Complex Regional Pain Syndrome Following Arthroscopic Shoulder Surgery

Marc E. Rankin, MD
and Akhil Andrews, MD

INTRODUCTION

According to the American Orthopedic Society of Sports Medicine, more than 1.4 million shoulder arthroscopies are performed annually.[1] Our understanding on the number of postoperative complications is less precise, relying mostly on anecdotes and subjective experience, including voluntary surveys from members of arthroscopic organizations and retrospective review studies with varying statistical significance. Neurovascular complications following shoulder surgery are rare, with neurologic injuries more common than vascular injuries with an incidence ranging from 0% to 30%.[2] While most of these neurologic injuries are transient, others such as complex regional pain syndrome (CRPS) can result in a protracted and incomplete postoperative recovery. CRPS is a painful and debilitating condition characterized by a constellation of sensory, motor, autonomic, skin, and bone maladies. It commonly arises after limb injury, but there is

Thompson TL, ed.
*Arthroscopic Shoulder Surgery:
Complications and Management* (pp 131-152).
© 2022 Taylor & Francis Group.

no relationship to the severity of trauma and in some cases no known precipitating trauma. Because CRPS remains poorly understood with imprecise terminology, it can lead to misdiagnosis, resulting in a delay in treatment and ultimately a poor outcome of the intended surgical procedure.

EPIDEMIOLOGY

The incidence of CRPS is uncertain, with the 2 best population-based studies yielding very different data: 5.5 cases per 100,000 person years in the United States and 26.2 per 100,000 person years in the Netherlands. The variation may result from the use of different diagnostic criteria. The results of 2 epidemiologic studies in the general population indicate that at least 50,000 new cases of CRPS type I occur annually in the United States alone. The incidence increases with age until 70 (most children diagnosed have a favorable prognosis), and women are affected 3 to 4 times more often.[3] There is a predilection for upper extremity involvement occurring in approximately 60% of cases and the leg in about 40%. Resolution rates differ greatly between studies, with many experiencing spontaneous remission, while in others, symptoms may persist for months or years, and some effects may be permanent.

The pernicious nature of CRPS as a postoperative complication rests in the fact that it remains a poorly understood and controversial diagnosis. CRPS is generally viewed as a chronic pain condition where complete manifestation of symptoms can take weeks, even months. The inherent problem in waiting on diagnostic confirmation is the disadvantage of having to treat the aspects of the syndrome that have become fully expressed and fixed. Early intervention is preferable and usually results in a more predictable outcome. CRPS is a condition that is characterized, in part, by impaired vasomotor function, usually affecting one limb after a traumatic incident. It is believed to be caused by damage or an impairment of the central and peripheral nervous systems. Its manifestations include excessive pain, hyperesthesia, swelling, changes in skin temperature, skin color, and joint stiffness. The delay in making an accurate diagnosis allows the syndrome to progress undetected, adding to its insidious and intransigent nature. By the time treatment is initiated, the syndrome can be far advanced in its destructive course, rendering it resistant to traditional pain management measures. As a result, the patient often experiences a protracted and incomplete recovery, often adversely affecting the outcome of the intended surgical procedure.

HISTORICAL PERSPECTIVE

The signs and symptoms of CRPS were originally reported in 1812 by British surgeon Dr. Demark following a supracondylar gunshot wound, naming the condition *algodystrophy*. The term *Sudeck's atrophy* referred to bony atrophy after certain injuries, which were visible on the newly popularized radiographs. In 1917, the first successfully surgical treated case of CRPS was documented. The procedure involved a periarterial sympathectomy performed by Rene Leriche, which provided complete resolution of symptoms. The success of this procedure supported the belief in the hypothesis that the sympathetic nervous system was key in the pathologic process. In 1936, James A. Evans introduced the term *reflex sympathetic dystrophy*. In the 1950s, John J. Bonica proposed staging criteria for CRPS.[4] In 1988, Amadio[5] described a pain dysfunction syndrome in his attempts to incorporate all related diagnoses under one heading. Merskey and Bogduk[6] are credited with grouping the former pain syndromes into a CRPS binary designation. In 1994, a consensus group of pain medicine specialists at the International Association for the Study of Pain (IASP) agreed on taxonomy based on the Orlando Criteria.[7] Although the IASP definition of CRPS is extremely sensitive, it has been criticized for leading to overdiagnosis of the condition. While a known traumatic event was required by the Orlando Criteria, the IASP itself noted that 5% to 10% of all patients will not have an inciting event or cause for immobilization and inferred that this criterion was not requisite for diagnosis. Recognizing this inherent dilemma in 2003, a panel of experts met in Budapest, Hungary, to find a resolution. Their modified criteria, published in 2007, are based on the grouping of signs and symptoms into 4 distinct categories, which were identified by factor analysis.[8] A CRPS severity score to monitor longitudinal changes was subsequently developed. Through the years, several attempts have been made to explain CRPS through a unified model. The pathogenesis was believed to be initiated by noxious stimuli from an injured region of the body sensitizing the peripheral and central neural circuits to an abnormal synapse, termed *ephapse* (Figure 9-1). This short-circuit would then enable a sympathetic discharge directly stimulating sensory nerves. It is this pathologic sensory nerve stimulation that was believed to be responsible for CRPS symptoms. The primary nociceptive pathway would follow, resulting in heightened sensation, spontaneous pain, and hyperalgesia. The central nervous system somatosensory processing would then misinterpret normal painful mechanical stimuli, resulting in both hyperalgesia and allodynia. Motor impairment was believed to arise secondary to a similar impairment of the central nervous system processing, causing weakness or tremor. The peripheral and central sensitization coupled with the impaired central nervous

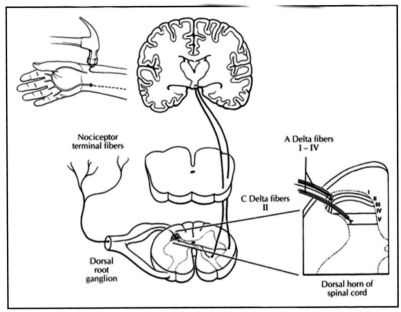

Figure 9-1. Abnormal central nervous system modulation of afferent sensory stimuli may contribute to the development of a dystrophic response after peripheral trigger (hammer striking superficial radial nerve). (Reproduced with permission from Patterson RW, Li Z, Smith BP, Smith TL, Koman LA. Complex regional pain syndrome of the upper extremity. *J Hand Surg Am.* 2011;36[9]:1553–1562.)

system processing leads to the proposed disturbances within the sympathetic nervous system. The protracted nature of the disease was believed to occur when this was coupled to the altered inflammatory response of healing. With the aforementioned process being the theorized pathway, CRPS was subsequently subdivided into 2 groups.

Complex Regional Pain Syndrome I

Previously termed reflex sympathetic dystrophy, CRPS I is a chronic neuropathic pain that follows soft tissue or bone injury in the absence of a defined nerve injury, followed by a period of immobilization, which leads to an exaggerated pain response. Traditionally, it was believed to be based on an inflammatory induction theory through an indirect defect of norepinephrine on sensory receptors.[9] The resulting inflammation from injury would sensitize the peripheral sensory nerve endings, which in turn would release norepinephrine and other inflammatory mediators. Prostaglandin is the end result and is released from the sympathetic terminals, stimulating the sensory nerves. It is now believed that some form of initial nerve injury is a key factor for the cascaded events, and neurogenic dysregulation may be a contributing factor.

Complex Regional Pain Syndrome II

The pathogenesis of CRPS type II, previously named *causalgia*, has the distinction of a known nerve injury. A neuroma forms in both the sensory nerve endings of the peripheral nerves as well as the central dorsal root ganglion. These nerve endings develop a sensitivity to catecholamine, which is increased through the expression of α2 receptors. The abnormal interaction within the sympathetic chain occurs when the sympathetic nerves, which normally innervate the blood vessels of the dorsal root ganglion, surround the injured nerve cell bodies. The newly expressed α2 receptors can be stimulated by circulating catecholamines as well as by sympathetic efferent nerves that grow into the neuroma. It is through these peripheral and central mechanisms that an abnormal coupling between the sensory pain nerves and the sympathetic nervous system occurs.[10]

LITERATURE REVIEW

Our review of the existing literature revealed a single reported case of CRPS II following shoulder arthroscopy,[11] suggesting either that the incidence of CRPS as a postoperative complication in this setting is rare or that the condition may be underdiagnosed. There are reported cases of peripheral nerve injury due to portal placement, requiring open neurolysis for return of function.[12] Nerve injury can range from transient self-limiting neurapraxias to focal injury to peripheral nerves requiring surgical intervention via tendon transfers.[13,14] Small,[15] in a retrospective review of arthroscopy cases performed by experienced arthroscopists, reported 2 cases of reflex sympathetic dystrophy that developed following subacromial space procedures. Martel et al[16] performed a retrospective single-center study of 287 patients who underwent surgery for extra-articular shoulder pathology and found 10% of the subjects developed CRPS. Comorbidities and preoperative clinical status were determined to be major contributing factors to the development of CRPS.

Current literature suggests that CRPS may be underdiagnosed,[17] and therefore, it is important to be cognizant of existing comorbidities that may precipitate neurapraxia in the setting of shoulder arthroscopy, especially cervical spine disorders. Connective tissue disorders with hypermobility in patients could be associated with an increased risk of nerve injury in the perioperative period, as reported by Stoler and Oaklander.[18]

Patient factors aside, various intraoperative factors have been hypothesized to contribute to perioperative nerve injury. The current view on patient positioning is that adoption of the beach chair position reduces strain on the brachial plexus.[19] Similarly, it has been discussed that, if used, traction should be applied in a direction perpendicular to the long axis of the humeral diaphysis, as opposed to a direction parallel to it. This has been described to not only accentuate any tear of the glenoid labrum but also virtually eliminate any traction neurapraxia. Careful and precise portal placement is imperative, both for adequate access to the glenohumeral joint as well as avoiding focal injury to nerve secondary to misplaced portals. Fluid extravasation during shoulder arthroscopy has been theorized to contribute to neurapraxia via local mass effect, and Pitman et al[20] looked at monitoring somatosensory evoked potentials during shoulder arthroscopy for the detection of neurapraxias and documented a case of total loss of SEP from all monitored peripheral nerves, after significant extravasation over the anterior aspect of the operative shoulder. Additionally, Andrews and Carson[21] recommended against the use of local anesthetic in the joint due to the theoretical risk of extravasation of intra-articular anesthetic into the soft tissues during manipulation of the joint intraoperatively, with resultant interference with nerve function and potential postoperative neurapraxia.

CONTEMPORARY CONCEPTS OF PATHOPHYSIOLOGY

The nervous system is a highly organized network of nerves whose purpose is to detect environmental changes that affect the body. That information is then interpreted and transmitted in tandem with the endocrine system, to respond to those stimuli. The nervous system comprises 2 main parts: the central nervous system, consisting of the brain and spinal cord, and the peripheral nervous system, consisting of the nerves and ganglia outside the spinal cord. The neural connections between the two that integrate the received information and both coordinate and influence the activities of all body parts. The peripheral nervous system is subdivided into the somatic nervous system and the autonomic nervous system. The autonomic nervous system is further subdivided into the sympathetic nervous system, which is responsible for "fight-or-flight" response and the parasympathetic nervous system, which is responsible for the "rest-and-digest" response. Much of what we have learned about CRPS is based on animal studies and remains both hypothetical and controversial. The leading theory is that CRPS is the result of an abnormal interplay between the central and peripheral nervous systems: exaggerated inflammation coupled with central reorganization.

The previous concept that the predominant problem was sympathetic dysfunction has now become obsolete. While multiple attempts have been made to reduce CRPS to a single pathophysiologic mechanism, currently it has become increasingly recognized that the causes are multifactorial. CRPS is not simply a sympathetically mediated peripheral pain condition but also a disease of the central nervous system.

One current area of research focuses on a genetic predisposition in the development of CRPS. While associations with known gene polymorphisms have been described, they have been demonstrated in smaller studies and not replicated in larger cohorts. As long as there is an absence of markers for subgrouping, the detection of genetic factors will remain a challenge. Additionally, association studies require a high statistical power for concordance, yet CRPS remains a rare disease.

The extreme psychologic distress exhibited by some patients with CRPS, as well as the unusual nature of its symptomatology, has led many to believe that the pathway was of a predominant or purely psychogenic mechanism. Current research suggests that there are some interactions between the psychologic and immunologic pathways. However, similar to the studies on the contributions of genetic inheritance, review of the existing literature has been limited to case series or cross-sectional psychologic comparisons between patients with CRPS and chronic pain patients as controls.

NEUROINFLAMMATORY PATHWAY

Of the several proposed pathophysiologic mechanisms believed to contribute to the development of CRPS, the inciting event by noxious stimuli to an extremity (no matter the magnitude) has the most support. This leads to the local release of proinflammatory cytokines and neuropeptides producing signs of inflammation and locally increased nociceptive responsiveness in a process known as central sensitization.[22] Central sensitization augments the function of neurons in nocioceptive pathways by enhancing membrane excitability, increasing synaptic efficacy, recruiting subthreshold synaptic inputs to nocioceptive neurons, and suppressing neural inhibition. This cascade of events results in an exaggerated action potential, which facilitates and amplifies the body's response to painful stimuli. This process is regulated by nociception-induced release of neuropeptides such as substance P and calcitonin gene–related peptide, which are known to have both neuromodulatory and immunomodulatory effects. Proinflammatory markers (interleukin [IL] A, IL-6, and tumor necrosis factor α) are elevated with a concomitant suppression of anti-inflammatory cytokines such as IL-4 and IL-10. The ongoing nociceptive input (resulting from sympatholytic efferent coupling) produces alterations in spinal nociceptive pathways, further increasing nociceptive responses. Peripheral sensitization occurs simultaneously where afferent fibers release pronociceptive neuropeptides (substance P, bradykinin), which directly trigger nociceptive firing and lower the firing threshold for thermal and mechanical stimuli. Therefore, both central and peripheral sensitization contribute to allodynia and hyperalgesia. Sympathetic dysregulation is partly responsible for the color and temperature changes seen in CRPS-affected limbs.

Historically, it was assumed that autonomic features of CRPS were the result of vasoconstriction reflecting excessive sympathetic nervous system outflow, and the pain was sympathetically maintained. This has been the rationale for the clinical use of selective sympathetic blockade as both a diagnostic tool and a therapeutic measure. While the findings regarding symptoms indicate that CRPS pain and other symptoms may in some instances be linked to sympathetic nervous system activity, it is not implicit that excessive sympathetic nervous system outflow is responsible. The 3 main discrepancies include the relatively low plasma concentration of catecholamines in CRPS-affected limbs, the discordant skin temperature with the activity of sympathetic vasoconstrictor neurons, and the fact that most patients do not obtain significant or lasting relief from sympathetic blocks.

There is no conclusive evidence in neuroimaging research to suggest there is a distinct "pain network" in the brain associated with neuropathic pain or a consistent brain activation pattern associated with the findings of CRPS. There are, however, several neuroimaging studies in patients with CRPS that suggest at least one consistent and specific brain alteration is associated with the condition: a reorganization of somatotopic maps.[23] Specifically, there is a reduction in size of the representation of the CRPS-affected limb in the lower somatosensory cortex, compared with the unaffected side. Consistent objective findings of patients with CRPS exhibiting signs of reorganization are impaired 2-point tactile discrimination and impaired ability to localize tactile stimuli, including preceding sensation outside of the nerve distribution port stimulated.

SHOULDER ANATOMY AND BIOMECHANICAL CONCERNS

The anatomy and biomechanics of the shoulder place nerves at particular risk for irritation and injury. The shoulder anatomy consists of a series of 4 joints and a total of 26 muscles that connect the axial skeleton to the humerus. In contrast to the hip joint, which has greater surface area coverage of the femoral head and where gravity provides a stabilizing force, the shallow glenoid has to suspend the weight of the upper extremity against the deforming force of gravity. With chronic shoulder disorders, the weak periscapular muscles result in a forward and inferior displacement of the glenohumeral joint, placing a sustained distraction force on the neighboring nerves. The close proximity of peripheral nerves around the shoulder increases their risk for irritation and injury. Movement of the arm during patient positioning and intraoperatively during repair places the nerves at risk for damage by traction or compression by the neighboring bones, rotator cuff, and periscapular musculature. The nerve supply to the upper limb is derived from the ventral rami of cranial nerves V, VI, VII, and VIII and a portion of the ventral ramus of the thoracic nerve. These rami unite to form the brachial plexus, which is further organized into trunks, divisions, and cords. It lays immediately medial and inferior to the glenohumeral joint, placing its branches at particular risk of injury from traction to penetration. Each cord ends in a terminal branch located at the inferior border of the pectoralis major muscle. The brachial plexus has 2 rigid points of fixation: the transverse process by the prevertebral fascia and in the arm by the axillary fascia. A traction injury (neurapraxia) can result from anything that increases the distance between these fixed points beyond their tolerance.[24] The plexus is also in close proximity to many freely mobile bony structures such as the clavicle and humeral head, rendering it susceptible to injury from malpositioning. The course of the suprascapular nerve around the scapula places it at particular risk to injury. As the nerve courses under the suprascapular ligament (separating from the artery), it is restricted in motion and vulnerable to traction or compression at the extremes of shoulder motion. The axillary nerve is vulnerable at a number of locations; it is superficial at the inferior aspect of the glenoid rim and as it courses around the proximal humerus through the quadrangular space, and its cutaneous branch emerges at the lateral deltoid. Complications can also occur secondary to patient positioning during arthroscopy. The lateral decubitus position has the advantage of joint distraction, which allows easier access to the inferior aspect of the glenoid during joint arthroscopy. This position distracts the arm placing a stretch on the underlying nerves. Traction neurapraxia has been reported to occur in up to 10%.[25] The beach chair position described in 1988 by Skyhar et al[19] has the advantage of easier airway access placing the patient in the standard upright position. While the risk of traction neurapraxia is decreased, more catastrophic complications have been reported, including stroke, vision loss, and ophthalmoplegia. These complications are thought to be attributable to variations in blood pressure reference points leading to decreased cerebral perfusion.

Numerous studies have evaluated the proximities of portal placement and suture anchors to neighboring nerves and recommendations for safe zones to avoid injury.[27,28] The posterior portal position approximately 2 cm inferior and 1 cm medial to the posterior lateral tip of the acromion increases the risk of injuring the axillary and suprascapular nerves. The anterior portal is lateral to the tip of the coracoid process and inferior to the anterolateral corner of the acromion, placing the musculocutaneous nerve at greatest risk for injury. The axillary nerve, which emerges cutaneously through the deltoid muscle 5 cm distal to the lateral acromion, is at the greatest risk with lateral portal placement. Superior portal placement exposes the suprascapular nerve, risking injury. Of the different shoulder surgical procedures, those performed for anterior instability are at the greatest risk for nerve injury.

CONTRIBUTING FACTORS

In addition to the anatomic factors, comorbidities and iatrogenic factors contribute to the increased likelihood of postoperative neurologic complications. Chronic cervical spine disorders may go unnoticed preoperatively as many develop insidiously, allowing the body the adapt, remaining asymptomatic. Neck and shoulder pain are common complaints in the primary care setting, with up to 30% to 50% of adults in the general population experiencing neck pain at least once per year.[29] Some cervical spine disorders may present to the patient as shoulder pain. Irritation of the C4 and C5 nerve roots can refer to pain in the dermatomal distribution that covers the shoulder and outer part of the upper arm. Thus, the resulting pain can present in the sensory distribution that the nerve serves, and a person does not have to experience neck pain for the problem to be emanating from the cervical spine. While this is not the same pain experienced in CRPS, it can sensitize the nerve, heightening its risk to injury, from even minor injury intraoperatively. A medical history of a stroke or seizure disorder increases risk for CRPS I. It is known to occur in the affected limbs of stroke patients in the recovery phase.

Diabetes mellitus is considered highly related to CRPS occurrence. Poorly controlled diabetes over a long period of time increases the risk for diabetic neuropathy. A retrospective study of 200 participants (108 diagnosed with CRPS; 92 diagnosed with non-CRPS) on the correlation between hemoglobin A1C level found a statistically significant increasing prevalence of CRPS with elevated hemoglobin A1C levels.[30] It is hypothesized that these elevated levels reflect increasing hyperglycemia through which proinflammatory cytokines and acute phase rectum proteins are elevated, which results in increased neuroinflammatory reactions leading to CRPS.

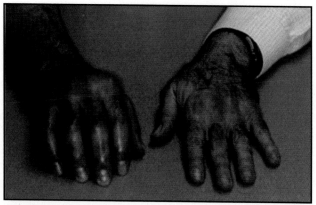

Figure 9-2. Clinical photograph demonstrating characteristic trophic changes and autonomic dysfunction in a right hand with CRPS. The contralateral hand is asymptomatic and is shown for comparison. (Reproduced with permission from Astifidis R. *Hand and Upper Extremity Rehabilitation*. Elsevier; 2016:151–158.)

Other comorbidities to consider are those that result in alteration in intraneural conductivity, thus increasing the risk of postoperative neuralgia. Vitamin B_{12} deficiency and pernicious anemia affect the dorsal root ganglion. Infectious diseases such as syphilis and HIV/AIDS can lead to neuropathy. Unlike peripheral neuropathy, which presents in a dermatomal distribution, they have a stocking glove appearance and can mimic CRPS.

CLINICAL PRESENTATION

In the acute phase, the injured limb is usually extremely painful, red, warm (although sometimes it quickly becomes relatively cold), and swollen (Figure 9-2). Other features, also confined to the injured limb but not confined to the distribution of a specific nerve or nerve root, include allodynia (in which usually nonpainful stimuli evoke pain) and hyperalgesia (in which painful stimuli evoke more intense pain than usual), changes in sweating, changes in hair and nail growth, and muscle weakness. Especially mechanical and thermal hyperalgesia are frequently present in CRPS. As the condition persists, pain does not subside but often spreads. Voluntary motor control can become impaired, and hyperpathia can develop, as well as negative sensory signs (hypoesthesia, hypoalgesia, hypothermesthesia). Thus, CRPS seems to be characterized by a mixture of noxious sensations ("positive symptoms") and sensory loss ("negative symptoms"). Over months, the relatively warm limb often becomes relatively cold. Dystonia, tremors, and myoclonus may also develop. Activity of the limb typically exacerbates the signs and symptoms. Over time, clinical features spread proximally (but not distally) and can even emerge on the opposite limb or the ipsilateral limb.

In chronic cases with longer disease durations (more than 5 years), other features are sometimes noted, such as urologic symptoms, syncope, and even mild cognitive deficits, although the latter probably is not specific for CRPS. Limb signs (such as swelling/sweating and color/temperature changes) usually reduce with time, even where pain and motor symptoms persist. However, such reduction of limb signs is in itself not necessarily considered a recovery. Where pain persists, the condition is considered active. However, without limb signs, a diagnosis of CRPS according to the Budapest Criteria can sometimes not be made.

DIAGNOSIS AND DIAGNOSTIC TOOLS

CRPS is a clinical diagnosis based on the patient's symptoms and signs elicited on physical examination. A thorough history and physical examination are instrumental in directing treatment by eliminating similar conditions on a differential diagnosis. Tests can be useful adjuncts, playing a supportive role in the diagnosis, primarily by ruling out of other differentials. Plain radiographs are an invaluable first tool in the diagnostic evaluation of CRPS. After shoulder arthroscopy, verifying anatomic alignment and eliminating the presence of a fracture or an infectious process are paramount as those abnormalities are high on the differential diagnoses. Radiographic characteristics of CRPS may be demonstrated relative to osteopenia and osteopathic changes in chronic and more severe cases. Bone scans and bone density scans may reveal earlier osteoporotic changes than plain film. In early postfracture CRPS, 3-phase bone scintigraphy has a higher sensitivity (97% vs 73%) and specificity (86% vs 57%) when compared to radiographs.[31] Its greatest value may be in differentiating CRPS from other pain syndromes in the first year. Similarly, magnetic resonance imaging (MRI) indicative of CRPS will reveal patchy areas of increased signal intensity (bone bruises) on T2-weighted imaging. Nerve conduction studies are diagnostic tests to consider, but their greatest utility may be in ruling out other neurologic conditions. Their limitation is that they only test large (fast-conducting) myelinated fibers in mixed peripheral nerves, which can reveal peripheral neuropathy. They do not test pain transmitting small A and C fibers, implicated in painful, small-fiber neuropathy. Nerve conduction studies and electromyography are normal in CRPS I but may be abnormal in CRPS II, reflecting the nerve damage that is associated with CRPS II. Punch skin biopsies are a useful tool; however, they are limited, revealing cutaneous sensory neuropathies and small-fiber and inheritable neuropathies but no findings that are specifically diagnostic to CRPS. Quantitative sensory testing in the assessment of CRPS is still primarily a research tool rather than a diagnostic clinical test. Thermography (digital thermal imaging) is a test that uses an infrared camera to detect heat patterns and blood flow and body tissues, and it is helpful in diagnosing the chronicity of the syndrome. Controversy remains concerning the efficacy of sympathetic blocks for diagnosis CRPS. A positive response is unpredictable but indicates sympathetically maintained pain, while an ineffective block suggests that the pain is sympathetically independent but does not rule out the diagnosis of CRPS.

MANAGEMENT

Early recognition of CRPS is paramount in resolving the condition and preserving the intended corrections made during the surgery. Implicit in the definition of CRPS is that the symptoms have been present for an extended period of time. This places the physician at a disadvantage, often playing catchup to mitigate the acute symptoms and addressing the underlying condition to prevent further deterioration, often complicating the success of the underlying surgical procedure. Identifying and treating all the protruding factors are important in resolving the symptoms. The goals of treatment for CRPS should be pain relief, functional restoration, and psychological stabilization.[32] Corradini et al[33] proposed a guideline for recognizing and treating CRPS in an orthopedic setting.

Physiotherapy

Physical and occupational therapy encompass a large swathe of various treatment modalities. The focus is in addressing the underlying pathology in the extremities and in the higher-functioning brain centers. Both have demonstrated efficacy in treating CRPS in patients exhibiting symptoms in less than a year. Therapeutic exercises include isometric strengthening exercises followed by active isotonic training in combination with sensory desensitization programs. Such programs involve the application of stimuli from different fabrics at varying pressures, including vibration, tapping, heat, or cold. With mirror therapy, a box has one mirror in the center, and on each side, the hands are placed in a manner that the affected limb is covered at all times and the unaffected limb is on the other side whose reflection can be seen on the mirror. The concept is using the mirror to create a reflective illusion of the unaffected arm in order to trick the brain into

TABLE 9-1. PHARMACOTHERAPEUTICS

MEDICATION	MECHANISM OF ACTION
Corticosteroids	Intracellular modulation of gene expression (anti-inflammatory)
Nonsteroidal anti-inflammatories	Cyclooxygenase inhibitor (anti-inflammatory)
Anticonvulsants	Suppresses pathologic electrical charges in central nervous system and peripheral nervous system
Antidepressants	Serotonin receptor inhibition
Calcium channel blockers	Smooth muscle relaxation; vasodilation
α-blockers	Sympathetic tone reduction
β-blockers	Vasodilation (peripheral); serotonin antagonist (central)
Bisphosphonates	Inhibits bone resorption

thinking movement has occurred in the affected limb without pain. Recent success has been found with the use of graded motor imagery (GMI). The 3 stages of GMI involve left/right discrimination, explicit motor imagery, and mirror therapy. Literature analyzing and comparing the data regarding the effectiveness of different physical therapy treatments concluded that GMI provided the greatest benefit in terms of pain reduction.

Other treatment modalities include whirlpool, acupuncture, ultrasound therapy, and kinesiotherapy.

Pharmacotherapy

There is no single medication to successfully treat CRPS; rather, they are useful adjuncts that hold their own side effects if not used appropriately (Table 9-1). Oral and topical medications have been useful in mitigating the acute symptoms as well as assisting in resolving the underlying condition. Intravenous regional anesthesia has demonstrated some efficacy with certain medications. In uncontrolled trials, calcium channel blocking agents such as nifedipine have been associated with pain reduction and improvement of the sympathetic dysfunction.

Nonsteroidal anti-inflammatory medications have been helpful in addressing mild cases of CRPS. The mechanism of action is to inhibit the enzyme cyclooxygenase, thereby reducing the release of prostaglandins. They likely are more helpful in addressing the symptoms of inflammation from the healing process of the given surgical procedure than of CRPS. Patients who are allergic to nonsteroidal anti-inflammatories or who have a history of gastroesophageal reflux disease or peptic ulcers, gastric bypass surgery, or chronic renal disease are not candidates.

Corticosteroids are particularly beneficial in the early stages of the disease. The anti-inflammatory effect is most pronounced when a clinical sign of redness, warmth, and swelling is present. A trial of short-acting oral corticosteroids after early onset can be highly efficacious in some instances, resulting in complete relief of the syndrome. Its repeated or continued use should be balanced against its potentially harmful effects and its contribution to osteopenia. The efficacy of chronic use of glucocorticoids in the treatment of CRPS is unproven, and there are numerous contraindications to their use.[34]

Controversy surrounds the use of opioid medications and treatment of CRPS. They can be helpful in addressing acute pain, but they are highly addictive, and their chronic use can lead to development of drug tolerance and opioid dependence. Opioids function on G protein–coupled receptors, which are not the primary culprit in CRPS, so they would have a mitigating affected best. A systematic review and medical analysis published in the *Lancet* emphasizes that the use of opioids for neuropathic pain is a reasonable second- or third-line treatment option to try, but tolerance and long-term toxicity of these agents remain unresolved issues, and long-term high-dose opioids might even worsen allodynia or hyperpathia.[35] As both mood disorders and chronic pain have interconnecting neurochemicals pathways, it has been hypothesized that some pharmacologic agents used to treat depression, such as tricyclic antidepressants and selective serotonin reuptake inhibitors, may have utility in treating neuropathic pain in CRPS.[36] Their mechanism of action is through blocking the outflow receptors that inhibit the presynaptic release of norepinephrine. While there are no clinical trials demonstrating efficacy in the treatment of the disease, they often provide the relief of burning pain and can help to ameliorate sleep disturbances (amitriptyline). The loading dose is generally less than the prescribed dose for depression, and the usual onset of action is within 2 to 3 weeks of the initial dose.

Anticonvulsants such as gabapentin and pregabalin interact with neuronal L-type calcium channels, reducing neurotransmitter release. Both medications are often used in the orthopedic setting for treating neuropathies, but in clinical trials, they have reliably demonstrated efficacy in treating the pain of trigeminal neuralgia, and little evidence exists to recommend their use for other neuropathic conditions.[37] The major advantages of gabapentin include the absence of significant drug interactions and the more tolerated side effect profile compared with antidepressants.[38]

Recently, bisphosphonates have been studied for the treatment of CRPS. They are potent inhibitors of osteoclast activity and have been used widely in the management of osteoporosis and other metabolic bone disease states. Several studies have demonstrated the efficacy of these medications compared to placebo in the treatment of CRPS. Oral or intravenous bisphosphonates have reduced pain and improved physical function with a good safety profile and tolerability.[39] While the patchy osteoporosis seen in CRPS is the result of osteoclast activity, its role in this condition is not well understood. A proposed secondary action could be the interference with inflammatory and nociceptive pathways in CRPS. It has been postulated that bisphosphonates could interfere with macrophage activation and may activate nociceptive acid-sensing receptors and the release of proinflammatory cytokines. In a randomized control trial on a population of 82 patients with CRPS I, the authors reported a significant decrease in visual analog scale score and other indices of pain and quality of life, and patients received 100-mg intravenous doses of neridronate vs placebo.[40]

Other treatment medications and modalities have included vitamin C and antihypertensives including α-blockers, β-blockers, and calcium channel blockers. A randomized, double-blind, placebo-controlled trial of vitamin C to prevent CRPS after wrist fractures was published. The authors demonstrated a statistically significant difference ($P = .03$) in the rate of development of CRPS in the vitamin C group vs the placebo group. The authors speculated there was likely a protective effect of vitamin C through its antioxidant properties.[41] Topically, clonidine, an α2 receptor agonist that inhibits the presynaptic release of norepinephrine, has been shown to reduce hyperalgesia. It has also been administered orally and by epidural injection in patients with CRPS with some efficacy.[42]

Interventional Techniques

When conservative measures fail, the next step usually involves interventional measures. Paravertebral sympathetic chain ganglion blockade techniques have been useful in both the diagnosis of CRPS and as a treatment modality. The goal of spinal cord stimulation in CRPS includes pain reduction, reversing muscle dysfunction, and improving blood circulation. Neuromodulation techniques including peripheral nerve stimulation and spinal cord stimulation are believed to work by 2 theories. In the gate control theory, stimulating large myelinated nerve fibers blocks transmission of the smaller pain nerve fibers. Another theory suggests that pain reduction is achieved because nerve stimulation promotes the release of endogenous opioids. Pain reduction and improved functional mobility after a block are considered a positive response, particularly when used in conjunction with physical and occupational therapy. Constant blockade through spinal cord stimulation consists of stimulating the dorsal columns of the spinal cord electrodes placed in the epidural space. Physical therapy is a necessary adjunct, and optimal dosage allows sensory and sympathetic blockade while permitting motor function, facilitating rehabilitation. Use in the upper extremity requires a stellate ganglion blockade that can produce Horner syndrome as a side effect. Other adverse effects of nerve blockade are decubitus ulcers, urinary retention, deep venous thrombosis, and permanent motor impairment. While controlled trials have demonstrated better results than placebo injections, there is a dearth of current literature supporting sympathetic blocks and sympathectomy techniques, and there are no practical guidelines regarding drug selection.

Surgical sympathectomy has been used in treating chronic unrelenting cases and has been met with mixed results. It is considered only when regional sympathetic blockade provides relief, but the effects are temporary. In addition to open surgical removal, ablation of the sympathetic chain and ganglia may be accomplished through percutaneous chemical ablation, radiofrequency percutaneous sympathectomy, and endoscopic sympathectomy. Relief after sympathectomy can be dramatic but incomplete, with many symptoms recurring within 2 to 5 years. There are a number of explanations as to why the effects are short-lived, and they usually include incomplete surgical removal of all sympathetic innervation to the extremity or secondary to collateral reinnervation from the contralateral ganglion. Contralateral sympathectomy, which is an option, carries the risk of interrupting sympathetic outflow to needed tissues, negatively affecting bowel and bladder function as well as causing sexual dysfunction.[43]

CASE PRESENTATION

History and Presentation

A 54-year-old woman with a medical history significant for a seizure disorder and depression presented with an insidious onset of a painful, stiff right shoulder. A nurse by profession, she found it increasingly difficult to carry out her work duties. Her clinical examination was suggestive of adhesive capsulitis and shoulder impingement. Initial attempts were made at conservative treatment, including a cortisone injection and physical therapy. Those measures failed, and an MRI was ordered, which revealed a torn supraspinatus tendon with minimal retraction. At this point, the decision was made to proceed with shoulder arthroscopy.

Surgery and Postoperative Course

Induction of anesthesia was performed, including both an interscalene block for regional analgesia and general endotracheal intubation. She was situated in a beach chair position (the senior author's preferred method). A full-thickness supraspinatus tendon tear with minimal retraction was confirmed and repaired with 2 suture anchors in a single-row fashion. The procedure was uncomplicated and lasted 70 minutes. She was discharged home in stable condition. The postoperative course initially was uneventful with good pain control and tolerating rehabilitation. A month later, she returned to the office for an urgent visit. Clearly in pain, she held her right arm by her side in a guarded position. The pain was of greater intensity and different characteristic from her preoperative level. The incision sites had healed nicely, with no signs of infection or acute trauma. The right upper extremity was notably cooler than the contralateral extremity, but there was no skin mottling. The was increasing elbow stiffness and allodynia of the proximal lateral forearm. She noted stiffness in her fingers and weakened grip strength. An MRI revealed patchy increased signal intensity in the proximal humerus and glenoid but with an intact rotator cuff repair. There were no abnormal laboratory values. She completed a short course of oral steroids, which reduced her pain by half, but it shortly returned to baseline once the course was completed. In consultation with her neurologist, a presumptive diagnosis of CRPS was made. She was referred to a pain management specialist who performed a stellate ganglia block. The patient's response was immediate and impressive, with an admitted 70% pain reduction. The discomfort that remained was centered on her shoulder. Five months from the onset of her postoperative symptoms, her pain improved to the point where she felt she could return to physical therapy. Over the next 7 months, her arm and elbow pain resolved, and her finger range of motion and grip strength improved. By 6 weeks, she was back to work full duty. She had no complaints of pain, mostly discomfort with prolonged used, for which she would on occasion treat with ibuprofen. Her last follow-up appointment was at 15 months, with her range of motion and strength nearly fully restored.

CONCLUSION

The diagnosis of CRPS after shoulder arthroscopy, while not common, it is a known complication that, if not diagnosed and treated early, can have an adverse and long-lasting effect on an elective procedure. Best practices dictate identifying patients who represent a particular at-risk group and initiating proactive treatment plan. Metha and Lindenfeld[44] designed an algorithm for the decision-making process once clinical suspicion has risen. A detailed history would include any prior trauma or surgical procedures to the shoulder, a thorough history of all comorbidities, and particular examination of the cervical spine. Underlying psychogenic factors can affect the intensity and duration of CRPS; therefore, it would be prudent to perform a thorough preoperative evaluation replete with an appropriate pain patient profile assessment. One a patient is deemed at increased risk for CRPS, a proactive preoperative treatment plan can minimize the risk. This plan should be comprehensive, and communication with the primary care physician is paramount, who, in addition to recognizing a patient at risk, is tailoring an individual treatment plan relative to the patient's medical history. This could save time and mitigate risk in choosing a treatment ineffective at best and possibly detrimental. Anesthesiology plays a pivotal role in determining the most appropriate induction method and perioperative medications to administer. It is crucial to involve physical therapy in the discussions regarding the timing of postoperative rehabilitation program and appropriate treatment modalities.

In addition to a preoperative risk assessment, it is critical to recognize the early warning signs postoperatively and the ability to intervene promptly. Implicit in its name is that the neuroinflammatory process is chronic, in which an actual diagnosis is not confirmed for several months. The inherent conflict in waiting to act until a definitive diagnosis is made is that significant damage to the system has already occurred, and your treatment options are therefore limited. The difference between early action to thwart the process and a protracted recovery with a suboptimal outcome is contingent upon having a high index of suspicion, recognizing warning signs and intervening swiftly. The future directions in diagnosing and treating CRPS after shoulder arthroscopy will undoubtably be shaped by advances in technology. The same genetic mapping technique that can identify regions responsible for eye color and personality traits will identify regions responsible for interpreting pain. This technology, coupled with an ever-growing intricate electronic health system, has the potential to assist in risk assessment, timely diagnosis, and prompt or even prophylactic intervention.

The selected case study is illustrative of the challenge presented in recognizing CRPS after shoulder arthroscopy. The patient's symptoms were not apparent immediately after surgery, and manifestation of her symptoms presented a month postoperatively, when progressing from one exercise routine to the next. This should reinforce the need to stay vigilant for weeks and even months postoperatively. Equally important is recognizing that CRPS does not have to be the sole diagnosis. In this instance, there was also an element of adhesive capsulitis remaining once her neuropathic symptoms resolved. It is prudent when treating CRPS to begin with the least invasive measures (medications, physical therapy), then advance to more invasive measures (nerve blocks) given the response. It is critical to know when to intervene with more proactive measures to thwart a protracted CRPS course to prevent intransigent symptoms. The case also highlights the importance of preoperative risk assessment and in collaborating with colleagues to formulate a treatment plan. Given the patient's medical history of an underlying seizure disorder and treatment for depression, she fell into the higher risk category. Collaborating preoperatively with her neurologist and physical therapist, a preventative plan might have been established reducing the risk of CRPS. It is also reassuring that given an early and accurate diagnosis followed by appropriate treatment in a timely manner, complete resolution of CRPS after shoulder surgery is possible.

REFERENCES

1. Bhaskar SA, Manjuladevi M. Shoulder arthroscopy and complications: can we afford to relax? *Indian J Anesthesiol.* 2015;59(6):335–337.
2. Rodeo SA, Foster RA, Weiland AJ. Neurological complications due to arthroscopy. *J Bone Joint Surg Am.* 1993;6:917–926.
3. de Mos M, de Bruijn AG, Huygen FJ, Dieleman JP, Dtricker BH, Sturkenboom MC. The incidence of complex regional pain syndrome: a population-based study. *Pain.* 2007;129(1–2):12–20.
4. Iolascon G, de Sire A, Morietti A, Gimigliano F. Complex regional pain syndrome (CRPS) type I: historical perspective and critical issues. *Clin Cases Miner Bone Metab.* 2015;12(suppl 1):4–10.
5. Amadio PC. Pain dysfunction syndromes. *J Bone Joint Surg Am.* 1988;70:944–949.
6. Merskey H, Bogduk N. *Classification of Chronic Pain: Descriptions of Chronic Pain Syndromes and Descriptions of Pain in Terms.* 2nd ed. IASP Press; 1994.
7. Stanton-Hicks M, Janig W, Hassenbusch S, Haddox JD, Boas R, Wilson P. Reflex sympathetic dystrophy: changing concepts and taxonomy. *Pain.* 1995;63(1):127–133.
8. Harden RN, Bruehl S, Stanton-Hicks M, Wilson PR. Proposed new diagnostic criteria for complex regional pain syndrome. *Pain Med.* 2007;6(4):326–331.
9. Schlereth T, Drummond P, Birklein F. Inflammation in CRPS: role of the sympathetic supply. *Autonomic Neurosci.* 2014;182:102–107.

10. Marinus J, Moseley GL, Birklein F, et al. Clinical features and pathophysiology of complex regional pain syndrome: current state of the art. *Lancet Neurol.* 2011;10(7):637–648.

11. Nunez FA, Papadonikolakis A, Liz A. Arthroscopic release of adhesive capsulitis of the shoulder complicated with shoulder dislocation and brachial plexus injury. *J Surg Orthop Adv.* 2016;25(2):114–116.

12. Bruno M, Lavanga V, Maiorano E, Sansone V. A bizarre complication of shoulder arthroscopy. *Knee Surg Sports Traumatol Arthrosc.* 2015;23(5):1426–1428.

13. Matthews LS, Zarins B, Michael RH, Helfet DL. Anterior portal selection for shoulder arthroscopy. *Arthroscopy.* 1985;1:33–39.

14. Stanish WD, Peterson DC. Shoulder arthroscopy and nerve injury: pitfalls and prevention. *Arthroscopy.* 1995;11(4):458–466.

15. Small NC. Complications in arthroscopic surgery performed by experienced arthroscopists. *Arthroscopy.* 1988;4(3):215–221.

16. Martel M, Laumonerie P, Pecourneau V, Ancelin D, Mansat P, Bonnevialle N. Type I complex regional pain syndrome after subacromial surgery: incidence and risk factor analysis. *Indian J Orthop.* 2020;54(suppl 1):210–215.

17. Quisel A, Gill JM, Witherell P. Complex regional pain syndrome underdiagnosed. *J Fam Pract.* 2005;54(6):524–532.

18. Stoler JM, Oaklander AL. Patients with Ehlers Danlos syndrome and CRPS: a possible association? *Pain.* 2006;123(1–2):204–209.

19. Skyhar MJ, Altchek DW, Warren RF, Wickiewicz TL, O'Brien SJ. Shoulder arthroscopy with the patient in the beach-chair position. *Arthroscopy.* 1988;4:256–259.

20. Pitman MI, Nainzadeh N, Ergas E, Springer S. The use of somatosensory evoked potentials for detection of neuropraxia during shoulder arthroscopy. *Arthroscopy.* 1988;4:250–255.

21. Andrews JR, Carson WG. Arthroscopic surgery of the shoulder. In: Parisien JS, ed. *Arthroscopic Surgery.* New York, NY: McGraw-Hill; 1988:23.

22. Goh EL, Chidambaram S, Ma D. Complex regional pain syndrome: a recent update. *Burns Trauma.* 2017;5:2.

23. Kuttikat A, Noreika V, Shenker N, Chennu S, Bekinschtein T, Brown CA. Neurocognitive and neuroplastic mechanisms of novel clinical signs in CRPS. *Front Hum Neurosci.* 2016;10:16.

24. Clausen EG. Postoperative ("anesthetic") paralysis of the brachial plexus. *Surgery.* 1942;12:933–942.

25. Pitman MI, Nainzedeh N, Ergas E, et al. The use of somatosensory evoked potentials for detection of neurophraxia during shoulder arthroscopy. *Arthroscopy.* 1988;4:250–255.

26. Noud PH, Esch J. Complications of arthroscopic shoulder surgery. *Sports Med Arthrosc Rev.* 2013;21(2):89–96.

27. Stanish W, Peterson DC. Shoulder arthroscopy and nerve injury: pitfalls and prevention. *Arthroscopy.* 1995;11(4):458–466.

28. Scully WF, Wilson DJ, Parada SA, Arrington ED. Iatrogenic nerve injuries in shoulder surgery. *J Am Acad Orthop Surg.* 2013;21(12):717–726.

29. Hogg-Johnson S, Velde G, Carroll LJ, et al. The burden and determinants of neck pain in the general population: results of the Bone and Joint Decade 2000–2010 Task Force on Neck Pain and Its Associated Disorders. *Spine.* 2008;33(suppl):39–51.

30. Choi JH, Yu KP, Yoon YS, Kim ES, Jeon JH. Relationship between HbA1c and complex regional pain syndrome in stroke patients with type 2 diabetes mellitus. *Ann Rehabil Med.* 2016;40(5):779–785.

31. Todorovic-Tirnanic M, Obradovic V, Han R, Goldner B, Stankovic D, Sekulic D. diagnostic approach to reflex sympathetic dystrophy after fracture: radiography or bone scintigraphy? *Eur J Nucl Med*. 1995;22(10):1187–1193.
32. Resmini G, Ratti C, Canton C, Murena L, Moretti, Lolascon G. Treatment of complex regional pain syndrome. *Clin Cases Miner Bone Metab*. 2015;12:26–30.
33. Corradini C, Bosizio C, Moretti A. Algodystrophy (CRPS) in minor orthopedic surgery. *Clin Cases Miner Bone Metab*. 2015;12(suppl 1):22–25.
34. Harden RN, Oaklander AL, Burton AW, et al. Complex regional pain syndrome: practical diagnostic and treatment guidelines 4th ed. *Pain Med*. 2013;14:180–229.
35. Finnerup NB, Attal N, Haroutounian S, et al. Pharmacotherapy for neuropathic pain in adults: a systematic review and medical analysis. *Lancet Neurol*. 2015;14(2):162–173.
36. Baltenberger EP, Buterbaugh WM, Martin BS, et al. Review of antidepressants in the treatment of neuropathic pain. *Mental Health Clinician*. 2015;5(3):123–133.
37. Van de Vusse AC, Stomp-van den Berg SG, Kessels AH, et al. Randomized control trial of gabapentin and complex regional pain syndrome type I. *BMC Neurol*. 2004;4:13.
38. Mellick GA, Mellick LB. Reflex sympathetic dystrophy treated with gabapentin. *Arch Phys Med Rehabil*. 1997;78:98–105.
39. Breuer B, Pappagallo M, Ongseng F, et al. An open-label pilot trial of ibandronate for complex regional pain syndrome. *Clin J Pain*. 2008;24:685–689.
40. Varenna M, Adami S, Rossini M, et al. Treatment of complex regional pain syndrome type I with neridronate: a randomized, double-blind, placebo controlled study. *Rheumatology (Oxford)*. 2013;52(3):534–542.
41. Amadio PC. Vitamin C reduced the incidence of RSD after wrist fracture. *J Bone Joint Surg Am*. 2000;82:873.
42. Davis KD, Treede RD, Raja SN, et al. Topical application of clonidine releases hyperalgesia in patients was sympathetically maintained pain. *Pain*. 1991;47:309–317.
43. Freedman M, Greis AC, Marino L, et al. Complex regional pain syndrome: diagnosis and treatment. *Phys Med Rehabil Clin North Am*. 2014;25:291–303.
44. Metha SH, Lindenfeld TN. Complex regional pain syndromes including reflex sympathetic dystrophy and causalgia. In: *DeeLee & Drez's Orthopaedic Sports Medicine Principles and Practice*. 2nd ed. Elsevier; 2003:441–457.

10

Postarthroscopic Glenohumeral Chondrolysis

Thomas X. Nguyen, MD; Abbas Naqvi, MD;
and Terry L. Thompson, MD

INTRODUCTION

Postarthroscopic glenohumeral chondrolysis (PAGHCL) is a rapid, destructive process of the articular cartilage, typically occurring within 12 months of a shoulder arthroscopic procedure. Chondrolysis occurs when chondrocytes lose the ability to maintain and produce cartilage matrix. It also occurs as a result of apoptosis. PAGHCL is distinguished from the more common glenohumeral osteoarthritis by its temporal relationship with an arthroscopic procedure.[1] The diagnosis is confirmed via a shoulder radiograph demonstrating a loss of normal glenohumeral joint space. The etiology can be divided into 3 broad categories as described by Solomon et al[2]: patient, surgical, and postoperative factors. Knowledge of the potential inciting causes is essential to avoid this devastating complication.

Thompson TL, ed.
Arthroscopic Shoulder Surgery:
Complications and Management (pp 153-160).
© 2022 Taylor & Francis Group.

EPIDEMIOLOGY

PAGHCL is rare. Most published reports describe a small number of cases,[3,4] but there are larger series.[5,6] Bailie and Ellenbecker[5] reported a series of 28 cases of PAGHCL. All patients had received an intra-articular bolus injection of 0.25% bupivacaine with epinephrine. Wiater et al[6] analyzed 375 shoulder cases in a single practice. Forty-nine of the cases were complicated by chondrolysis, all of which were associated with intra-articular infusion of a local anesthetic. Solomon et al[2] performed a systematic review to identify causative factors of chondrolysis. Most patients were male, and the mean age was 27.9 years. The most frequent preoperative diagnoses were instability and superior labrum anterior to posterior (SLAP) lesions. The inciting factors were thermal, chemical, and mechanical. There are no well-designed epidemiologic studies that examine PAGHCL.

ETIOLOGY

Patient Factors

Patient factors that contribute to chondrolysis include a history of collagen disorders and/or processes affecting the synovium and/or synovial fluid. These factors could potentially affect chondrocytes and increase risk for chondrolysis.[2] Previous traumatic shoulder injuries, such as dislocations, may increase the susceptibility of articular cartilage to intraoperative injury.[7] Single and repetitive traumatic events may also cause chondrolysis.[8] Additionally, an increased time interval between injury and surgical intervention has been shown to increase the risk for postoperative chondrolysis.[7,9] Instability (32%) and SLAP lesions (23%) were the most frequent surgical diagnoses associated with surgical procedures that resulted in postoperative chondrolysis.[2]

Surgical Factors

Surgical techniques, implants, and irrigating solutions can also cause harm to the articular cartilage. Inadvertent trocar trajectory can result in iatrogenic cartilaginous injury.[5,10] The use of a radiofrequency device adjacent to articular cartilage has been attributed to a 45% incidence of chondrolysis.[2] In a case series, thermal capsulorrhaphy in shoulder arthroscopy caused 8 patients to develop glenohumeral chondrolysis.[4] In another case series, 7 of 23 patients developed chondrolysis at a mean of 9 months after being subjected to an arthroscopic thermal probe for capsular laxity.[5]

Bioabsorbable implants have also been reported to cause chondrolysis.[8] In one case series, 2 of 6 patients developed cartilage damage after SLAP repairs with poly-L-lactic acid bioabsorbable tacks.[11] In another case series, 14 of 23 patients developed chondrolysis at a mean of 9 months after labral repair with bioabsorbable devices (suture anchors and/or tacks).[5] In the same study, 5 of 14 had Bankart tears and 9 of 14 had SLAP tears.

In a basic science study, hypotonic irrigating solutions (distilled water) were found to potentially decrease chondrocyte viability with an established scalpel trauma to the articular cartilage. On the other hand, hypertonic irrigating solutions may have a protective effect.[12] The results of the study suggest that the osmolarity of irrigation solutions could be manipulated to reduce chondrocyte death resulting from mechanical injury during arthroscopic surgery.

Postoperative Factors

Local anesthetics have been studied as a possible cause of chondrocyte cell death. The use of postoperative pain pumps with constant infusion of local anesthetics is chondrotoxic. In a case series, 7 of 23 patients developed chondrolysis at a mean of 9 months after use of an intra-articular pain pump with 250 to 300 mL of 0.25% bupivacaine for 48 hours after arthroscopic surgery.[5] In another study, intra-articular pain pumps with bupivacaine 0.25% or 0.5% with or without epinephrine were the main factors contributing to 37 out of 40 patients developing chondrolysis.[13] The effect of epinephrine in combination with local anesthetics on chondrocyte viability is unclear.[14,15] Postoperatively, extensive periods of immobilization limiting cartilage nutrition via synovial diffusion may be detrimental to cartilage health. Inflammatory responses generated by absorbable sutures have been hypothesized to increase the susceptibility of articular cartilage to chondrolysis.[2] Postoperative infection can also lead to an inflammatory cascade that can cause permanent destruction of articular cartilage.[8]

PATHOPHYSIOLOGY

In a basic science in vitro study, Lo et al[16] cultured bovine articular disks in different concentrations of 0.25% bupivacaine, 1% lidocaine, and 0.5% ropivacaine (0%, 2.5%, 5%, 10%, 25%, 50%, 100%) with different time points (1 hour, 3 hours, 5 hours, 8 hours, 12 hours). They showed that chondrocyte cell death occurred with increasing concentrations and/or duration of these local anesthetics on fluorescence microscopy. Chondrocyte nuclear morphology and chromatin organization were also disrupted, as seen on transmission electron microscopy. At 5 hours, chondrocyte viability was less than 50% for all 3 types of anesthetics. Epinephrine alone did not cause cytotoxicity. However, when it was added to the 0.25% bupivacaine (1:200,000 epinephrine), there was an enhanced cytotoxicity effect. When epinephrine was added to lidocaine and ropivacaine, there was no added cytotoxicity. The authors cautioned against the use of high-dose, long-term intra-articular administration of local anesthetics.

Tissues are heated to 65°C or higher with radiofrequency probes during thermal capsulorrhaphy, chondroplasty, and tissue debridement. This subsequently increases the joint fluid temperature and can cause chondrocyte death. There is a decrease in cell viability at a minimum of 45°C.[17]

Dislodgement and fragmentation of bioabsorbable tacks into loose bodies can cause mechanical irritation and articular damage. However, it is not the bioabsorbability of the tacks that is causing the chondrolysis.[11] Proud suture anchors can cause abrasion of the articular cartilage during glenohumeral articulation and subsequent destruction.[10] In addition, knots on the articular surface can result in cartilaginous scuffing with glenohumeral articulation.[3,18]

SIGNS AND SYMPTOMS

Patients will experience loss of shoulder motion over time. The onset of pain may be delayed pain 8 to 12 months after shoulder arthroscopy. Some patients experience worsening pain usually in the evening and after activity. Others notice crepitus with range of motion, deteriorating function, and new mechanical symptoms after the index procedure. Constitutional symptoms are not present. The index procedure typically alleviates their pain, and they develop a new, different type of pain months later.[5]

DIAGNOSIS

Diagnosis can be made with serial radiographs demonstrating rapid, diffuse loss of glenohumeral joint cartilage, subchondral cysts, and erosions (Figure 10-1). Magnetic resonance imaging can be obtained to confirm diagnosis showing cartilage loss and subchondral cysts.[13] In addition, broken or dislodged tacks can be identified on magnetic resonance imaging.[11] A second-look shoulder arthroscopy can also confirm loss of articular cartilage (Figure 10-2). Arthrocentesis, white blood cell count, sedimentation rate, and C-reactive protein should be done to rule out infection, as the clinical presentation may be similar.

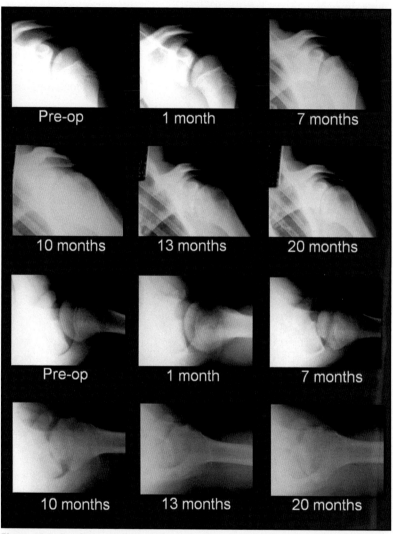

Figure 10-1. Serial true anteroposterior and axillary-lateral radiographs showing progression of chondrolysis over a 20-month period in a 16-year-old patient. (Reproduced with permission from Hasan SS, Fleckenstein CM. Glenohumeral chondrolysis: part I—clinical presentation and predictors of disease progression. *Arthroscopy.* 2013;29[7]:1135–1141.)

Figure 10-2. Arthroscopic photograph of a right shoulder viewed from the posterior portal. Significant chondrolysis of the humeral articular surface developed after an index arthroscopic shoulder procedure. This patient continued to have pronounced pain and disability after the index procedure, prompting reexploration. (Reproduced with permission from Noud PH, Esch J. Complications of arthroscopic shoulder surgery. *Sports Med Arthrosc Rev.* 2013;21[2]:89–96.)

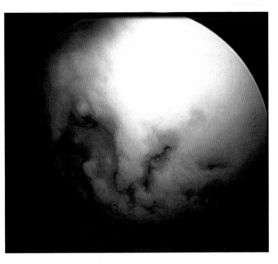

TREATMENT

Nonoperative

Nonoperative treatment can be performed with corticosteroid injections, nonsteroidal anti-inflammatory drugs, and physical therapy. However, all nonoperative treatments eventually fail.[5]

Operative

Arthroscopic debridement and/or capsular release followed by aggressive rehabilitation was successful in 14 of 23 patients, as reported by Bailie and Ellenbecker.[5] Arthroscopy can also be performed to remove tack fragments, evaluate superior labral healing, and repair SLAP lesions with suture anchors.[11] Shoulder arthroplasty may be the final option if all other treatments have been exhausted. After failure of conservative treatment, 9 of 23 patients underwent cementless humeral head resurfacing arthroplasty.[5] In a study by Hasan and Fleckenstein,[19] 27 of 40 patients (67.5%) eventually underwent shoulder arthroplasty (humeral head resurfacing, stemmed hemiarthroplasty, or total shoulder arthroplasty) after an index surgery to treat chondrolysis. The mean interval from the index surgery to arthroplasty was 32 months.

Prevention

Careful placement of trocars and arthroscopic instruments, preferably under direct visualization, is advised to prevent iatrogenic cartilaginous injury.[5,10] While using a radiofrequency probe in shoulder arthroscopy, the joint fluid temperature should be under the threshold of 45°C with the use of fluid pump flow rate of 50% to 100% rather than no flow.[17] The heat also disperses faster with higher flow rates vs no flow. Caution should also be taken with the placement of suture anchors and knots such that they do not result in cartilage scuffing during glenohumeral articulation.[5,10] Finally, do not use high-dose, long-term intra-articular administration of local anesthetics like those found in postoperative pain pumps.[16]

REFERENCES

1. Yeh PC, Kharrazi FD. Postarthroscopic glenohumeral chondrolysis. *J Am Acad Orthop Surg.* 2012;20(2):102–112.
2. Solomon DJ, Navaie M, Stedje-Larsen ET, Smith JC, Provencher MT. Glenohumeral chondrolysis after arthroscopy: a systematic review of potential contributors and causal pathways. *Arthroscopy.* 2009;25(11):1329–1342.
3. Athwal GS, Shridharani SM, O'Driscoll SW. Osteolysis and arthropathy of the shoulder after use of bioabsorbable knotless suture anchors: a report of four cases. *J Bone Joint Surg Am.* 2006;88(8):1840–1845.
4. Good CR, Shindle MK, Kelly BT, Wanich T, Warren RF. Glenohumeral chondrolysis after shoulder arthroscopy with thermal capsulorrhaphy. *Arthroscopy.* 2007;23(7):797.e1–797.e7975.
5. Bailie DS, Ellenbecker TS. Severe chondrolysis after shoulder arthroscopy: a case series. *J Shoulder Elbow Surg.* 2009;18(5):742–747.
6. Wiater BP, Neradilek MB, Polissar NL, Matsen FA III. Risk factors for chondrolysis of the glenohumeral joint: a study of three hundred and seventy-five shoulder arthroscopic procedures in the practice of an individual community surgeon. *J Bone Joint Surg Am.* 2011;93(7):615–625.
7. Buscayret F, Edwards TB, Szabo I, Adeleine P, Coudane H, Walch G. Glenohumeral arthrosis in anterior instability before and after surgical treatment: incidence and contributing factors. *Am J Sports Med.* 2004;32(5):1165–1172.
8. Noud PH, Esch J. Complications of arthroscopic shoulder surgery. *Sports Med Arthrosc Rev.* 2013;21(2):89–96.
9. Cameron ML, Kocher MS, Briggs KK, Horan MP, Hawkins RJ. The prevalence of glenohumeral osteoarthrosis in unstable shoulders. *Am J Sports Med.* 2003;31(1):53–55.
10. McNickle AG, L'Heureux DR, Provencher MT, Romeo AA, Cole BJ. Postsurgical glenohumeral arthritis in young adults. *Am J Sports Med.* 2009;37(9):1784–1791.
11. Sassmannshausen G, Sukay M, Mair SD. Broken or dislodged poly-L-lactic acid bioabsorbable tacks in patients after SLAP lesion surgery. *Arthroscopy.* 2006;22(6):615–619.
12. Amin AK, Huntley JS, Bush PG, Simpson AH, Hall AC. Osmolarity influences chondrocyte death in wounded articular cartilage. *J Bone Joint Surg Am.* 2008;90(7):1531–1542.

13. Hasan SS, Fleckenstein CM. Glenohumeral chondrolysis: part I—clinical presentation and predictors of disease progression. *Arthroscopy*. 2013;29(7):1135–1141.
14. Hashimoto K, Hampl KF, Nakamura Y, Bollen AW, Feiner J, Drasner K. Epinephrine increases the neurotoxic potential of intrathecally administered lidocaine in the rat. *Anesthesiology*. 2001;94(5):876–881.
15. Gomoll AH, Yanke AB, Kang RW, et al. Long-term effects of bupivacaine on cartilage in a rabbit shoulder model. *Am J Sports Med*. 2009;37(1):72–77.
16. Lo IK, Sciore P, Chung M, et al. Local anesthetics induce chondrocyte death in bovine articular cartilage disks in a dose- and duration-dependent manner. *Arthroscopy*. 2009;25(7):707–715.
17. Good CR, Shindle MK, Griffith MH, Wanich T, Warren RF. Effect of radiofrequency energy on glenohumeral fluid temperature during shoulder arthroscopy. *J Bone Joint Surg Am*. 2009;91(2):429–434.
18. Barber FA, Snyder SJ, Abrams JS, Fanelli GC, Savoie FH III. Arthroscopic Bankart reconstruction with a bioabsorbable anchor. *J Shoulder Elbow Surg*. 2003;12(6):535–538.
19. Hasan SS, Fleckenstein CM. Glenohumeral chondrolysis: part II—results of treatment. *Arthroscopy*. 2013;29(7):1142–1148.

11

Recurrent Anterior Instability After Arthroscopic Repair

James E. Carpenter, MD, MHSA

INTRODUCTION

Arthroscopic anterior labral repair and capsulorrhaphy (also know as arthroscopic Bankart repair) is the most commonly performed procedure for recurrent anterior instability of the shoulder. The procedure has been refined significantly over the past 30 years but continues to have a rate of failure from recurrent instability that is higher than open repairs. When recurrence of instability does occur, revision surgery is generally necessary. Identification of the underlying cause(s) for failure of the index procedure is the key to planning revision surgery. A thorough understanding of the pathomechanics of shoulder instability and the risk factors for failure of arthroscopic capsulorrhaphy allows for a systematic evaluation of the patient with recurrent instability after surgery. Understanding normal shoulder anatomy and biomechanics is the first step in recognizing the etiology of anterior shoulder instability.

Thompson TL, ed.
Arthroscopic Shoulder Surgery:
Complications and Management (pp 161-190).

Stability of the glenohumeral joint is conferred by a complex combination of structural and functional elements. Concavity of the glenoid is established by the shape of the bone and is deepened by the attached labrum. Compression of the humeral head into this glenoid concavity achieved by the synchronized actions of the shoulder muscles creates the functional stability. Stability is further supported by the capsular ligaments, especially the inferior glenohumeral ligament, at the extremes of motion. These mechanisms establish joint stability while allowing for a large range of motion necessary for complex upper extremity tasks. Disruptions to this complex balance from loss of any one of these components can lead to symptomatic shoulder instability. In anterior instability, this is recognized to generally be from detachment of the anterior, inferior labrum, and tearing of capsule but can also include bony injury.

Surgical treatment of anterior shoulder instability is indicated to treat recurrent episodes of shoulder subluxation or dislocation as well as after a single dislocation in some circumstances. The goals of surgical repair are to restore normal joint function and return individuals to preinjury level of activity while eliminating episodes of instability and reducing the risk for long-term joint dysfunction. Toward this goal, reestablishment of a pain-free shoulder range of motion and full strength, while minimizing surgical morbidity, is desired. Restoration of the injuries' structures to normal anatomy and function has been the hallmark of surgical repair. As the pathologic lesions became understood to be at the level of the glenohumeral labrum and capsular ligaments (not in the rotator cuff or more superficial structures), there has been a desire to directly address these lesions without disrupting the subscapularis, typical of open repairs.

Minimally invasive, arthroscopic approaches have been developed in the hope to achieve with these goals less risk for the complications seen in open surgical techniques. Over the past 30 years, there have been improvements in understanding of the pathophysiology of shoulder instability as well as in arthroscopic techniques and tools, but failures of arthroscopic techniques due to recurrence of instability continue to occur. When recurrence does occur, identification and correction of the underlying cause for failure are critical to successful revision surgery. While repeat shoulder trauma is the most common factor, structural anatomic factors or technical errors in the initial surgical procedure may also be identified in a patient with a failed repair. This chapter will explore the issues of recurrent of instability after arthroscopic surgery for shoulder instability, evaluate a systematic approach for identifying the etiology of failures, and provide pearls on how to manage revision surgery for recurrence of instability.

EPIDEMIOLOGY

Few topics in sports medicine surgery have been as controversial as whether arthroscopic or open techniques are better for treating anterior shoulder instability. These arthroscopic techniques have become the predominant approach to surgical care in the United States, comprising 90% of surgical procedures done for shoulder instability.[1] It is well established that neither open nor arthroscopic surgical repairs are uniformly successful in preventing recurrently instability. While arthroscopic techniques have low rates of other complications, such as infection, stiffness, and rotator cuff weakness, arthroscopic repairs have generally been reported to have a higher rate of recurrence of instability symptoms than open repairs.[3] Reported rates of surgical failure due to recurrence of instability vary widely. This is the case due, in part, because failure is variably defined in the literature as repeat dislocation only, dislocation or subluxation, or any symptoms of instability, including apprehension. The lack of a universally accepted definition across studies has led to inconsistency in reports of outcome from arthroscopic repairs.[4] These rates range from 3% to 30% in arthroscopic repairs with suture anchors (the currently preferred technique) with a mean of 9%, slightly higher than for open repairs.[3]

Comparative studies, even randomized trials, have generally shown no significant differences in recurrence between open and arthroscopic approaches but typically suffer from lack of power and short-term follow-up.[5] In a larger, prospective, randomized trial, Mohtadi et al[6] reported, "Recurrence rates at 2 years were significantly different: 11% in the open group and 23% in the arthroscopic group ($P = .05$)." The debate on the best surgical technique for anterior shoulder instability continues, and the approach is best tailored to the individual patient's anatomy and activity. An important way to improve results of arthroscopic repair, as well as to manage failures due to recurrent instability, is to understand the etiologies of failure of arthroscopic repair. These factors must be considered and, when possible, addressed at the time of surgery, at times choosing a different surgical technique, such as an open repair or bone augmentation procedure.

ETIOLOGY FOR RECURRENCE

Multiple studies have explored the causes for recurrence of instability after arthroscopic repair. The findings have typically been separated into patient factors, anatomic factors, and technical errors (Table 11-1). The patient factors identified consistently include age, activity level (eg, competitive sports), and number of dislocations prior to initial surgery. Anatomic

TABLE 11-1. ETIOLOGY OF RECURRENT INSTABILITY FOLLOWING ARTHROSCOPIC REPAIR

PATIENT FACTORS

Age (under 25)

Sex (male)

Activity (competitive sports)

Number of dislocations (3 or more)

ANATOMIC FACTORS

Bony:

- Glenoid deficiency (greater than 20%)
- Humeral head defect (engaging or off-track)
- Combined defects (increased effect)

Soft tissue:

- Humeral avulsion of the glenohumeral ligament (HAGL lesion)
- Shoulder hyperlaxity

TECHNICAL ERRORS

Anchor placement (too high, too medial)

Too few anchors (fewer than 3)

Inadequate soft tissue tensioning

Rehabilitation error (premature return to sports)

factors include soft tissue factors (joint hyperlaxity, humeral avulsion of the glenohumeral ligament [HAGL] lesion) and bony factors (glenoid, humeral, and combined defects). Technical factors include inappropriate location and number of suture anchors, failure to address capsular laxity, and insufficient postoperative activity restriction. Other technical factors suggested by some authors are the use of absorbable (vs nonabsorbable) anchors and the use of knotted (vs knotless suture techniques), but these have not consistently been found to be significant. To help quantify the risk of failure when multiple factors are present, Balg and Boileau[7] have introduced the Instability Severity Score to help predict if patients are at a high risk for recurrent instability with an arthroscopic repair. The factors they determined to be important include both patient factors, including age younger than 20 years (2 points), sports participation at a competitive level (2 points), and contact or overhead sports (1 point), as well as anatomic factors, including hyperlaxity (1 point), humeral head defect (2 points), and glenoid defect (2 points). They found that patients with a score of 6 or more had a 70% chance of failure with an arthroscopic approach and recommended an open approach for these patients (open capsulorrhaphy or Latarjet). In the situation of revising a failed arthroscopic repair, these factors are likely to be even more significant predictors of failure. A clear understanding of these factors is critical to decision making and achieving good outcomes in revision shoulder instability surgery.

PATIENT FACTORS

The patient factors that have been linked to an increased risk for recurrent instability after arthroscopic repair are important to recognize because they may help explain the high recurrence rate in some studies and, if identified, may lead to the selection of a different surgical approach (ie, open repair) or a modification in an arthroscopic repair (eg, addition of a remplissage into a humeral head defect). When possible, these factors should be identified prior to initial surgical intervention, and they may also help to explain why an arthroscopic repair has failed. Age and sex have been the most consistent patient characteristics associated with recurrence rates. Younger patients (under 20 to 25 years old) and male sex consistently have a higher rate of recurrent instability following arthroscopic repair.[8-10] This is not surprising as this same group has a higher incidence of recurrent instability with nonoperative treatment and even with open surgical repair. This may be related to frequency of exposure to at-risk activities, which is common in this group. While age is highly correlated with activity, certain activities are known to result in a higher rate of recurrence. These activities generally include competitive sports such as football, wrestling, and rugby.[10,11] Some studies report a high rate of success and return to activities with arthroscopic repairs even in contact athletes.[12] It seems that level of involvement (competitive vs recreational) may be more predictive of recurrence than the type of sport.

The number of dislocations prior to initial surgery also has had a strong association with an increased risk for failure of arthroscopic repairs in anterior instability.[13-15] As few as 3 dislocations have been associated with an increased rate of failure of arthroscopic repair. It is likely that this factor in a patient's history is associated with more extensive soft tissue and/or bony damage from cumulative injury. Thus, the number of dislocations might not be an independent predictor for risk of recurrence but certainly should trigger a search for additional anatomic factors.

ANATOMIC FACTORS

Soft Tissues

Successful arthroscopic capsulorrhaphy requires adequate soft tissue integrity to support a repair. Soft tissue conditions that can predispose arthroscopic repair to failure include ligamentous hyperlaxity and untreated disruption of the glenohumeral ligament from the humerus.[16-18] These issues should be assessed prior to initial surgery but are especially critical to identify in the setting of a failed arthroscopic repair. Recurrent anterior dislocations can occur in patients who also have joint hyperlaxity, but it is important to realize that they have an increased rate of failure from arthroscopic repair.[7] Joint hyperlaxity is a feature that can be best assessed on physical examination. In the shoulder, this is typically identified as a positive sulcus sign as well as an increase in anteroposterior joint translation with a load and shift test.[19] This condition is almost always bilateral and can often be best assessed in the asymptomatic shoulder. Hyperlaxity may also be generalized and present in multiple joints. When present, these patients generally require a more extensive capsular plication at arthroscopic surgery or an open capsular shift procedure.

Another soft tissue factor that might predispose an arthroscopic repair to failure is the presence of an avulsion of the inferior glenohumeral ligament from the neck of the humerus, rather than from the glenoid. This condition has been coined as a HAGL lesion.[20] While relatively rare, this injury is found more commonly in certain types of dislocations, classically in hyperabduction injuries. It can be present in addition to labral tears and capsular stretching. The lesion cannot be diagnosed on physical examination but can be seen on magnetic resonance imaging (MRI) or, more reliably, on a magnetic resonance (MR) arthrogram (Figure 11-1). It is important to assess for the presence or absence of a HAGL lesion at the time of arthroscopy during a thorough diagnostic evaluation (Figure 11-2). Most authors recommend addressing repair of this lesion through an open technique, but arthroscopic repairs have been described.[21] In the small set of series that have been published, there have not been significant differences in outcome between open and arthroscopic techniques.[16] The important point is that, if found, it should be addressed as a part of the initial surgical repair. When a failure of arthroscopic capsulorrhaphy does occur, the presence of an untreated HAGL lesion as a contributing factor to recurrence should be considered and addressed if present.

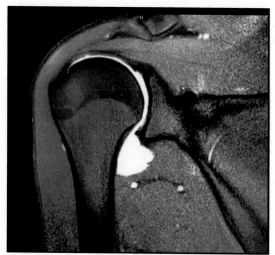

Figure 11-1. Coronal view of an MR arthrogram of the shoulder demonstrating a HAGL lesion.

BONY FACTORS

Bony lesions associated with anterior shoulder instability are common and have come to be recognized as the most frequent cause for recurrent instability after arthroscopic repair. These lesions occur at the anterior-inferior portion of the glenoid, the posterior-superior aspect of the humeral head, or as a combination of the two. In 2000, Burkhart and De Beer[22] reported in a landmark study a 11% overall recurrence rate of arthroscopic capsulorrhaphy, but most important, they stratified the outcomes according to those with and without significant bone loss. They found 4% failure in those without bone loss and a 67% failure rate in those with bone loss. This finding has led to a large body of work critically assessing the role of bony deficiency in anterior instability. There is debate in the literature on how much bone loss is critical as well as on how the location of the defects impacts their significance and how they should alter surgical planning. It is generally accepted that, if not treated, 20% to 25% isolated loss of bone from the anterior-inferior edge of the glenoid is associated with a high rate of failure of arthroscopic repairs.[8,10] Clinical studies suggest that even a 15% glenoid bone loss can increase the rate of surgical failures.[23] It follows that glenoid defects in the setting of a failed arthroscopic repair must be considered and may be significant even if small.

Figure 11-2. Arthroscopic image of a HAGL lesion from an anterior portal in the lateral decubitus position.

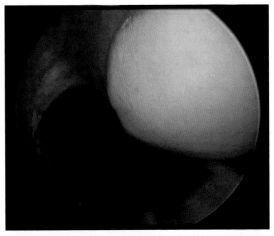

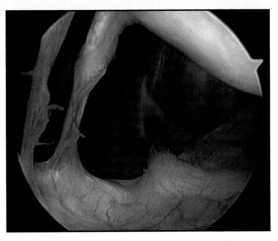

Acute injuries with displaced glenoid bone defects of this size can often be addressed with an arthroscopic approach.[24] With these acute glenoid rim fractures, fixation of a small, mobile bony fragment along with the labrum can generally be achieved arthroscopically with a low incidence of recurrence. In chronic cases, or in the settings of a previously failed arthroscopic repair, the bone fragment from a glenoid rim fracture is often resorbed or malunited to the glenoid in a medial position. If it is present and can be mobilized to reestablish its anatomic location, an arthroscopic refixation technique may be successful.[25] However, large bony defect lesions cannot be simply managed with soft tissue repairs alone, and one of several options for bony restoration is indicated.

Humeral bone lesions (also known as *Hill-Sachs lesions*) are also very common in anterior shoulder instability and can be found in isolation or in combination with glenoid lesions. The critical degree of humeral loss that must be treated is less well understood than it is for the glenoid. The significance of a defect is more dependent on the location of rather than on the depth or volume of the defect. Humeral lesions that extend further anteriorly on the articular surface, to where they might engage with the anterior rim of the glenoid as the shoulder reaches an abducted, externally rotated position, will increase the risk for failure of a soft tissue repair unless they are also addressed.[8,10] In 2007, Yamamoto et al[26] presented the concept of the "glenoid track" to help identify critical humeral bone defects. They defined the glenoid track as the portion of the humeral head that remains posterior to the edge of the anterior glenoid rim throughout range of motion. If the humeral head defect does not extend beyond this track, then it should not engage the anterior glenoid with normal motion. However, if a defect extends anteriorly beyond this track, it will engage in some arm positions and increase the risk for dislocation. With an intact glenoid rim, this track has been reported to extend approximately 18 mm, or 83% of the width of the glenoid, from the insertion of the rotator cuff onto the humeral head. As long as the glenoid rim does not come into contact with this glenoid track, the humeral defect will not have an impact on the risk for surgical failure. Logically, if there is a coexisting loss of bone from the glenoid rim, the significance of a humeral defect is greater than the same defect in isolation. The glenoid track concept had been extended to consider these combined lesions. With associated glenoid defects, the glenoid track narrows. Lesions in which the humeral head defect does not reach the anterior glenoid rim (with the arm in abduction and internal rotation) are considered to be "on-track" and would not be considered at increased risk for failure of an arthroscopic repair, while lesions in which the humeral defect extends to or beyond the rim of the anterior glenoid are "off-track" and at higher risk for surgical failure.[27] A thorough understanding of how humeral head and glenoid bone defects impact the risk for failure in arthroscopic capsulorrhaphy for anterior instability is crucial in the management of failed repairs. Failure of previous arthroscopic surgery due to bony deficiency generally cannot be managed by soft tissue repair alone.

TECHNICAL FACTORS

Another category of factors associated with failure of arthroscopic capsulorrhaphy are technical factors in the performance of the initial surgical procedure. The most commonly recognized errors in these procedures are inappropriate placement of the suture anchor fixation points, incomplete repair of labral tears that extend to the posterior-inferior aspect of the glenoid, and the use of fewer than 3 anchors and failure to adequately address pathologic laxity in the inferior glenohumeral ligament.[8,10]

INCORRECT ANCHOR PLACEMENT

Ideally, placement of anchors into the glenoid rim during arthroscopic capsulorrhaphy facilitates repair of the glenoid labrum and capsule to restore normal anatomy. Since pathologic injury in anterior dislocations is recognized to be most common at the anterior-inferior portion of the labrum, typically extending to the 6-o'clock position, the most inferior anchor placement should approximate this location. The anchors also should be placed lateral onto the rim (slightly onto the articular face) to recreate the effect of the labrum to increase the depth of the glenoid cavity (sometimes termed the *bumper*). Anchors placed more medially on the glenoid will fail to recreate this effect. Anchors are generally placed through a portal located superior to the upper edge of the subscapularis tendon, which can make it difficult to reach the ideal position for the anchor on the inferior aspect of the glenoid. The furthest inferior anchor is the most difficult to place accurately, and this position may not be achieved. Failure to adequately repair the anterior, inferior labrum and capsule can be a cause for failure of arthroscopic surgery. A trans-subscapularis portal has been described to place the most inferior anchor but is not often utilized.[28]

INCOMPLETE SOFT TISSUE REPAIR

Extensile Labral Lesions

While it is well accepted that anterior instability is associated with tears of the anterior-inferior labrum (2- to 6-o'clock), tears can extend beyond the most inferior point to the posterior-inferior portion of the glenoid (past the 6-o'clock position). Such tears are generally continuous with the anterior separation between the labrum and the glenoid. The biomechanical significance of these tears is not well understood, except that they are pathologic and related to the instability. They may represent a multidirectional component to the patient's instability, even in the setting of recurrent anterior dislocation and subluxation. If present, an extensile labral tear should be repaired at the time of arthroscopic capsulorrhaphy.[29] Failure to repair these lesions may increase the risk for recurrent instability after surgery. Repairs require an extension of the anterior repair to the posterior inferior labrum through a posterior portal (while viewing from anterior), often using a small posterior-inferior portal for anchor placement. With this technique, the repair can be extended as far along the posterior glenoid as necessary to repair the lesion.

CAPSULAR LAXITY

In addition to a separation of the labrum from the glenoid rim, injury to the anterior-inferior portion of the joint capsule, specifically the anterior portion of the glenohumeral ligament, is considered an essential component of anterior instability. In cadaver studies, it has been shown that labral tears in isolation do not create enough joint laxity to allow for glenohumeral dislocations.[30] In addition, arthroscopy of acute anterior dislocations has frequently identified capsular injuries.[31,32] Because these injuries are interstitial stretch injuries, they can be hard to detect. Arthroscopic descriptions, such as the "drive-through" sign and a patulous anterior-inferior pouch, have been used to help identify this pathologic finding. It should be assumed that some degree of pathologic capsular laxity is present in all cases of recurrent anterior dislocations and addressed at the time of arthroscopic repair. However, the degree of anterior-inferior capsular laxity may be hard to assess. In addition, anterior instability can occur in patients with preexisting hyperlaxity and excessive laxity in this area of joint capsule. In nearly all cases of anterior instability, capsular laxity should be addressed surgically by advancing the inferior glenohumeral ligament tissue from inferior to superior as well as reducing the medial to lateral capsular length with plication of the capsule to restore normal tension. The degree to which capsular plication should be done to remove the laxity of the anterior-inferior capsule is variable on an individual patient basis, and it is a judgment made at the time of surgery. Failure to address pathologic capsular laxity can be a reason for failure of arthroscopic repair even if a labral repair heals successfully. In the setting of a failure of arthroscopic repair, the degree of capsular laxity present must be assessed and managed.

INADEQUATE POSTOPERATIVE REHABILITATION

A potential technical error in arthroscopic capsulorrhaphy is an inadequate period for recovery postoperatively. Most studies support the inclusion of an initial period of postoperative immobilization followed by progressive mobilization and rehabilitation prior to return to activities.[33]

Errors in the postoperative period include too much motion or excessive joint loading in the early phase of recovery or a premature return to at-risk activities. A period of relative immobilization is recommended during the initial 4 to 6 weeks postoperatively to establish initial soft tissue healing. During this time, only a limited range of motion is allowed (especially no abduction–external rotation). Also, there should be no loading that might produce translation of the glenohumeral joint in this phase of recovery. After initial healing is established, recovery of a full functional range of motion should be achieved. This typically occurs in the 6- to 12-week time frame but is not always achieved by the 3-month mark. The final phase of recovery, from 12 to 24 weeks, includes recovery of muscle strength and sport-specific functional training. A return to at-risk activities and sports is typically not recommended until the 6-month point. Excessive early motion and loading during these phases or lack of compliance with postoperative restrictions can increase the risk for recurrent instability even when there are no other risk factors for failure.

A thorough understanding of the factors that are known to increase the risk for failure of arthroscopic capsulorrhaphy for anterior instability, as detailed above, will help to diagnose the etiology of failure when it presents. When none of these factors are present or they are appropriately addressed at the time of initial surgery, the rate of failure can be minimized (to a rate of 10% or less).[34] In the face of a failed arthroscopic repair, a critical assessment for the presence of one or more of these etiologic factors is an essential step in the planning of revision surgery. Once identified, these factors either can be addressed as a part of a revision arthroscopic repair or can guide selection of alternative operative approaches.

EVALUATION OF FAILED ARTHROSCOPIC REPAIRS

An evaluation of a patient with a known or suspected recurrence of instability after an arthroscopic capsulorrhaphy should follow a systematic approach, first to confirm the diagnosis of recurrent anterior instability and, second, to identify the reasons for surgical failure. This evaluation includes a history of the indications for initial surgery, an understanding of the postsurgical outcome prior to recurrence (level of return to activity), details of the subsequent events leading to the recurrence (eg, recurrent trauma), a focused physical examination, and imaging studies to assess the anatomic or technical factors for failure. While most poor outcomes from arthroscopic capsulorrhaphy for anterior instability are due to recurrent anterior instability, it is critical to confirm that there is not another reason for the symptoms. It is possible for patients to have symptoms of shifting or catching in the shoulder due to causes other than instability. An accurate diagnosis is the critical first step in the postcapsulorrhaphy patient. If a radiograph confirming recurrent anterior dislocation is available, that is the most definitive diagnostic evidence for recurrent instability, but this is not always available.

Physical examination signs consistent with anterior instability should be present. Assessment for hyperlaxity and specifically for symptomatic posterior instability (jerk test) may indicate that the symptoms are not from anterior instability alone and that a different treatment approach is needed. Similarly, imaging should rule out other diagnoses such as posttraumatic arthritis, loose bodies, acromioclavicular injury, and so on.

HISTORY

Recurrent instability after arthroscopic repair is most commonly attributed to a new traumatic event, but atraumatic recurrences are not uncommon.[35,36] It is not surprising that a repeat injury might result in a recurrent shoulder dislocation in the same way that initial dislocations are generally due to traumatic events. Many individuals who have had shoulder instability attempt to return to the activities that caused the condition in the first place, especially competitive sports. In some cases, such an injury should be considered a new injury after a successful surgery, essentially repeating the initial instability injury. In such cases, the recurrence can often be treated much as an initial dislocation might be treated. This is more likely to be the case when the individual has had a significant period of normal function after initial surgery, returns to sports or other high-level activity, has no other identifiable causes for failure, and has sustained a significant recurrent injury. On the other hand, a postrepair instability event from a low-energy or no injury should be considered a surgical failure and needs to be managed with that in mind. Surgical failure due to recurrent instability requires a thorough evaluation to assess potential causes for surgical failure detailed in this chapter. It is often unknown which of these scenarios is present, and thus, even in cases where a recurrent dislocation or subluxation was clearly due to a traumatic event, a workup for predisposing anatomic factors or technical surgical deficiency is important.

TABLE 11-2. PHYSICAL EXAMINATION IN PATIENTS WITH FAILED ARTHROSCOPIC CAPSULORRHAPHY

Range of motion (may be limited by apprehension)

Strength

Provocative tests:

- Apprehension (crank test)
- Relocation test (supine)
- Jerk test (posterior instability)

Joint laxity:

- Load and shift (anteroposterior translation)
- Sulcus (inferior translation)
- Hyperabduction (>105 degrees)
- Generalized laxity (Beighton score)

PHYSICAL EXAMINATION

A thorough, focused physical examination should be performed on both the injured and the uninjured shoulder (Table 11-2). Once out of the acute injury phase, the diagnosis of recurrent instability is generally associated with a near-normal range of motion, normal strength, and no localizing tenderness. Lack of active motion, especially elevation and external rotation, may be related to fear of instability and seems to have an association with significant bone defects. A better degree of relaxation is often achieved by examination of the contralateral, uninjured shoulder using the same maneuvers, especially during the acute or subacute phases as well as examining in the supine position. The reproduction of apprehension symptoms on provocative testing is expected in cases of anterior instability. These provocative tests include anterior loading in abduction, external rotation (crank test), and the relocation test (stabilization of the shoulder in abduction, external rotation, typically in the supine position).[37] Reproduction of apprehension with these tests helps to confirm the diagnosis of recurrent anterior instability. If these tests do not reproduce the patient's symptoms, then other causes for the shoulder dysfunctions should be sought. An important assessment on physical examination in the setting of recurrent instability symptoms after arthroscopic capsulorrhaphy includes the assessment for posterior instability and hyperlaxity.[38] Posterior instability is most readily detected through the jerk test. Symptomatic shifting of the humerus from a subluxated position to a reduced position (as the arm is brought posteriorly from an anterior position at 90 degrees of extension) may confirm that posterior instability is present. Hyperlaxity, which often is present in patients with posterior instability, can be detected with the presence of a sulcus sign as well as with anteroposterior hypermobility during a load-and-shift maneuver.[19] More specific for the inferior capsule is the hyperabduction test. Shoulders with greater than 105 degrees of range of passive abduction are associated with instability and increased laxity of the inferior glenohumeral ligament.[39]

Generalized ligamentous laxity can help to establish an individual's inherent soft tissue quality. It is typically assessed by examination at the elbows, hands, and knees and quantified using the Beighton score.[40] In this 9-point scheme, 1 point is assessed for hypermobility at each elbow (10 degrees or more of hyperextension), each thumb (ability to touch to forearm), each small finger (90 degrees or more of metacarpophalangeal extension), each knee (10 degrees or more of hyperextension), and the ability to touch one's palms to the floor with the knees straight. Generalized joint mobility is assessed as 0 to 4 points = normal, 5 to 6 points = increased range of motion, and 7 to 9 points = hypermobility. In the general population, only 3% to 4% of individuals are considered to be hypermobile using this scale. It should be recognized that there is not always a perfect correlation between generalized laxity and shoulder-specific laxity.[41] Thus, while generalized ligamentous laxity may be a factor, hypermobility of the shoulder is the more important finding. Increased laxity might be present in an individual with anterior instability, but it is also often associated with multidirectional and posterior laxity. Thus, identification of this on examination in a patient with instability symptoms is an important factor that may lead to change in diagnosis and/or treatment plan. The presence of hyperlaxity does not preclude a diagnosis of recurrent anterior instability but should raise the question about whether the symptoms are due to posterior or multidirectional instability. If symptoms are not isolated to the anterior-inferior direction, then further consideration of a different treatment approach, often nonoperative, should be undertaken.

IMAGING

Imaging in the setting of recurrent symptoms following arthroscopic capsulorrhaphy for anterior instability provides an essential guide toward understanding the pathoanatomy and the planning of treatment (Table 11-3). In some cases, imaging will confirm that a repeat dislocation or subluxation event has occurred. Thus, the finding of an anterior dislocation on an injury film

TABLE 11-3. IMAGING IN PATIENTS WITH FAILED ARTHROSCOPIC CAPSULORRHAPHY

RADIOGRAPHS
Injury films (may document anterior dislocation)
Glenoid abnormality (demonstrates need for 3-D imaging)
Humeral head defect (anteroposterior view in internal rotation)
Arthritis (postcapsulorrhaphy arthrosis)

CT SCANNING (WITH 3-D RECONSTRUCTION)
Glenoid fracture
Glenoid deficiency:
• Linear method
• Surface area method
Humeral head defect:
• Engaging vs nonengaging
• Off-track vs on-track
Combined defects
Anchor placement from prior surgery

MRI SCANNING
Bone defects (3-D MR could be valuable)
HAGL (MR arthrogram)
Capsular laxity (MR arthrogram)

or an acute bone bruise on the posterior aspect of the humeral head by MRI verifies that an instability event has taken place. However, the greatest value of imaging is to establish the cause for failed surgery or to document a new traumatic injury. Plain radiographs are useful to detect abnormalities of the glenoid rim, humeral head defects, periarticular fractures, and osteoarthritis but are usually not adequate to quantify the extent of these lesions. Thus, some form of 3-dimensional (3-D) imaging is important to guide in decision making in planning treatment of postcapsulorrhaphy recurrences.

Bony defects are the most common anatomic patient factor in failure of arthroscopic repair. It is critical to accurately assess the degree of bony injury in the setting of surgical failure. Methods of assessing bone loss have established the value of 3-D imaging, especially computed tomography (CT) scanning with 3-D reconstructions as a preferred method of imaging these lesions.[42,43] However, these CT scans are generally not as useful for assessment of the periarticular soft tissues as MRI. As 3-D MRI methods become more available and refined, this method may allow for preferred assessment of both soft tissue and bone.[44] While several methods of measurement of bone loss have been described, the simplest and most commonly used method involved the fitting of a circle to the lower aspect of the glenoid and measuring the proportion of radius lost in the anterior portion, known as the *linear method*. This method overestimates the proportion of glenoid surface area that is lost but is most frequently used in the literature. Another approach is to estimate the proportion area of the glenoid lost in the best-fit circle. There are challenges to the reproducibility of either of these techniques,[45] but either one can provide valuable information to guide decision making. In the setting of failure of an arthroscopic repair, even a 10% to 15% defect of the glenoid should be considered significant and often needs to be treated with some sort of bony augmentation procedure such as a Latarjet operation. Glenoid defects above 30% may be too big to be managed with a coracoid transfer (Latarjet) and require glenoid reconstruction with either iliac crest autograft or an osteoarticular allograft.

Imaging methods for assessment of humeral head defects have been less well established than for glenoid defects. The significance of defects of the humeral head is best evaluated by how far they extend anteriorly onto the articular surface rather than their depth alone. As previously described, defects that extend anteriorly and are considered "off-track" need to be addressed. The presence of a humeral head defect can be fairly well reliably detected on plain radiographs, most commonly on anteroposterior view with the shoulder in internal rotation. However, the specific depth and location on the humeral head are more difficult to assess without advanced imaging. The 3-D imaging with CT has been evaluated for detecting humeral head defects and has been found to be sensitive and specific in locating these defects.[46,47] The specific degree of humeral bone defect that requires treatment during surgery for recurrent anterior instability has not been well established. Defects that engage with the anterior edge of the glenoid rim during a functional arc of motion are important to address (off-track). A rough guide is that isolated lesions of the humeral head that extend less than 15% of the width of the glenoid from the rotator cuff insertion can be ignored; these lesions are considered "on-track." While lesions larger than this can be considered at risk for engaging, or are "off-track," they should be addressed surgically.

Another important use of 3-D imaging in the setting of a failed arthroscopic repair is to identify the location of the anchors placed at the index surgery. As previously described, it is important to achieve appropriate anchor placement along the anterior-inferior portion of the glenoid rim. Many times, the most inferior anchor will not reach this location, demonstrating

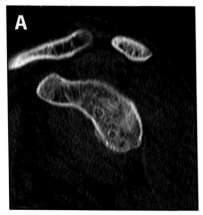

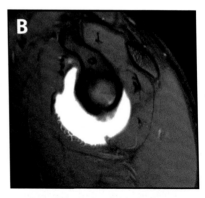

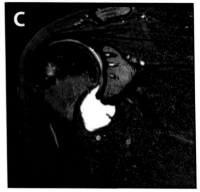

Figure 11-3. (A) CT scan demonstrating appropriate anchor placement. (B, C) MRI demonstrating anchors placed too high on the glenoid.

that an anatomic repair was never achieved. This can be the reason for surgical failure (Figure 11-3). On the other hand, appropriate placement of anchors should prompt further evaluation for other factors responsible for recurrence of instability. In some cases, there can be a fracture through the holes from anchor placement, creating a deficient anterior glenoid (Figure 11-4). Unlike acute glenoid rim fractures seen without prior surgery, these lesions are unlikely to heal closed or with arthroscopic repair and are best managed with a bony procedure at the glenoid (typically a Latarjet procedure).

While CT scans with 3-D reconstructions have been preferred for imaging the bony anatomy of the glenoid and humeral head, they do not effectively allow assessment of the periarticular soft tissues. The presence of ligamentous hyperlaxity of the shoulder can generally be assessed on physical examination, but the diagnosis of a HAGL lesion cannot. This lesion is best identified on an MR arthrogram.[16] Thus, in the setting of failed anterior capsulorrhaphy with normal bony anatomy and appropriate anchor placement on CT scanning, an MR arthrogram may be valuable in identifying soft tissue lesions

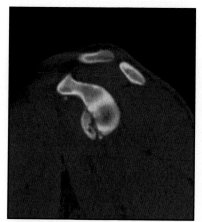
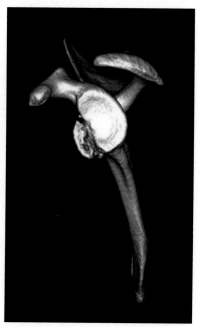

Figure 11-4. CT scan with 3-D reconstruction demonstrating a fracture through previous drill holes.

such as a HAGL. Of course, these lesions can also be identified at the time of arthroscopic surgery. Arthroscopic repair of HAGL lesions has also been described, but most authors preferred to address these lesions with an open approach when they are identified preoperatively. Thus, knowledge about the presence of HAGL lesions is very valuable in planning surgical management.

AUTHOR'S PREFERRED TREATMENT

The treatment of recurrence of instability following arthroscopic capsulorrhaphy should be based on a thorough understanding of the etiology for failure, the individual patient's pathoanatomy, and the patient's goals. A flowchart outlining decision-making steps in this process is presented (Figure 11-5). Once a thorough history, physical examination, and imaging studies are completed, the diagnosis of and the etiology for recurrent instability following arthroscopic capsulorrhaphy for anterior dislocations should be evident. Depending on the degree of bone and soft tissue defects present, as well as the patient factors in each case, the most appropriate revision procedure can be determined. Clinically significant bony defects of the glenoid are very common in the setting of failure surgery and are often associated with humeral head lesions. They should be highly suspected

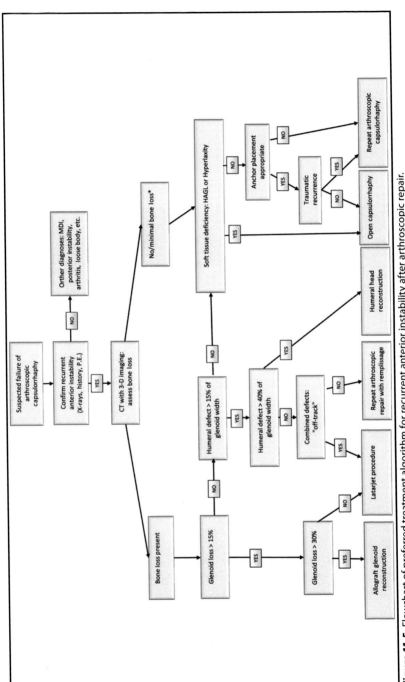

Figure 11-5. Flowchart of preferred treatment algorithm for recurrent anterior instability after arthroscopic repair.

when an arthroscopic soft tissue procedure fails. Even when small (15%), these glenoid defects should be considered significant. Thus, every case of recurrent instability following repair requires advanced imaging with CT or MRI to assess the bony anatomy of the glenoid and humerus.

When present, glenoid defects at 15% or more (but less than 30% to 40%) are best managed with a coracoid transfer (Latarjet) procedure. There is a high rate of success for this procedure, even when there are associated humeral head defects.[48,49] The author's preference is to perform the coracoid transfer procedure through a split in the subscapularis muscle as described by Young et al.[49] In this method, 2 parallel screws are placed to secure the coracoid fragment. The inferior drill hole in the glenoid is placed first, directly visualizing its location on the glenoid to best ensure proper positioning. The superior screw is placed directly through the previously created upper coracoid hole. The capsular ligament is reattached to the glenoid rim inside (deep) to the coracoid process (with suture anchors or with sutures placed around the screws); the stump of the coracoacromial ligament on the coracoid fragment is sutured to the capsule.

Unusual cases of very large glenoid bony defects (greater than 30%) require autograft or allograft glenoid reconstruction. Small series have reported good results with both approaches.[50,51] Allografts from the distal tibia have been shown to match the contour of the glenoid and are the preferred graft if available.[50] This procedure is performed much the same as the Latarjet operation. A subscapularis splitting approach or tenotomy approach can be used depending on the size of the defect and patient anatomic factors. Good results in small series have been reported. It has also been demonstrated that iliac crest grafts can be used with comparable results when an allograft is not available or an autograft is preferred.[52]

Humeral lesions large enough to be of concern, without coexisting glenoid bone loss, can be addressed with a revision arthroscopic capsulorrhaphy with the addition of a remplissage procedure.[53] In this procedure, the posterior aspect of the rotator cuff and capsule is sutured into the humeral defect (after preparation of the bone surface). Typically, 2 suture anchors are placed into the center of the prepared defect, and sutures are passed through the infraspinatus tendon and posterior capsule; these are tied outside the rotator cuff but deep to the deltoid. Combined with a standard repair of the anterior labrum and appropriate capsular plication, remplissage has been an effective way to reduce the rate of recurrence in the setting of humeral head defects.[54] Generally, it is easiest to visualize and address the humeral head defect, placing the anchors and passing the sutures without tying the sutures down, before repairing the anterior inferior capsule. Then, once the anterior labral repair and capsulorrhaphy are complete, the posterior sutures can be tied deep to the deltoid on the outside of the infraspinatus. Laboratory studies have suggested that the remplissage procedure can reduce external rotation motion, but most studies have not found a clinically significant loss of motion in this position.[55-57]

In combined defects of the humeral head with glenoid loss, treatment of the glenoid defect takes precedent. Thus, combined defects of small to medium size are generally treated with a Latarjet procedure alone as previously described. Large glenoid lesions may require autograft or allograft glenoid reconstruction. In these cases, it does not seem to be necessary to address the humeral head lesion. However, very large humeral lesions that approach 40% to 50% of the head may not be adequately managed by glenoid-sided reconstruction only, and something must be done to address the humeral head defect. Allograft or prosthetic reconstruction can be considered in these settings.[58] An open approach with takedown of the subscapularis and full external rotation can make it possible to access the posterior aspect of the humeral head as well as repair anterior bone and/or soft tissue deficiencies. Fortunately, these lesions are uncommon and typically associated with major trauma or seizures. They are addressed on an individual basis depending on the patient's age, function, and associated injuries.

When soft tissue deficiency (hyperlaxity or HAGL lesion) is evident in a failed arthroscopic repair, revision surgery is generally best approached through an open capsulorrhaphy approach with an anatomic restoration of capsular laxity (plus labral repair if necessary). Open repairs can be most easily achieved with a takedown of the subscapularis from the lesser tuberosity; at times, with HAGL lesions, it is possible to leave the upper portion of the subscapularis tendon intact.[21] With a humeral head retractor in place, a labral detachment can be repaired at the same time if present. The glenohumeral ligament detachment from the humerus is identified and repaired directly to the anatomic neck with suture anchors as well as restoring normal capsular tension. Results from open HAGL repair have been good.[16,17] At times, these HAGL lesions are discovered at arthroscopy for a planned capsulorrhaphy. In this situation, the procedure can be converted to an open operation or the avulsion can be repaired arthroscopically with suture anchors placed through an accessory anterior-inferior portal.[59]

Cases without bony defects, but with technical errors in the initial surgery, such as poor anchor placement, inadequate soft tissue tensioning, or a premature return to activity in the postoperative period, are candidates for revision arthroscopic capsulorrhaphy. On occasion, the evaluation finds no evidence of bony defects, soft tissue deficiency, or technical errors from the index procedure. If there is a clear history of recurrent trauma, these cases may represent true traumatic reinjuries and can be treated much as an initial dislocation with an arthroscopic or open anterior labral repair and capsulorrhaphy. In these selected cases, the results for revision arthroscopic repair

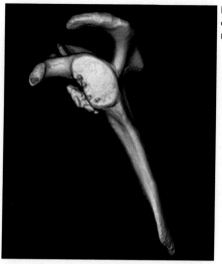

Figure 11-6. Case 1. 3-D reconstruction of CT scan demonstrating anterior glenoid bone loss.

have been reported to be good.[35] However, if recurrence occurs without a traumatic event and with no identifiable risk factors for surgical failure, then one should be concerned that a repeat arthroscopic surgery will have an increased risk for failure. In these cases, an MR arthrogram to look for capsular abnormalities such as a HAGL can be valuable. An open capsulorrhaphy is often the best surgical option for revision surgery in this situation.

CASE PRESENTATIONS

Case 1: Latarjet for Bone Loss

An 18-year-old male, recreational athlete presents with a history of recurrent anterior shoulder dislocations. He underwent an arthroscopic capsulorrhaphy 2 years ago. He successfully returned to full activity but sustained a repeat dislocation 1 year ago. This was due to a traumatic event playing basketball. Nonoperative treatment has not been successful, and he has sustained 2 additional dislocations and several subluxation events. He would like to return to basketball in college. On examination, he has a full, symmetric range of motion and strength. He has a positive crank test and relocation test causing apprehension. He does have a degree of hyperlaxity and a Beighton score of 5 (increased generalized laxity) but a negative jerk test. His imaging demonstrates a chronic, displaced fracture of the anterior glenoid through the drill holes made for anchor placement during his arthroscopic repair (Figure 11-6). The bone loss is between 15% and 30%.

A Latarjet procedure is recommended for this problem and is completed through a subscapularis splitting approach. He recovered successfully with full range of motion and normal strength and has been able to return to basketball. An alternative approach could have been an arthroscopic mobilization, reduction, and stabilization of the glenoid fragment with a repeat capsulorrhaphy. Reduction and fixation have a good record for small acute fractures of the glenoid for initial surgeries. However, in the face of poor bone quality, due to the holes from previous anchor placement, the rate of healing is likely to be lower in this setting. Also, his desire to return to competitive sports makes a revision arthroscopic repair less attractive.

Case 2: Revision Capsulorrhaphy With Remplissage

A 30-year-old woman with a prior arthroscopic capsulorrhaphy 2 years previously presents with a history of recurrent instability. There has been no significant injury, but when she reaches overhead, she has apprehension and has had many subluxation events. Recently, she has had 2 dislocations requiring reduction under sedation. On examination, she has internal rotation to T10 and external rotation at her side of 60 degrees, equal to her uninjured shoulder. She has active forward elevation to 120 degrees (vs 170 degrees). Passive elevation is to 150 degrees but with apprehension. Strength and sensation are symmetric and normal. There is no evidence of shoulder or generalized hyperlaxity. Imaging studies demonstrate a large humeral head defect and no glenoid bone loss, with adequate placement of her previous anchors (Figures 11-7A through 11-7D). In this case, the predominant feature is the humeral head defect. Since there is no associated glenoid bone loss and no evidence of hyperlaxity, it was elected to perform a repeat arthroscopic capsulorrhaphy combined with a remplissage procedure (Figures 11-7E through 11-7H). Her rehabilitation was progressed more slowly due to the revision nature of the case. She recovered well with a return to full function and no instability events. Her motion was slightly limited in external rotation (40 degrees) and elevation (160 degrees). This case could also have been managed with a Latarjet procedure (despite no glenoid bone loss). In fact, a Latarjet procedure would have been preferred if she had been planning to return to competitive sports.

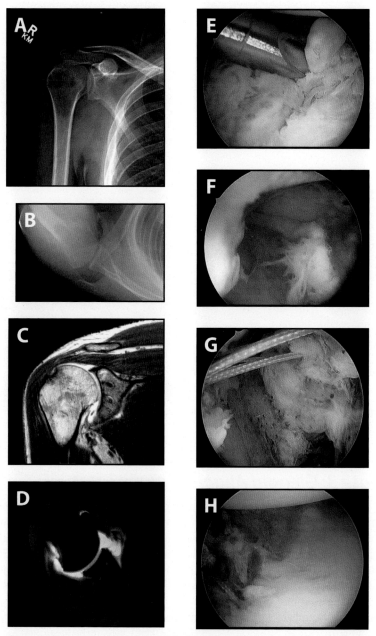

Figure 11-7. Imaging of Case 2. (A, B) Radiographs demonstrating a humeral head defect without an associated glenoid lesion. (C, D) MR arthrogram images. (E-H) Arthroscopic views: (E) anterior labrum, (F) humeral head defect, (G) remplissage sutures in place, (H) anterior capsulolabral repair complete.

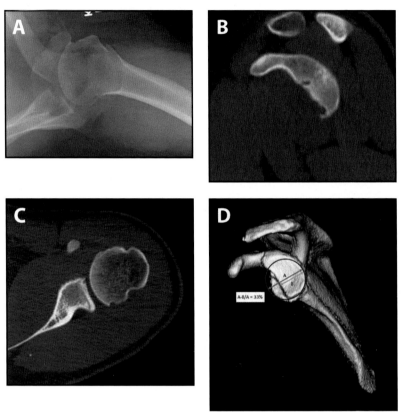

Figure 11-8. Case 3 evaluation imaging. (A) Axillary view demonstrating glenoid defect. (B) Sagittal reconstruction of CT scan with glenoid defect. (C) CT scan showing humeral head defect. (D) 3-D reconstruction of CT scan with large glenoid defect.

Case 3: Glenoid Allograft Augmentation

A 25-year-old man with a history of an arthroscopic repair 5 years previously for shoulder dislocations presents with multiple recurrent dislocations. He is unable to elevate his arm above 90 degrees while experiencing a subluxation or dislocation. He is able to self-reduce his dislocations. He has symmetric strength and internal/external rotation with his arms at his side. He actively elevates to 90 degrees and is resistant to passive motion beyond this point with apprehension. He has no increased joint laxity. Images demonstrate a large anterior glenoid defect (33%) with a small humeral defect (Figure 11-8). Given the large size of his glenoid defect, it was felt that a restoration of the anterior articular surface was indicated. This was achieved with the use of a distal tibia allograft

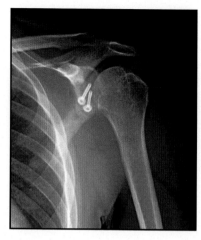
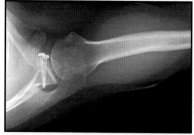

Figure 11-9. Case 3 postoperative imaging of allograft reconstruction.

reconstruction through a subscapularis tenotomy approach. The graft is fashioned to restore the glenoid with a few millimeters of extension and a repair of the capsule to the newly created rim of glenoid (Figure 11-9). At 12 months postoperatively, he has regained a near full range of motion (170 degrees of elevation, 50 degrees of external rotation at side, internal rotation to L1) and resumed normal daily activities.

REFERENCES

1. Riff AJ, Frank RM, Sumner S, Friel N, Bach BR Jr, Verma NN, Romeo AA. Trends in shoulder stabilization techniques used in the United States based on a large private-payer database. *Orthop J Sports Med.* 2017;5(12):2325967117745511.
2. Owens BD, Harrast JJ, Hurwitz SR, Thompson TL, Wolf JM. Surgical trends in Bankart repair: an analysis of data from the American Board of Orthopaedic Surgery certification examination. *Am J Sports Med.* 2011;39(9):1865–1869.
3. Hobby J, Griffin D, Dunbar M, Boileau P. Is arthroscopic surgery for stabilisation of chronic shoulder instability as effective as open surgery? A systematic review and meta-analysis of 62 studies including 3044 arthroscopic operations. *J Bone Joint Surg Br.* 2007;89(9):1188–1196.
4. Kennedy MI, Murphy C, Dornan GJ, et al. Variability of reporting recurrence after arthroscopic Bankart repair: a call for a standardized study design. *Orthop J Sports Med.* 2019;30;7(5):2325967119846915.
5. Godin J, Sekiya JK. Systematic review of arthroscopic versus open repair for recurrent anterior shoulder dislocations. *Sports Health.* 2011;3(4):396–404.
6. Mohtadi NG, Chan DS, Hollinshead RM, et al. A randomized clinical trial comparing open and arthroscopic stabilization for recurrent traumatic anterior shoulder instability. *J Bone Joint Surg Am.* 2014:353–360.
7. Balg F, Boileau P. The instability severity index score: a simple pre-operative score to select patients for arthroscopic or open shoulder stabilisation. *J Bone Joint Surg Br.* 2007;89(11):1470–1477.

8. Ho AG, Gowda AL, Michael Wiater J. Evaluation and treatment of failed shoulder instability procedures. *J Orthop Traumatol.* 2016;17(3):187–197.

9. Porcellini BG, Campi F, Pegreffi F, Castagna A, Paladini P. Predisposing factors for recurrent shoulder dislocation after arthroscopic treatment. *J Bone Joint Surg Am.* 2009;91(11):2537–2542.

10. Randelli P, Ragone V, Carminati S, Cabitza P. Risk factors for recurrence after Bankart repair a systematic review. *Knee Surg Sports Traumatol Arthrosc.* 2012;20(11):2129–2138.

11. Torrance E, Clarke CJ, Monga P, Funk L, Walton MJ. Recurrence after arthroscopic labral repair for traumatic anterior instability in adolescent rugby and contact athletes. *Am J Sports Med.* 2018;46(12):2969–2974.

12. Dickens JF, Rue JP, Cameron KL, et al. Successful return to sport after arthroscopic shoulder stabilization versus nonoperative management in contact athletes with anterior shoulder instability: a prospective multicenter study. *Am J Sports Med.* 2017;45(11):2540–2546.

13. Kandziora F, Ja A, Bischof F, Herresthal J, Starker M, Mittlmeier T. Arthroscopic labrum refixation for post-traumatic anterior shoulder instability: suture anchor versus transglenoid fixation technique. *Arthroscopy.* 2000;16(4):359–366.

14. Lee SH, Lim KH, Kim JW. Risk factors for recurrence of anterior-inferior instability of the shoulder after arthroscopic Bankart repair in patients younger than 30 years. *Arthroscopy.* 2018;34(9):2530–2536.

15. Wasserstein D, Dwyer T, Veillette C, et al. Predictors of dislocation and revision after shoulder stabilization in Ontario, Canada, from 2003 to 2008. *Am J Sports Med.* 2013;41(9):2034–2040.

16. Bozzo A, Oitment C, Thornley P, Yan J, et al. Humeral avulsion of the glenohumeral ligament: indications for surgical treatment and outcomes: a systematic review. *Orthop J Sports Med.* 2017;5(8):2325967117723329.

17. Longo UG, Rizzello G, Ciuffreda M, et al. Humeral avulsion of the glenohumeral ligaments: a systematic review. *Arthroscopy.* 2016;32:1868–1876.

18. Voos JE, Livermore RW, Feeley BT, et al. Prospective evaluation of arthroscopic Bankart repairs for anterior instability. *Am J Sports Med.* 2010;38(2):302–307.

19. Bahk M, Keyurapan E, Tasaki A, Sauers EL, McFarland EG. Laxity testing of the shoulder: a review. *Am J Sports Med.* 2007;35:131–144.

20. Wolf EM, Cheng JC, Dickson K. Humeral avulsion of glenohumeral ligaments as a cause of anterior shoulder instability. *Arthroscopy.* 1995;11(5):600–607.

21. Provencher MT, McCormick F, Leclere L, et al. Prospective evaluation of surgical treatment of humeral avulsions of the glenohumeral ligament. *Am J Sports Med.* 2017;45(5):1134–1140.

22. Burkhart SS, De Beer JF. Traumatic glenohumeral bone defects and their relationship to failure of arthroscopic Bankart repairs: significance of the inverted-pear glenoid and the humeral engaging Hill-Sachs lesion. *Arthroscopy.* 2000;16(7):677–694.

23. Shin SJ, Kim RG, Jeon YS, Kwon TH. Critical value of anterior glenoid bone loss that leads to recurrent glenohumeral instability after arthroscopic Bankart repair. *Am J Sports Med.* 2017;45(9):1975–1981.

24. Sugaya H, Kon Y, Tsuchiya A. Arthroscopic repair of glenoid fractures using suture anchors. *Arthroscopy.* 2005;21(5):635.e1–635.e5.

25. Kitayama S, Sugaya H, Takahashi N, et al. Clinical outcome and glenoid morphology after arthroscopic repair of chronic osseous Bankart lesions: a five to eight-year follow-up study. *J Bone Joint Surg Am.* 2015;97(22):1833–1843.

26. Yamamoto N, Itoi E, Abe H, et al. Contact between the glenoid and the humeral head in abduction, external rotation, and horizontal extension: a new concept of glenoid track. *J Shoulder Elbow Surg.* 2017;16(5):649–656.

27. Di Giacomo G, Itoi E, Burkhart SS. Evolving concept of bipolar bone loss and the Hill-Sachs lesion: from "engaging/non-engaging" lesion to "on-track/off-track" lesion. *Arthroscopy.* 2014;30(1):90–98.

28. Resch H, Wykypiel HF, Maurer H, Wambacher M. The antero-inferior (transmuscular) approach for arthroscopic repair of the Bankart lesion: an anatomic and clinical study. *Arthroscopy.* 1996;12(3):309–319.

29. Tokish JM, McBratney CM, Solomon DJ, LeClere L, Dewing CB, Provencher MT. Arthroscopic repair of circumferential lesions of the glenoid labrum: surgical technique. *J Bone Joint Surg Am.* 2010;92(suppl 1, pt 2):130–144.

30. Speer KP, Deng X, Borrero S, Torzilli PA, Altchek DA, Warren RF. Biomechanical evaluation of a simulated Bankart lesion. *J Bone Joint Surg Am.* 1994;76(12):1819–1826.

31. Baker CL, Uribe JW, Whitman C. Arthroscopic evaluation of acute initial anterior shoulder dislocations. *Am J Sports Med.* 1990;18(1):25–28.

32. Taylor DC, Arciero RA. Pathologic changes associated with shoulder dislocations: arthroscopic and physical examination findings in first-time, traumatic anterior dislocations. *Am J Sports Med.* 1997;25(3):306–311.

33. Gaunt BW, Shaffer MA, Sauers EL, Michener LA, Mccluskey GM, Thigpen CA. The American Society of Shoulder and Elbow Therapists' consensus rehabilitation guideline for arthroscopic anterior capsulolabral repair of the shoulder. *J Orthop Sports Phys Ther.* 2010;40(3):155–168.

34. Leroux TS, Saltzman BM, Meyer M, et al. The influence of evidence-based surgical indications and techniques on failure rates after arthroscopic shoulder stabilization in the contact or collision athlete with anterior shoulder instability. *Am J Sports Med.* 2017;45(5):1218–1225.

35. Abouali JAK, Hatzantoni K, Holtby R, Veillette C, Theodoropoulos J. Revision arthroscopic Bankart repair. *Arthroscopy.* 2013;29:1572–1578.

36. Tauber M, Resch H, Forstner R, Raffl M, Schauer J. Reasons for failure after surgical repair of anterior shoulder instability. *J Shoulder Elbow Surg.* 2004;13(3):279–285.

37. Hippensteel KJ, Brophy R, Smith MV, Wright RW. Comprehensive review of provocative and instability physical examination tests of the shoulder. *J Am Acad Orthop Surg.* 2019;27(11):395–404.

38. Bernhardson AS, Murphy CP, Aman ZS, LaPrade RF, Provencher MT. A prospective analysis of patients with anterior versus posterior shoulder instability: a matched cohort examination and surgical outcome analysis of 200 patients. *Am J Sports Med.* 2019;47(3):682–687.

39. Gagey OJ, Gagey N. The hyperabduction test. *J Bone Joint Surg Br.* 2001;83(1):69–74.

40. Beighton P, Horan F. Orthopaedic aspects of the Ehlers-Danlos syndrome. *J Bone Joint Surg Br.* 1969;51(3):444–453.

41. Whitehead NA, Mohammed KD, Fulcher ML. Does the Beighton score correlate with specific measures of shoulder joint laxity? *Orthop J Sports Med.* 2018;6(5):1–7.

42. Saliken DJ, Bornes TD, Bouliane MJ, Sheps DM, Beaupre LA. Imaging methods for quantifying glenoid and Hill-Sachs bone loss in traumatic instability of the shoulder: a scoping review. *BMC Musculoskeletal Disorders.* 2015;16(1):164.

43. Walter WR, Samim M, LaPolla FWZ, Gyftopoulos S. Imaging quantification of glenoid bone loss in patients with glenohumeral instability: a systematic review. *AJR Am J Roentgenol.* 2019;1–10.

44. Vopat BG, Cai W, Torriani M, et al. Measurement of glenoid bone loss with 3-dimensional magnetic resonance imaging: a matched computed tomography analysis. *Arthroscopy.* 2018;34(12):3141-3147.

45. Parada SA, Eichinger JK, Dumont GD, et al. Accuracy and reliability of a simple calculation for measuring glenoid bone loss on 3-dimensional computed tomography scans. *Arthroscopy.* 2018;34(1):84-92.

46. Matsumura N, Oki S, Kitashiro M, et al. Three-dimensional quantitative analysis of humeral head and glenoid bone defects with recurrent glenohumeral instability. *J Shoulder Elbow Surg.* 2017;26(9):1662-1669.

47. Ozaki R, Nakagawa S, Mizuno N. Hill-Sachs lesions in shoulders with traumatic anterior instability evaluation using computed tomography with 3-dimensional reconstruction. *Am J Sports Med.* 2014;42(11):2597-2605.

48. Gwathmey FW, Warner JJP. Management of the athlete with a failed shoulder instability procedure. *Clin Sports Med.* 2013;32(4):833-863.

49. Young AA, Maia R, Berhouet J, Walch G, Specialists SS, Wales NS. Open Latarjet procedure for management of bone loss in anterior instability of the glenohumeral joint. *J Shoulder Elbow Surg.* 2011;20(2):S61-S69.

50. Provencher MT, Frank RM, Golijanin P, et al. Distal tibia allograft glenoid reconstruction in recurrent anterior shoulder instability: clinical and radiographic outcomes. *Arthroscopy.* 2017;33(5):891-897.

51. Warner JJP, Gill TJ, O'Hollerhan JD, Pathare N, Millett PJ. Anatomical glenoid reconstruction for recurrent anterior glenohumeral instability with glenoid deficiency using an autogenous tricortical iliac crest bone graft. *Am J Sports Med.* 2006;34(2):205-212.

52. Moroder P, Schulz E, Wierer G, et al. Neer Award 2019: Latarjet procedure vs. iliac crest bone graft transfer for treatment of anterior shoulder instability with glenoid bone loss: a prospective randomized trial. *J Shoulder Elbow Surg.* 2019;28(7):1298-1307.

53. Boileau P, O'Shea K, Vargas P, Pinedo M, Old J, Zumstein M. Anatomical and functional results after arthroscopic Hill-Sachs remplissage. *J Bone Joint Surg Am.* 2012;94(7):618-626.

54. Franceschi F, Papalia R, Rizzello G, et al. Remplissage repair-new frontiers in the prevention of recurrent shoulder instability: a 2-year follow-up comparative study. *Am J Sports Med.* 2012;40(11):2462-2469.

55. Buza JA, Iyengar JJ, Anakwenze OA, Ahmad CS, Levine WN. Arthroscopic Hill-Sachs remplissage: a systematic review. *J Bone Joint Surg Am.* 2014;96(7):549-555.

56. Lazarides AL, Duchman KR, Ledbetter L, Riboh JC, Garrigues GE. Arthroscopic remplissage for anterior shoulder instability: a systematic review of clinical and biomechanical studies. *Arthroscopy.* 2019;35(2):617-628.

57. Rashid MS, Crichton J, Butt U, Akimau PI, Charalambous CP. Arthroscopic "Remplissage" for shoulder instability: a systematic review. *Knee Surg Sports Traumatol Arthrosc.* 2016;24(2):578-584.

58. Kropf EJ, Sekiya JK. Osteoarticular allograft transplantation for large humeral head defects in glenohumeral instability. *Arthroscopy.* 2007;23(3):322.e1-5.

59. Flury M, Rickenbacher D, Audigé L. Arthroscopic treatment of anterior shoulder instability associated with a HAGL lesion—a case series. *J Shoulder Elbow Surg.* 2016;25(12):1989-1996.

12

Recurrent Rotator Cuff Tear After Repair

Timothy S. Johnson, MD
and Alexander R. M. Bitzer, MD

INTRODUCTION

Rotator cuff repair is one of the most commonly performed outpatient orthopedic procedures in the United States.[1] The national rate has steadily risen over the past decade, with dramatic increases in arthroscopically assisted cases as surgeon preference has shifted from open to arthroscopic techniques.[2] Several studies show equivalent or even better results with arthroscopic rotator cuff repairs compared to mini–open repairs.[3,4] The overall trend leading to a higher volume of rotator cuff repair surgeries is multifactorial. One important driver is the increased ability to use minimally invasive arthroscopic techniques at a reasonable cost that provide positive and reproducible outcomes. The advantages of arthroscopically performed rotator cuff repairs include smaller incisions, improved soft tissue handling, improved ability to address intra-articular pathology, and less postoperative pain.[5] Several studies demonstrate the improved functional outcomes of patients who undergo arthroscopic rotator cuff repair.[6-8]

Thompson TL, ed.
Arthroscopic Shoulder Surgery:
Complications and Management (pp 191-220).
© 2022 Taylor & Francis Group.

Despite the positive effects seen by the increased application of minimally invasive techniques, no surgery is perfect, and complications can occur after arthroscopic rotator cuff repair. One of these complications is a recurrent tear of the rotator cuff after a previous arthroscopic repair. Retear rates have been reported over a wide range from 24% to 90%.[9,10] The causes of recurrent tears vary, but several risk factors and modes of failure have been identified. Risk factors for retears include larger tear size, older patient age, poor tendon quality, fatty degeneration and atrophy of the rotator cuff muscles, suboptimal surgical technique, and inappropriate rehabilitation.[11,12]

The diagnosis of a recurrent rotator cuff tear is challenging. Often, the patient's postoperative clinical history is unclear, and a repeat injury cannot be identified. Instead, many patients will describe that the pain they had before surgery has returned after an initial period of improvement during the immediate postoperative period. A thorough shoulder examination should be performed with emphasis on specialized rotator cuff tests, strength, and range of motion. Positive provocative maneuvers and decreased strength and range of motion are common with recurrent rotator cuff tears.[13] Useful imaging modalities typically consist of magnetic resonance imaging (MRI) and ultrasound evaluations, although the quality of ultrasound evaluation is heavily user dependent. Consequently, MRI remains the gold standard.[14] After diagnosis, the following challenge is management. The recurrent tear portends a somewhat poor prognosis, as retear rates are higher in revision cases compared to primary cases.[15] This is largely secondary to larger tear size, inferior tendon quality, decreased tissue mobility, decreased footprint surface area available for implants, and decreased neovascularization potential in revision cases.[16] Despite the increased complexity, several options do exist and are available to address recurrent tears after previous arthroscopic rotator cuff repair and will be discussed in detail.

EPIDEMIOLOGY

Rotator Cuff Tears

The incidence of rotator cuff tears in the United States has increased over the past few decades as a result of an aging population.[17] Yamaguchi and colleagues[18] performed a prospective study in 588 patients and found a high correlation between the occurrence of rotator cuff tears and advancing age, with a 50% chance of bilateral rotator cuff tear after the age of 66 years.

Teunis et al[19] performed a systematic review of 6112 shoulders and found an age-dependent increase in rotator cuff abnormalities with less than 10% in patients aged 20 years and younger, while 62% of those 80 years and over had rotator cuff abnormalities. Thus, as a population's age increases, so does the incidence of rotator cuff tears and consequently the number of arthroscopic repairs that are performed. Given the direct proportionality of cuff tears to surgery and surgery to complications, one can conclude that retears are also increasing over time as more repairs are being performed. Reported rotator cuff retear rates are quite variable, but even retear rates at the lower end of the spectrum mean there is a large prevalence of retears given the high volume of rotator cuff repairs that are performed annually.

Rotator Cuff Retears

Several studies on clinical outcomes after arthroscopic rotator cuff repair have reported varying rates of retears, which provide insight regarding how often these actually occur. Importantly, one must keep in mind that there is a fair amount of heterogeneity within these studies in regards to the tear types, repair techniques, and how the retears are diagnosed. Additionally, patient-specific risk factors will affect the survival of the repair and should be kept in mind when interpreting and comparing the data.

Rotator cuff retear rates after arthroscopically performed rotator cuff repair range from 5% to 94% according to recent studies.[20-27] Table 12-1 provides a brief summary of retear rates, including the type of tear that was repaired, the technique used, and diagnostic criteria. Interestingly, the study by Lee and colleagues[25] reported one of the lowest retear rates at 8%, while Galatz et al[28] reported retear rates as high as 94%. Primary tear types differed significantly between these 2 studies given that the entire cohort in Galatz et al[28] was made up of massive rotator cuff tears with greater than 2-cm defects and involving at least 2 tendons. Meanwhile, the Lee et al[25] cohort did not include any massive tears, and repairs were performed on full-thickness and partial-thickness tears. Another finding is that rates are higher in studies that diagnosed retears using ultrasound rather than MRI or computed tomography arthrogram (CTA). It is unclear why since studies show that ultrasound has a high sensitivity and specificity for diagnosing full-thickness tears, partial-thickness tears, and retears after previous repair.[29,30]

Table 12-1. Rotator Cuff Retear Rates After Previous Arthroscopically Performed Rotator Cuff Repair

FIRST AUTHOR	NO. OF SHOULDERS	PRIMARY TEAR TYPE	REPAIR TECHNIQUE AND RETEAR RATES		DIAGNOSTIC IMAGING	TIME TO DIAGNOSIS
Cho[11]	180	FTT	SRT	23%	MRI	Min. 6 months
			SBT	28%		
Kim[21]	201	FTT	SRT	48%	MRI	Min. 6 months
			SBT	23%		
			KSBT	36%		
Cho[22]	87	FTT	SBT	33%	MRI	Min. 6 months
Mihata[23]	195	FTT	SRT	11%	MRI	Min. 6 months
			DRT	26%		
			SBT	5%		
Miller[24]	22	FTT/MT	SBT	41%	US	24 months
Lee[25]	417	FTT/HGPT	SR	8%	MRI	Min. 6 months
			SBT	8%		
Lafosse[27]	105	FTT/MT	DRT	11%	MRI/CTA	Min. 6 months
Boileau[26]	65	FTT	SBT	29%	MRI/CTA	Min. 6 months
Galatz[28]	18	MT	UK	94%	US	Min. 12 months

DR, double-row technique; FTT, full-thickness tear; KSBT, knotless suture bridge technique; MT, massive tear; SBT, suture bridge technique; SRT, single-row technique; UK, unknown; US, ultrasound.

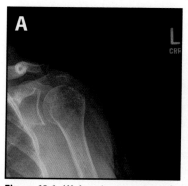
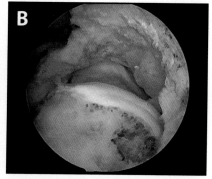

Figure 12-1. (A) Anterior-posterior radiograph of left shoulder with poor bone quality at the greater tuberosity. (B) Arthroscopic image of left shoulder from the lateral portal in the beach chair position demonstrating cystic changes and osteoporotic bone of the greater tuberosity in the setting of a large, retracted, atrophied rotator cuff tear.

RETEAR RISK FACTORS

Much to the chagrin of shoulder and sports medicine surgeons, recurrent tears of the rotator cuff after previous arthroscopic surgery are not uncommon. Several factors have been found to increase one's risk for retears, which has allowed surgeons to better identify patients at risk and improve patient–physician communication in managing expectations. Risk factors can be thought of as patient specific, which are typically nonmodifiable and surgeon related, which usually are modifiable.

Tashjian et al[31] analyzed 49 shoulders after double-row arthroscopic rotator cuff repairs and identified several risk factors for retears. These included advanced age at the time of surgery, higher number of years of postoperative follow-up, and more tendons torn at the time of surgery. Rashid et al[32] found that a massive tear is an independent risk factor even when controlling for age. Chung et al[33] later found that lower bone mineral density, increased fatty infiltration, and amount of retraction were all independent factors for failure after multivariate analysis, whereas age was not (Figure 12-1). This finding suggests that patient characteristics that change with age may have a larger influence on retears than age itself. It also emphasized that tissue quality is a critical component for a successful repair as higher failures are seen in tendons with severe retraction and poor quality. Larger and chronic rotator cuff tears lead to increased retraction, larger gaps between the footprint on the humerus and the distal tendon stump, and fatty degeneration of the rotator cuff muscles. Meyer et al[34] studied 33 shoulders and found that the length of the tendon stump, the amount of tendon retraction, and increased fatty infiltration of the supraspinatus all led to increased failure rates. They reported failure rates of

33% when the tendon length was 15 mm or more while failure rates increased dramatically when the tendon length was less than 15 mm, with retear rates up to 92%. Retracted and shortened tendon tissue becomes harder to mobilize during repair, which causes undue tension on the final repair, which can lead to failure. Kim et al[35] used a tensiometer while performing 132 arthroscopic repairs and found a mean repair tension of 28.5 N with an inverse relationship between tendon healing and tension. Elevated tension has biomechanical and biologic implications as it puts increased stress at the suture–tendon interface and can injure muscle sarcomeres via excessive stretch of cell membranes.[36]

Surgeon repair technique is considered an important modifiable risk factor whose contribution to repair integrity and outcomes has become somewhat controversial over the past few years. The gold standard in the 1990s was a transosseous open or mini–open repair as this technique allowed one to use bone-to-suture fixation along with a modified Mason-Allen suture technique, which provided favorable biomechanical fixation.[37] Over time, arthroscopic repairs became popular, and several techniques have evolved since. The arthroscopic techniques most commonly used today are the single-row technique, the double-row technique, and the suture bridge technique. Biomechanically, double-row techniques are stronger than single-row techniques.[38,39] Kim et al[38] performed a cadaveric study in which 9 double-row repairs were compared to 9 single-row repairs. The double-row repair significantly increased both strength and stiffness and decreased strain over the repaired footprint compared to the single-row repair. When comparing double-row to suture bridge techniques, Park and colleagues[39] showed that the arthroscopically performed transosseous equivalent suture bridge technique is stronger compared to the double-row technique. Despite biomechanical assessment by Park et al,[39] the suture bridge technique and double-row modified Mason-Allen technique have similar clinical outcomes regarding retear rates and functional scores.[40] Finally, several biomechanical cadaveric studies have compared traditional transosseous to suture bridge technique and found no statistical difference in elongation, load failure, stiffness, or initial fixation strength.[41,42] The benefit of double-row and suture bridge technique is increased restoration of the rotator cuff footprint coverage with a larger contact surface area of tendon to bone. This increase in tendon-footprint contact area is thought to facilitate healing by decreasing strain and increasing the available tendon–bone biological interface that is involved in restoring the enthesis at the repair site. The literature on the biomechanical properties of various repairs clearly favors a double-row or suture bridge construct compared to a single-row technique, but controversy persists on whether these techniques actually affect patient retear outcomes clinically. Franceschi and colleagues[43] performed a randomized controlled trial with 60 patients and found no significant difference between UCLA scores, range of motion, and retear rates between single-row and double-row repairs at 2-year follow-up. Charousset et al[44] similarly performed a prospective trial comparing single-row vs double-row repairs and again found no clinical outcomes difference but did see a difference in anatomic healing evaluated with CTA. Systematic reviews and meta-analyses have shown similar findings, with higher retear rates in single-row vs double-row techniques but no significant clinical difference in outcomes between the two.[45,46] The decision to use one technique over another ultimately depends on surgeon preference, intraoperative findings, and cost sensitivity as suture bridge and double-row constructs are more expensive compared to single-row repairs.[47] Also, sometimes it is not possible to perform a suture bridge or double-row repair as a consequence of the available tissue quality, especially in the revision setting. The repair technique will influence not only the biomechanical strength and retear rates but also how and where the repair fails.

MODES OF FAILURE

The types of retears and modes of failure are specific to the surgical repair technique employed. Suture anchors are commonly used when rotator cuff repairs are performed arthroscopically, and one must consider several points of failure specific to the anchors. Potential sites of failure are between the tendon and suture, the suture and anchor, and the anchor and the bone. Failure between the suture and anchor typically occurs at the eyelet of the suture anchor.[48] Generally speaking, the entire suture anchor–rotator cuff construct typically fails, causing a retear via 3 mechanisms, as failure between the suture and anchor is uncommon. These include failures at the tendon–suture interface, suture anchor pullout from the bone, and a tear in a new location.

Cummins and Murrell[49] performed a prospective study of 81 primary rotator cuff repairs using suture anchor fixation and found the predominant mode of failure (86%) to be failure at the tendon–suture interface at the time of revision surgery. Reed and colleagues[50] performed a biomechanical cadaver study in which they found that repairs performed with suture anchors failed predominantly due to suture breakage. Still, some failures occur as a result of anchor pullout from the bone, and this is influenced by the patient's bone quality. Studies have shown a significant correlation between cortical volumetric bone mineral density and metal anchor pullout strength.[51,52] This may explain why clinical studies have shown decreased bone mineral density to be an independent risk factor for retears after surgery. Retears in new locations are typically medial to the repair, resulting in

Figure 12-2. Large rotator cuff retear with suture anchor artifact in the humeral head. A stump of repaired tendon remains healed and attached to the greater tuberosity. The retear has occurred medial to the suture–tendon interface.

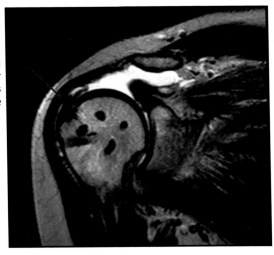

an intact repair site with a well-fixed lateral tendon stump to the tuberosity with the remaining medial portion of the tendon significantly retracted. These are considered type 2 failures and are associated with nonanatomic, medially placed suture knots, tendon strangulation, and increased focal areas of stress medially[53] (Figure 12-2). Decreased vascular perfusion at the repair site has gained some attention as certain repair techniques may lead to possible tissue strangulation. Kim and colleagues[54] performed an animal study using immunofluorescence to detect postrepair perfusion and found inferior repair site perfusion in suture bridge technique compared to transosseous repair. One clinical study also noted the reduction in blood flow after suture bridge technique fixation and suggested that the resulting ischemia may be responsible for the type 2 medial row failures.[55] Finally, arthroscopic rotator cuff repairs performed via a transosseous tunnel technique have been show to primarily fail at the bone–suture interface in biomechanical and clinical studies.[50,56,57]

TIMELINE OF RETEARS

It is important to know when rotator cuff repairs fail as this information can facilitate patient education, help manage patient expectations, and establish guidelines for therapists in the postoperative setting. Retears are more common in the early postoperative period as sufficient time is needed for the repaired tendon to heal to the footprint through the various stages of inflammation, proliferation, and repair. Once healed, it is unlikely for retears to occur. Kim and colleagues[58] studied 61 shoulders with rotator cuff tears following repair with single-row and suture bridge techniques and obtained an MRI preoperatively, 3 months postoperatively, and 1 year postoperatively. They determined that repairs that appeared healed at 3 months were unlikely to tear at 1 year, with their study having a total retear rate of 6.6%. Other studies, however, show that the healing process takes longer than 3 months, and repairs are still at risk for failure for up to 15 months. Koike et al[59] performed an animal study to determine the timeline from surgical repair to mature enthesis formation of the supraspinatus in rabbits. They found that only at 24 weeks was the extracellular matrix and collagen spatial orientation complete, but even at that time point, there was continued reorganization of fibrils. A meta-analysis performed by Chona et al[60] showed that the risk for retears increased up to 12 months after arthroscopic repair of medium and large full-thickness rotator cuff tears using single-row, double-row, suture bridge, and surface-holding techniques. After the 12-month period, the retear rate leveled out. Thus, it is likely prudent to develop a rehabilitation program that progresses patients throughout the duration of a year with return to full activity roughly at the 1-year mark.

IMAGING THE PRE- AND POSTOPERATIVE ROTATOR CUFF

The diagnostic imaging for evaluation of the rotator cuff has evolved over time due to a better understanding of the pathologic processes and the progression of rotator cuff tears, alongside advances in imaging techniques and modalities. Traditional radiographs are useful screening tools to evaluate whether bony elements, such as subacromial spurs or a calcific enthesopathy, may be contributing to pathologic processes of the rotator cuff. However, traditional radiographs are limited in their ability to adequately assess the quality and integrity of soft tissue structures. MRI and more recently ultrasound have filled this gap in soft tissue visualization and evaluation over the past few decades. Consequently, MRI and ultrasound have become the most frequently used modalities for diagnosis of rotator cuff tears given the consistent diagnostic accuracy of both modalities in the literature.[14,29,30]

Iannotti and colleagues[61] evaluated the glenohumeral joint and rotator cuff tendons of 91 shoulder MRIs of patients who subsequently had surgery. They compared the preoperative MRI images to intraoperative findings and found that a 1.5T MRI was 100% sensitive and 95% specific in the diagnosis of complete rotator cuff tears. Magnetic resonance arthrography (MRA) is another popular modality for the diagnosis of rotator cuff tears. It is able to distend the joint with contrast and considered to provide more information specific to labral pathology. An MRA allows one to see if intra-articularly placed contrast is able to extravasate through deficient glenohumeral joint structures like torn rotator cuff tendons, capsular defects, or ligamentous injuries. One study by Flannigan et al[62] performed noncontrast MRI and MRA on 23 patients followed by intraoperative diagnostic arthroscopy and, when comparing the sensitivities and specificities between the 2 modalities, found that MRA was superior to noncontrast MRI for evaluation of glenoid and rotator cuff pathology. De Jesus et al[63] performed a meta-analysis using 65 previous studies and compared the reported accuracy of noncontrast MRI, MRA, and ultrasound for detecting partial-thickness and full-thickness rotator cuff tears and found that MRA was superior to both MRI and ultrasound in sensitivity and specificity. There was no significant difference in the sensitivity or specificity between noncontrast MRI and ultrasound in the meta-analysis. Aside from MRI and MRA, the diagnostic accuracy of ultrasound has also been validated in several studies. A systematic review by Smith et al[64] found that ultrasound had a sensitivity of 0.96 and a specificity of 0.93 for full-thickness rotator cuff tears and a sensitivity of 0.84 and a specificity of 0.89 for partial-thickness rotator cuff tears. Despite the statistical benefit of MRA over noncontrast MRI and ultrasound, surgeons must weigh its superior accuracy against the added invasiveness/discomfort of a glenohumeral injection, the need for an experienced and skilled radiologist, and the risk of infection or allergic reaction to the contrast agent. Ultrasound has the benefit of low cost and dynamic evaluation of both tendon and muscle, but its diagnostic accuracy is very user dependent. Thus, many surgeons prefer to use noncontrast MRI as the workhorse for diagnosis of rotator cuffs given the low risk with high accuracy and patient satisfaction.

Imaging the postoperative rotator cuff is a lot more challenging as repaired tendons appear abnormal for a considerable amount of time on both MRI and ultrasound.[65] The repaired rotator cuff tends to have a higher signal intensity and appears thinner compared to a native uninjured tendon on MRI. It is also common to see a moderate degree of fluid signal within the subacromial space as this compartment communicates with the glenohumeral joint during surgery and for several weeks afterward until the repair has healed. Importantly, the person evaluating the postoperative imaging should be knowledgeable about the specifics of the index surgery given that some repairs cannot be repaired anatomically, and thus any postoperative imaging may appear irregular as a result of the surgery itself and not a retear. A true retear is typically seen as a full-thickness defect with separation between the site of repair and the retracted tendon. The gap is

TABLE 12-2. SUGAYA CLASSIFICATION FOR THE REPAIRED ROTATOR CUFF BASED ON MRI

TYPE	DESCRIPTION
Intact Repairs	
Type I	Cuff repair with sufficient thickness and low-intensity homogeneous signal
Type II	Cuff repair with sufficient thickness but area of partial high-intensity signal
Type III	Cuff repair with insufficient thickness (< 50%) but without discontinuity
Retears	
Type IV	Cuff repair with presence of minor discontinuities in 1 or 2 images
Type V	Cuff repair with presence of major discontinuities in more than 2 images

Adapted from Sugaya H, Maeda K, Matsuki K, Moriishi J. Repair integrity and functional outcome after arthroscopic double-row rotator cuff repair: a prospective outcome study. *J Bone Joint Surg Am.* 2007;89(5):953–960.

filled with fluid, which produces a high signal intensity that is most evident at the level of the repaired tendon.[66] Tendon healing vs retears can be accurately evaluated with MRI or ultrasound with good intra- and interobserver reliability, although ultrasound has been shown to be slightly less sensitive compared to MRI.[67] The ambiguity of the postoperative cuff evaluation has led authors to seek classification systems to standardize the radiologic findings of the postoperative rotator cuff. These have helped determine what findings are considered normal vs abnormal, which, in turn, has led to improved communication between researchers and surgeons.

Sugaya and colleagues[68] performed a prospective cohort study of 86 shoulders that underwent double-row technique repair of full-thickness rotator cuff tears. In this study, they described 5 types of T2-weighted MRI findings of postoperative cuff repairs, which has subsequently allowed surgeons to better communicate regarding postoperative cuff integrity evaluated with MRI. The classification system is outlined in Table 12-2, and an MRI example of the Sugaya type II repair is shown in Figure 12-3. This classification scheme possesses diagnostic value and improves communication as it has been shown to have very good interobserver reliability in several studies.[67,69] It is yet to be determined if Sugaya's classification system

Figure 12-3. Postoperative MRI scan image of supraspinatus tendon repair consistent with Sugaya-type classification. The image demonstrates an intact repair with sufficient thickness but area of partial high-intensity signal.

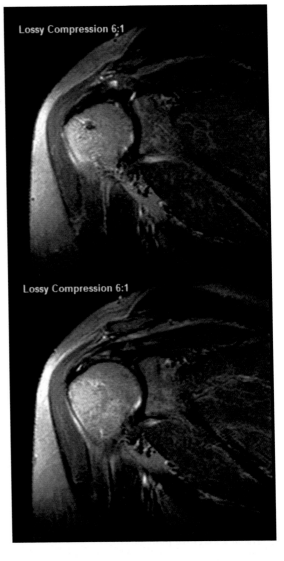

provides insight regarding patients' postoperative clinical results based on clinical outcome measures. Yoshida and colleagues[69] prospectively followed 62 patients who underwent arthroscopically repaired full-thickness supraspinatus and/or infraspinatus tears and performed MRI at 24 months postoperatively and found no correlation between Sugaya's classification and Constant outcome scores but did notice a correlation with abduction muscle strength in the scapular plane. Similarly, Malavolta et al[70] prospectively

TABLE 12-3. CHAROUSSET CLASSIFICATION FOR THE REPAIRED ROTATOR CUFF BASED ON CTA

STAGE	DESCRIPTION
Intact Repairs	
Stage I	Cuff repair that is watertight with anatomic healing (no leakage of contrast material into the SA bursa, perfectly healed tendon)
Stage II	Cuff repair that is water tight with partial defect healing (no leakage of contrast material into SA bursa, defective tendon healing in sagittal plane or defective deep-tissue healing)
Retears	
Stage III	Retear (leakage of contrast material into the SA bursa, FTT)

FTT, full-thickness tear; SA, subacromial.

Adapted from Charousset C, Grimberg J, Duranthon LD, Bellaïche L, Petrover D, Kalra K. The time for functional recovery after arthroscopic rotator cuff repair: correlation with tendon healing controlled by computed tomography arthrography. *Arthroscopy.* 2008;24(1):25–33.

followed 54 patients who underwent arthroscopically performed repairs for full-thickness supraspinatus tears who were evaluated with MRI at 3, 6, and 12 months and found no correlation with Constant and UCLA outcome scores but did see a correlation between classification type and visual analog scale (VAS) scores. Another classification scheme available that is used somewhat less frequently to evaluate postoperative rotator cuff repair integrity was proposed by Charousset and colleagues[71] and is based on CTA findings.[72] There are a total of 3 stages, with stages 1 and 2 considered globally as intact vs stage 3, which are considered retears (Table 12-3). To know whether Sugaya's, Charousset's, or some other classification scheme will be useful for predicting clinical outcomes remains to be seen. For now, they are a good starting point so that at least everyone is speaking the same language.

CLINICAL OUTCOMES OF RETEARS

Thus far in this chapter, the focus has been on the epidemiology, etiology, and diagnostics of retears, but one important question remains: *do retears even matter?* Sure, a retear strikes a moderate blow to the surgeon's technical ego and another thud to the patient's psyche, but do patients with retears fare worse clinically compared to their healed counterparts? Several studies show improved postoperative shoulder strength, range of motion, and functional outcome after arthroscopic rotator cuff repair compared to preoperative values, regardless of whether the repair remains intact or fails postoperatively.[22,23,26,27] However, these same studies also report that there are significant differences in clinical outcomes between patients when they are subdivided into healed and retear subgroups. The healed groups in each study consistently scored statistically significantly better in functional outcome measures. These outcome scores included the Constant, the American Shoulder and Elbow Surgeons (ASES), and the UCLA shoulder scores. Aside from outcome measures, objective physical examination findings like shoulder abduction strength are also superior in the healed groups compared to the retear groups. Meanwhile, the difference in pain relief between healed and retear groups is inconsistent throughout the literature while statistically significant differences in range of motion have not been shown between healed and retear groups. Yang et al[72] performed a large meta-analysis with strict inclusion and exclusion criteria that included 29 primary articles with over 5000 patients and compared several outcome metrics between patients with a structurally intact repair vs those with a full-thickness retear. They found that the intact repair group had higher ASES, Constant, and UCLA scores and better shoulder abduction strength compared to the full-thickness group; these findings were statistically significant. The only measure that was noted not to differ between the groups was pain relief. These findings are not only consistent throughout several studies but also persistent over time. Heuberer et al[73] found that Constant scores, particularly in the strength subscore, remained significantly higher in patients with intact repairs at 10 years compared to patients with retears. This is an important finding as the literature on long-term repair integrity is scarce, and few involve evaluation with high-accuracy diagnostic imaging like MRI.

There is clear statistical evidence that by and large, healed repairs have better functional outcomes compared to retears. Nevertheless, and as mentioned previously, postoperative clinical measures of patients with retears after arthroscopic repair are still better compared to preoperative values. This information argues that patients who undergo arthroscopic rotator cuff repairs do better than nonoperative patients, regardless of whether the repairs remain structurally intact or not at follow-up. Dodson and colleagues[74] evaluated 13 shoulders with known retears at an average follow-up of 7.9 years. They found that functional outcomes measures, such as the ASES, L'Insalata, and Simple Shoulder Test (SST), were similar at long- and short-term follow-up and overall improved compared to preoperative outcome scores.[74] The tear size was noted to increase over time, although pain scores did not differ significantly. Predictably, shoulder abduction strength was significantly weaker in patients with retears compared to those without.

The suspicion of a rotator cuff retear after surgery should initiate a thorough workup, including a detailed physical examination and imaging to include radiographs and some form of advanced imaging, whether it be CTA, MRI, or ultrasound. If confirmed, an important discussion should be had between patient and surgeon to decide how best to move forward. Several factors need to be considered when determining if a revision surgery is appropriate. A few critical ones include the patient's willingness to undergo a revision surgery, the patient's ability to tolerate a revision surgery from a general health standpoint, the ability to adequately follow postoperative rehabilitation protocols, and the probable success of a revision surgery. After weighing all options, an appropriate plan is to be developed. If nonoperative management is chosen, future care may consist of a physical therapy rehabilitation program, nonsteroidal anti-inflammatory medicine, steroid injections, and close follow-up to monitor for degenerative changes that may occur secondary to a nonfunctional rotator cuff. If operative management is chosen, there are several options based on the current biological state of the patient's shoulder. These include the rotator cuff tendon quality and amount of retraction, how many tendons are involved, the presence of muscle atrophy, glenoid and humeral bone quality, concomitant labral or ligamentous pathology, and the presence and/or degree of glenohumeral chondromalacia. It is important that patients are made aware that, like many other types of revision surgeries, a revision rotator cuff repair typically has worse outcomes when compared to a primary procedure. Shamsudin et al[75] compared arthroscopically performed primary vs revision rotator cuff repairs and found that the primary group had significantly better pain relief, range of motion, and shoulder strength at 2-year follow-up. Interestingly, preoperative shoulder satisfaction was higher in revision cases vs primary ones, again demonstrating a postoperative benefit in surgically treated patients even when they required a reoperation. Not surprisingly, the retear rate was higher in the revision group, 21% vs 40%, but it is important to note that this group was significantly older and had larger tears compared to the primary group. Despite the inferior outcomes in patients with revision surgeries compared to primary ones, the revision patients still achieved improvements in pain relief and overall shoulder satisfaction compared to their prerevision baseline.

SURGICAL OPTIONS AND RESPECTIVE OUTCOMES FOR RETEARS

A revision arthroscopic repair of a retear after a primary arthroscopic or open primary rotator cuff repair is challenging. Typically, this is due to factors that are inherent to any type of revision surgery, which includes distorted anatomy due to the primary surgery, scar tissue deposition, and hardware interference left over from the previous surgery, which affects both visualization and available "real estate" within the repair surface area. One must also consider the increased operative time spent on previously placed implants that necessitate removal during the revision procedure. Challenges specific to rotator cuff rerepairs are tendon quality, degree of tendon retraction, fatty muscle atrophy, size of tendon retear, and difficulty with visualization of the anterior and posterior cuff leaflets as they are typically scarred and adhered to bursal tissue and deltoid fibers. From a technical standpoint, one's ability to perform a double-row repair in revision cases is unpredictable and less likely to occur as often the tendons are shorter and the remaining medial leaflets are in close proximity to the musculotendinous junction. Traditionally, revision repairs were performed as open procedures, but the advancement of arthroscopic techniques and technology has led more surgeons to employ arthroscopic methods in revision cases. There are several advantages that arthroscopy may provide over open techniques, which include improved visualization that allows a more detailed and thorough assessment of intra-articular pathology, the ability to operate in multiple planes and angles, decreased surgical trauma to the soft tissues, and smaller incisions. Disadvantages include fewer fixation options, complications due to fluid extravasation, and more difficulty with tendon mobilization.

Despite facing these challenges in a compromised biologic environment, arthroscopically performed revision repair of rotator cuff retears has been shown to provide significant pain relief and functional outcomes that are superior to that found in patients with retears preoperatively. One of the first studies to look at functional outcomes in patients after arthroscopic revision rotator cuff repair was a case series by Lo and Burkhart.[76] Their study included 14 patients with large retears diagnosed via clinical symptoms and MRI. Importantly, 11 of the total 14 retears were massive and only amenable to single-row repairs. They found statistically significant improvements in UCLA, pain scores, overall shoulder function scores, and shoulder range of motion, including forward flexion and external rotation, at a minimum of 2-year follow-up. In another study, Piasecki et al[77] performed a retrospective study of 54 shoulders with full-thickness retears of one or more tendons. They were able to arthroscopically repair 21 shoulders with double-row fixation, and the other 33 were with single row, with only 11% of revision cases deemed "failures," defined as patients who required additional surgical intervention within the follow-up period or if patients had an ASES score of 50 or less. It is important to note that patients were not evaluated with MRI or arthrography postoperatively unless clinically warranted. They found statistically significant improvements in several outcome scores, including ASES, SST, and VAS pain scale, along with improvement in forward elevation. Keener and colleagues[78] went one step further and, in addition to functional outcomes, also evaluated the integrity of revision repairs at 1 year using ultrasound of 21 shoulders. They were able to repair most retears using a double-row technique (18/21) while only a few (3/21) were repaired with a single-row technique, which is likely due in part to the fact that roughly half were only single-tendon retears. They found improved Constant, SST, and VAS pain scores as well as increased range of motion in active forward flexion and external rotation postoperatively. The revision retear rate was found to be 52% and was associated with the preoperative number of torn tendons and the patient's age. The intact revision repair group had statistically significant better Constant scores and scapular plane abduction strength compared to the revision repairs retear group, which is consistent with findings in intact vs failure groups after primary rotator cuff repair.[72-74] The current evidence on outcomes after arthroscopic revision rotator cuff is somewhat scarce, but what is available suggests that revision repairs consistently improve range of motion, function, and pain despite a high retear rate at short-term follow-up. Additionally, revision repairs that remain intact benefit from larger improvements in abduction strength and functional scores. Thus, arthroscopic revision repairs are a good option in the hands of experienced arthroscopists when the tissue quality permits. Unfortunately, there are situations when revision cuff repairs are just not possible due to poor tendon and tissue quality. In these cases, one can perform tendon augmentation procedures, tendon transfers, or a superior capsular reconstruction (SCR).

Tendon augmentation procedures with allografts or autografts have shown promise when repairing large to massive rotator cuff tears when the available tissue is of poor quality. The thought is to use as much native tendon possible and then additionally incorporate a graft into the repair that will act as a scaffold for repopulation of native cells and collagen fibers. Barber et al[79] performed a randomized controlled trial of 42 patients with large (> 3 cm and 2 tendon involvement) primary cuff tears and found improved UCLA, Constant, and ASES scores in the group with a GraftJacket (Wright Medical) acellular human dermal matrix graft vs the group without an augment graft. The repairs were performed as a single-row technique, and the graft was augmented with an onlay technique. Additionally, the repair integrity of the graft group was 85% at the time of follow-up evaluated with gadolinium MRI vs 40% in the nongraft group. A biomechanical study using fascia lata graft supports these clinical findings as the authors found decreased gap formation and less failures after multiple testing cycles in human cadaveric repairs performed with patch augmentation vs those without.[80] Clinical studies have also shown success when using autografts, such as fascia lata and biceps tendon, for patch augmentation.[81,82]

When there is very little healthy rotator cuff tissue available for repair and what is left is highly nonmobile, an SCR can be performed rather than an attempted partial cuff repair with a patch graft. The idea of repairing the superior capsule comes from the belief that it helps maintain the humeral head centered "down and in" on the glenoid, and it provides a roof across the superior glenohumeral interval, preventing superior escape of the humerus. One important feature to recognize is that it likely does not provide any dynamic stability given the minimal or absent muscular attachments, but it does provide static stability in multiple planes. Mihata et al[83] performed a retrospective study on 24 shoulders with rotator cuff tears that were deemed irreparable, defined by the inability to move the tendon to the original footprint, and performed SCR using fascia lata autograft. They found that 83% of reconstructions remained intact at almost 3 years, and all outcome scores, including ASES, UCLA, and Japanese Orthopedic Association, were significantly improved compared to preoperative scores. Active range of motion was also significantly improved. Importantly, the acromial humeral distance was significantly higher postoperatively, showing that SCR is capable of preventing superior migration of the humeral head and helps keep the humeral head located within the glenoid. Other authors have used acellular dermal allografts to perform SCRs and have had similar success in patient clinical outcomes.[84,85] The promising data above pertain largely to SCR and patch augmentation in the setting of primary irreparable tears that are not amenable to traditional single-row or double-row repairs. Meanwhile, there are currently little to almost no data on outcomes specific to the use of SCR or patch augmentation in the revision setting. However, the tear characteristics of recurrent rotator cuff tears after previous repair and primary massive irreparable tears are similar in terms of tissue quality, tendon retraction, and fatty degeneration. Thus, one can hypothesize that some of the preliminary data on outcomes after SCR for primary massive tears might look similar when performing SCR or patch augmentation for revision surgery of failed primary repairs. The decision to perform an arthroscopic revision SCR or partial repair with patch augmentation procedure vs a reverse arthroplasty after a previously failed cuff repair is contingent on multiple factors. Age is important to consider as arthroplasty is traditionally reserved for older lower-demand individuals while arthroscopic repair is favored in younger active patients. The presence of glenohumeral arthritis is also important as its presence favors arthroplasty over arthroscopic repair or reconstruction. Finally, tendon transfers, including latissimus dorsi and pectoralis major, are large invasive procedures, which carry a high degree of morbidity and risk. The next sections will discuss the authors' decision-making process for when to repair or reconstruct, preferred treatments, and a useful algorithm for addressing patients with recurrent rotator cuff tears after previous arthroscopic primary repair.

AUTHORS' PREFERRED TREATMENTS

Many patients with retear of the rotator cuff can be successfully treated with nonsurgical methods. We use a rehabilitation regimen that de-emphasizes exercise of the torn tendons and focus primarily on dynamic stabilizers that remain intact.[86] Corticosteroid injection can be helpful, but we avoid repeat injection if relief is short-lived and if the patient is an otherwise good surgical candidate.

We prefer arthroscopic repair to open repair. The visualization of the anatomy and the pathology with a high-definition camera is unrivaled in comparison to the naked eye. We prefer double-row, transosseous equivalent rotator cuff repair of rotator cuff tears when possible. Our goal for every repair is to anatomically reapproximate the tendons to their insertions on the humerus without tension. Patients with small retears without retraction, good tissue quality, and good bone quality are good candidates for revision repair without tissue augmentation. Even larger, retracted tears are amenable to revision repair without tissue augmentation. If the tendon can be mobilized back without tension and the tissue quality is good enough to hold sutures, anatomic repair is straightforward. We always assess tension on the repair with the arm in adduction. We also perform a dynamic arthroscopic assessment of the repaired tendon after repair. Arthroscopic examination of the repair through passive range of motion prior to wound closure is a good predictor of the tears that will fail. If the tendon repair remains uncompromised during passive range of motion, it is likely to survive. On the other hand, if the shoulder needs to be abducted to alleviate tension on the repair, we find the possibility of retear likely.

In the setting of a retear, diagnostic imaging is helpful. However, the physical examination and the examination under anesthesia are critical to our decision making. Fixed superior subluxation of the head that limits passive shoulder elevation on physical examination bodes poorly for direct repair, patch augmentation SCR, or any other soft tissue procedure. We find the arthroscopic assessment of the tissue quality and retraction critical to deciding the surgical approach to revision surgery. Its worthwhile spending some time on arthroscopic assessment of the tear shape, the tissue quality, and mobility of the torn tendons. We find that many failed repairs are amenable to revision repair without augmentation. This is especially true if the original repair was performed in a nonanatomic manner. Many times in this setting, tissue of adequate quality remains present and healthy enough for primary repair. Margin convergence of longitudinal splits between the supraspinatus and infraspinatus is helpful in restoring the anatomy. When it is avulsed from the greater tuberosity, securing the anterior cable of the supraspinatus to its anatomic footprint is critical to repair survival under

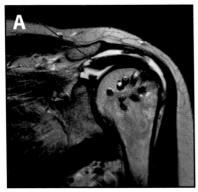 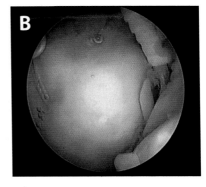

Figure 12-4. (A) MRI scan coronal image of a failed superior capsular reconstruction. The dermal allograft is no longer attached to the superior glenoid. (B) Arthroscopic image of failed glenoid anchor. The anchor has been dislodged from the glenoid. It remains attached to the dermal allograft and is floating within the glenohumeral articulation.

rotational loads. We prefer double-row, transosseous equivalent rotator cuff repair of rotator cuff retears when the tendon can be mobilized back without tension, the tissue quality is good enough to hold sutures, and the bone quality is good enough to hold anchors. When tissue quality is compromised but the tendon can be mobilized to the tuberosity without tension, augmenting the tendon with an onlay allograft patch can be effective.

Tensionless, anatomic repair of massive chronic retracted retears is sometimes impossible. For massive chronic, retracted tears/retears with poor tissue quality, with little to no radiographic evidence of arthrosis and good bone quality, we prefer SCR. The subscapularis tendon must be intact or at least capable of being primarily repaired for the SCR to survive. The most common location of failure for an SCR is on the glenoid at the anchor–bone interface (Figure 12-4). Hence, solid anchor fixation of the allograft tissue to the glenoid is critical to success. We use 3 anchors on the glenoid to secure a dermal allograft to the superior glenoid. We use a double-row, transosseous equivalent suture bridge technique to secure the dermal allograft to the greater tuberosity. Any tendon that can be repaired to the periphery of the dermal graft posteriorly is repaired using side-to-side stitches.

In the older patient with multiple medical comorbidities and persistent pain despite nonsurgical treatment, simple arthroscopic debridement can sometimes go a long way toward controlling pain.

CASE PRESENTATIONS

Case 1 (Figure 12-5)

This is a 49-year-old man following shoulder rotator cuff repair 12 years prior to recent recurrence of pain. He denies acute injury. Pain with activities of daily living persisted despite nonsteroidal anti-inflammatory drugs, activity modification, and physical therapy for more than 12 weeks. He denies acute injury at that time.

- **Active motion**: Forward flexion 180 degrees/abduction: 180 degrees/ external rotation: 80 degrees/internal rotation: T12
- **Scapular dyskinesis**: Positive
- **Passive motion**: External rotation motion is 90 degrees with the humerus at the side as well as abducted 90 degrees. Internal rotation is 40 degrees with the arm abducted. Active range of motion is less than passive motion, particularly in forward elevation and abduction.
- **Strength**: Deltoid 5/5, supraspinatus 4/5, infraspinatus 4/5

Provocative maneuvers/special testing:

- Neer's impingement maneuver: Positive
- Hawkins impingement maneuver: Positive
- Cross-chest adduction pain testing: Negative
- Speed test: Positive
- O'Brien's maneuver/adduction compression test: Negative
- Yergason's test: Negative
- Liftoff test: Equivocal
- Belly press test/abdominal compression test: Negative
- External rotation lag sign: Negative
- Drop arm test: Negative
- Bear hug test: Positive for pain

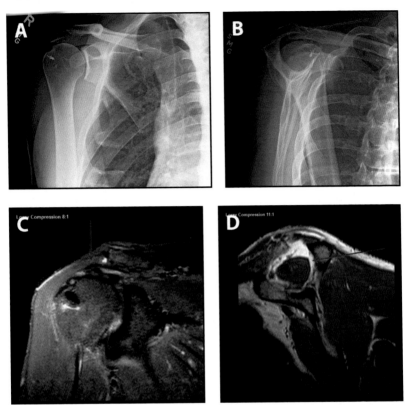

Figure 12-5. (A, B) Right shoulder radiographs. (A) AP Grashey view in external rotation revealing elevation of the humeral head relative to the glenoid with a metallic suture anchor in the greater tuberosity from a prior, failed rotator cuff repair. (B) The supraspinatus outlet view reveals extrinsic narrowing of the outlet secondary to type III acromion (red arrow). There is metallic suture in the greater tuberosity consistent with prior single-row rotator cuff repair. (C, D) Right shoulder MRI scan. (C) There is a full-thickness tear of the supraspinatus tendon with retraction. There is metallic suture anchor artifact in the greater tuberosity prior to repair. (D) There is mild supraspinatus muscle atrophy demonstrated on the sagittal T1-weighted image. *(continued)*

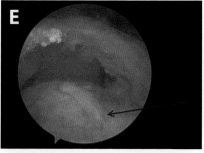
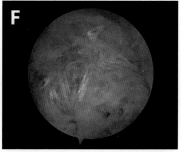

Figure 12-5 continued. (E, F) Arthroscopic images before and after revision repair without allograft augmentation. (E) Before: Image of a right shoulder full-thickness supraspinatus tendon retear viewed from the lateral portal in the beach chair position. Residual suture from the original single-row supraspinatus tendon repair is marked by the arrow. (F) After: A revision double-row suture bridge transosseous equivalent repair of the torn tendon was performed.

Case 2 (Figure 12-6)

Case 2 is a 62-year-old woman following primary rotator cuff repair 23 years prior to the recurrence of pain without trauma. Pain with activities of daily living persisted despite nonsteroidal anti-inflammatory drugs, activity modification, and physical therapy for more than 12 weeks. She complains of pain with arm elevation and reaching.

- **Active motion**: Forward flexion 120 degrees/abduction: 70 degrees/external rotation: 80 degrees/internal rotation: T12
- **Scapular dyskinesis**: Positive
- **Passive motion**: External rotation motion is 85 degrees with the humerus at the side as well as when passively abducted at 90 degrees. Internal rotation is 40 degrees with the arm abducted. Active range of motion is less than passive motion, particularly in forward elevation and abduction.
- **Strength**: Deltoid 5/5, supraspinatus 3/5, infraspinatus 4/5
  Provocative maneuvers/special testing:
  - Neer's impingement maneuver: Positive
  - Hawkins impingement maneuver: Positive
  - Cross-chest adduction pain testing: Negative
  - Speed test: Positive
  - O'Brien's maneuver/adduction compression test: Painful
  - Yergason's test: Negative

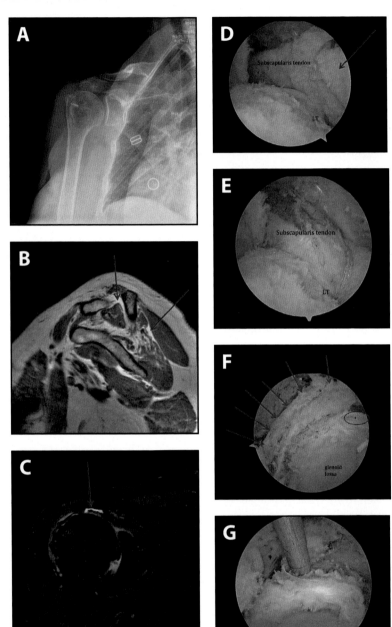

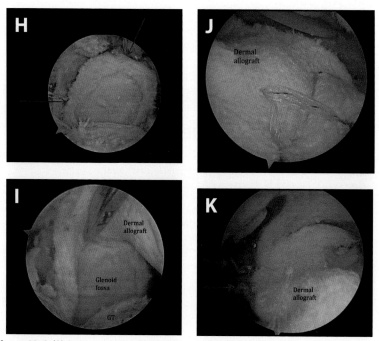

Figure 12-6. (A) Anteroposterior Grashey view in external rotation radiograph demonstrating a residual metallic suture anchor in the humeral head from prior single-row rotator cuff repair. (B) Right shoulder MRI scan: T1-weighted MRI scan, sagittal view of supraspinatus and infraspinatus atrophy. (C) Right shoulder MRI scan. T2-weighted MRI scan, coronal view of supraspinatus tear with retraction and elevation of the humeral head relative to the glenoid. (D) Arthroscopic view of right shoulder viewed from the subacromial space through lateral portal in the beach chair position. The subscapularis is partially torn from the lesser tuberosity (LT). (E) Arthroscopic view of right shoulder viewed from the subacromial space through lateral portal in the beach chair position. The subscapularis tendon repaired to the lesser tuberosity with a suture anchor. (F) Arthroscopic view of right shoulder viewed from the subacromial space through the lateral portal in the beach chair position demonstrating a massive, chronic supraspinatus and infraspinatus retear with retraction to the level of the glenoid (red arrows) after biceps tenotomy.* (G) Arthroscopic view of right shoulder viewed from the subacromial space through the lateral portal in the beach chair position demonstrating suture anchor insertion onto the superior glenoid. (H) Arthroscopic view of right shoulder viewed from the subacromial space through the lateral portal in the beach chair position demonstrating 2 of 3 suture anchors placed in the glenoid in preparation for fixing a dermal allograft patch to the glenoid. (I) Arthroscopic view of right shoulder viewed from the subacromial space through the lateral portal in the beach chair position demonstrating an allograft patch well fixed to the glenoid. A grasper is used to elevate the dermal allograft and inspect the fixation of the graft to the glenoid. (J) Arthroscopic view of right shoulder viewed from the subacromial space through the lateral portal in the beach chair position. The dermal allograft is fixed to the greater tuberosity with a double-row, transosseous equivalent suture bridge technique. (K) Arthroscopic view of right shoulder viewed from the subacromial space through the lateral portal in the beach chair position demonstrating a superior capsular reconstruction. The patch is fixed to the glenoid and the humerus. The residual cuff has been sutured to the posterior edge of the patch.

- Liftoff test: Equivocal
- Belly press test/abdominal compression test: Negative
- External rotation lag sign: Negative
- Drop arm test: Positive
- Bear hug test: Painful

REFERENCES

1. SDI. *Free-standing Outpatient Surgery Centers (FOSC) Database.* 2009. https://www.health.state.mn.us/data/economics/hccis/data/foscdata.html
2. Colvin AC, Egorova N, Harrison AK, Moskowitz A, Flatow EL. National trends in rotator cuff repair. *J Bone Joint Surg Am.* 2012;94(3):227–233.
3. Köse KC, Tezen E, Cebesoy O, Karadeniz E, Guner D, Adiyaman S, Demirtas M. Mini-open versus all-arthroscopic rotator cuff repair: comparison of the operative costs and the clinical outcomes. *Adv Ther.* 2008;25(3):249–259.
4. Severud EL, Ruotolo C, Abbott DD, Nottage WM. All-arthroscopic versus mini-open rotator cuff repair: a long-term retrospective outcome comparison. *Arthroscopy.* 2003;19(3):234–238.
5. Yamaguchi K, Levine WN, Marra G, Galatz LM, Klepps S, Flatow EL. Transitioning to arthroscopic rotator cuff repair: the pros and cons. *Instr Course Lect.* 2003;52:81–92.
6. DeFranco MJ, Bershadsky B, Ciccone J, Yum JK, Iannotti JP. Functional outcome of arthroscopic rotator cuff repairs: a correlation of anatomic and clinical results. *J Shoulder Elbow Surg.* 2007;16(6):759–765.
7. Bhatia S, Greenspoon JA, Horan MP, Warth RJ, Millett PJ. Two-year outcomes after arthroscopic rotator cuff repair in recreational athletes older than 70 years. *Am J Sports Med.* 2015;43(7):1737–1742.
8. Novoa-Boldo A, Gulotta LV. Expectations following rotator cuff surgery. *Curr Rev Musculoskelet Med.* 2018;11(1):162–166.
9. Calvert PT, Packer NP, Stoker DJ, Bayley JIL, Kessel L. Arthrography of the shoulder after operative repair of the torn rotator cuff. *J Bone Joint Surg Br.* 1986;68:147–150.
10. Gazielly DF, Gleyze P, Montagnon C. Functional and anatomical results after rotator cuff repair. *Clin Orthop Rel Res.* 1994;304:43–53.
11. Cho NS, Yi JW, Lee BG, Rhee YG. Retear patterns after arthroscopic rotator cuff repair: single-row versus suture bridge technique. *Am J Sports Med.* 2010;38(4):664–671.
12. Saccomanno MF, Sircana G, Cazzato G, Donati F, Randelli P, Milano G. Prognostic factors influencing the outcome of rotator cuff repair: a systematic review. *Knee Surg Sports Traumatol Arthrosc.* 2016;24(12):3809–3819.
13. Jain NB, Wilcox RB, Katz JN, Higgins LD. Clinical examination of the rotator cuff. *PM R.* 2013;5(1):45–56.
14. Nazarian LN, Jacobson JA, Benson CB, et al. Imaging algorithms for evaluating suspected rotator cuff disease: Society of Radiologists in Ultrasound consensus conference statement. *Radiology.* 2013;267(2):589–595.
15. Provencher MT, Kercher JS, Galatz LM, ElAttrache NS, Franke RM, Cole BJ. Evolution of rotator cuff repair techniques: are our patients really benefitting? *AAOS Instructions Course Lecture.* 2011;60:123–136.
16. Keener JD. Revision rotator cuff repair. *Clin Sports Med.* 2012;31(4):713–725.
17. Sambandam SN, Khanna V, Gul A, Mounasamy V. Rotator cuff tears: an evidence based approach. *World J Orthop.* 2015;6(11):902–918.

18. Yamaguchi K, Ditsios K, Middleton WD, Hildebolt CF, Galatz LM, Teefey SA. The demographic and morphological features of rotator cuff disease: a comparison of asymptomatic and symptomatic shoulders. *J Bone Joint Surg Am.* 2006;88(8):1699–1704.
19. Teunis T, Lubberts B, Reilly BT, Ring D. A systematic review and pooled analysis of the prevalence of rotator cuff disease with increasing age. *J Shoulder Elbow Surg.* 2014;23(12):1913–1921.
20. Cho NS, Yi JW, Lee BG, Rhee YG. Retear patterns after arthroscopic rotator cuff repair: single-row versus suture bridge technique. *Am J Sports Med.* 2010;38(4):664–671.
21. Kim KC, Shin HD, Cha SM, Park JY. Comparisons of retear patterns for 3 arthroscopic rotator cuff repair methods. *Am J Sports Med.* 2014;42(3):558–565.
22. Cho NS, Lee BG, Rhee YG. Arthroscopic rotator cuff repair using a suture bridge technique: is the repair integrity actually maintained? *Am J Sports Med.* 2011;39(10):2108–2116.
23. Mihata T, Watanabe C, Fukunishi K, Ohue M, Tsujimura T, Fujiwara K, Kinoshita M. Functional and structural outcomes of single-row versus double-row versus combined double-row and suture-bridge repair for rotator cuff tears. *Am J Sports Med.* 2011;39(10):2091–2098.
24. Miller BS, Downie BK, Kohen RB, et al. When do rotator cuff repairs fail? Serial ultrasound examination after arthroscopic repair of large and massive rotator cuff tears. *Am J Sports Med.* 2011;39(10):2064–2070.
25. Lee YS, Jeong JY, Park CD, Kang SG, Yoo JC. Evaluation of the risk factors for a rotator cuff retear after repair surgery. *Am J Sports Med.* 2017;45(8):1755–1761.
26. Boileau P, Brassart N, Watkinson DJ, Carles M, Hatzidakis AM, Krishnan SG. Arthroscopic repair of full-thickness tears of the supraspinatus: does the tendon really heal? *J Bone Joint Surg Am.* 2005;87(6):1229–1240.
27. Lafosse L, Brzoska R, Toussaint B, Gobezie R. The outcome and structural integrity of arthroscopic rotator cuff repair with use of the double-row suture anchor technique. *J Bone Joint Surg Am.* 2008;90(suppl 2, pt 2):275–286.
28. Galatz LM, Ball CM, Teefey SA, Middleton WD, Yamaguchi K. The outcome and repair integrity of completely arthroscopically repaired large and massive rotator cuff tears. *J Bone Joint Surg Am.* 2004;86(2):219–224.
29. Read JW, Perko M. Shoulder ultrasound: diagnostic accuracy for impingement syndrome, rotator cuff tear, and biceps tendon pathology. *J Shoulder Elbow Surg.* 1998;7(3):264–271.
30. Naqvi GA, Jadaan M, Harrington P. Accuracy of ultrasonography and magnetic resonance imaging for detection of full thickness rotator cuff tears. *Int J Shoulder Surg.* 2009;3(4):94–97.
31. Tashjian RZ, Hollins AM, Kim HM, et al. Factors affecting healing rates after arthroscopic double-row rotator cuff repair. *Am J Sports Med.* 2010;38(12):2435–2442.
32. Rashid MS, Cooper C, Cook J, et al. Increasing age and tear size reduce rotator cuff repair healing rate at 1 year. *Acta Orthop.* 2017;88(6):606–611.
33. Chung SW, Oh JH, Gong HS, Kim JY, Kim SH. Factors affecting rotator cuff healing after arthroscopic repair: osteoporosis as one of the independent risk factors. *Am J Sports Med.* 2011;39(10):2099–2107.
34. Meyer DC, Wieser K, Farshad M, Gerber C. Retraction of supraspinatus muscle and tendon as predictors of success of rotator cuff repair. *Am J Sports Med.* 2012;40(10):2242–2247.
35. Kim DH, Jang YH, Choi YE, Lee HR, Kim SH. Evaluation of repair tension in arthroscopic rotator cuff repair: does it really matter to the integrity of the rotator cuff? *Am J Sports Med.* 2016;44(11):2807–2812.

36. Consolino CM, Brooks SV. Susceptibility to sarcomere injury induced by single stretches of maximally activated muscles of mdx mice. *J Appl Physiol (1985)*. 2004;96(2):633-638.

37. Gerber C, Schneeberger AG, Beck M, Schlegel U. Mechanical strength of repairs of the rotator cuff. *J Bone Joint Surg Br*. 1994;76(3):371-380.

38. Kim DH, Elattrache NS, Tibone JE, et al. Biomechanical comparison of a single-row versus double-row suture anchor technique for rotator cuff repair. *Am J Sports Med*. 2006;34(3):407-414.

39. Park MC, Tibone JE, ElAttrache NS, Ahmad CS, Jun BJ, Lee TQ. Part II: biomechanical assessment for a footprint-restoring transosseous-equivalent rotator cuff repair technique compared with a double-row repair technique. *J Shoulder Elbow Surg*. 2007;16(4):469-476.

40. Lee KW, Yang DS, Lee GS, Ma CH, Choy WS. Clinical outcomes and repair integrity after arthroscopic full-thickness rotator cuff repair: suture-bridge versus double-row modified Mason-Allen technique. *J Shoulder Elbow Surg*. 2018;27(11):1953-1959.

41. Behrens SB, Bruce B, Zonno AJ, Paller D, Green A. Initial fixation strength of transosseous-equivalent suture bridge rotator cuff repair is comparable with transosseous repair. *Am J Sports Med*. 2012;40(1):133-140.

42. Bisson LJ, Manohar LM. A biomechanical comparison of transosseous-suture anchor and suture bridge rotator cuff repairs in cadavers. *Am J Sports Med*. 2009;37(10):1991-1995.

43. Franceschi F, Ruzzini L, Longo UG, et al. Equivalent clinical results of arthroscopic single-row and double-row suture anchor repair for rotator cuff tears: a randomized controlled trial. *Am J Sports Med*. 2007;35(8):1254-1260.

44. Charousset C, Grimberg J, Duranthon LD, Bellaiche L, Petrover D. Can a double-row anchorage technique improve tendon healing in arthroscopic rotator cuff repair? A prospective, nonrandomized, comparative study of double-row and single-row anchorage techniques with computed tomographic arthrography tendon healing assessment. *Am J Sports Med*. 2007;35(8):1247-1253.

45. Duquin TR, Buyea C, Bisson LJ. Which method of rotator cuff repair leads to the highest rate of structural healing? A systematic review. *Am J Sports Med*. 2010;38(4):835-841.

46. Millett PJ, Warth RJ, Dornan GJ, Lee JT, Spiegl UJ. Clinical and structural outcomes after arthroscopic single-row versus double-row rotator cuff repair: a systematic review and meta-analysis of level I randomized clinical trials. *J Shoulder Elbow Surg*. 2014;23(4):586-597.

47. Bisson L, Zivaljevic N, Sanders S, Pula D. A cost analysis of single-row versus double-row and suture bridge rotator cuff repair methods. *Knee Surg Sports Traumatol Arthrosc*. 2015;23(2):487-493.

48. Meyer DC, Fucentese SF, Ruffieux K, Jacob HA, Gerber C. Mechanical testing of absorbable suture anchors. *Arthroscopy*. 2003;19(2):188-193.

49. Cummins CA, Murrell GA. Mode of failure for rotator cuff repair with suture anchors identified at revision surgery. *J Shoulder Elbow Surg*. 2003;12(2):128-133.

50. Reed SC, Glossop N, Ogilvie-Harris DJ. Full-thickness rotator cuff tears: a biomechanical comparison of suture versus bone anchor techniques. *Am J Sports Med*. 1996;24(1):46-48.

51. Tingart MJ, Apreleva M, Lehtinen J, Zurakowski D, Warner JJ. Anchor design and bone mineral density affect the pull-out strength of suture anchors in rotator cuff repair: which anchors are best to use in patients with low bone quality? *Am J Sports Med*. 2004;32(6):1466-1473.

52. Tingart MJ, Apreleva M, Zurakowski D, Warner JJ. Pullout strength of suture anchors used in rotator cuff repair. *J Bone Joint Surg Am.* 2003;85(11):2190–2198.
53. Millett PJ, Hussain ZB, Fritz EM, Warth RJ, Katthagen JC, Pogorzelski J. Rotator cuff tears at the musculotendinous junction: classification and surgical options for repair and reconstruction. *Arthrosc Tech.* 2017;6(4):e1075–e1085.
54. Kim SH, Cho WS, Joung HY, Choi YE, Jung M. Perfusion of the rotator cuff tendon according to the repair configuration using an indocyanine green fluorescence arthroscope: a preliminary report. *Am J Sports Med.* 2017;45(3):659–665.
55. Christoforetti JJ, Krupp RJ, Singleton SB, Kissenberth MJ, Cook C, Hawkins RJ. Arthroscopic suture bridge transosseus equivalent fixation of rotator cuff tendon preserves intratendinous blood flow at the time of initial fixation. *J Shoulder Elbow Surg.* 2012;21(4):523–530.
56. Zheng N, Harris HW, Andrews JR. Failure analysis of rotator cuff repair: a comparison of three double-row techniques. *J Bone Joint Surg Am.* 2008;90(5):1034–1042.
57. Aramberri-Gutiérrez M, Martínez-Menduiña A, Valencia-Mora M, Boyle S. All-suture transosseous repair for rotator cuff tear fixation using medial calcar fixation. *Arthrosc Tech.* 2015;4(2):e169–e173.
58. Kim JH, Hong IT, Ryu KJ, Bong ST, Lee YS, Kim JH. Retear rate in the late postoperative period after arthroscopic rotator cuff repair. *Am J Sports Med.* 2014;42(11):2606–2613.
59. Koike Y, Trudel G, Uhthoff HK. Formation of a new enthesis after attachment of the supraspinatus tendon: a quantitative histologic study in rabbits. *J Orthop Res.* 2005;23(6):1433–1440.
60. Chona DV, Lakomkin N, Lott A, et al. The timing of retears after arthroscopic rotator cuff repair. *J Shoulder Elbow Surg.* 2017;26(11):2054–2059.
61. Iannotti JP, Zlatkin MB, Esterhai JL, Kressel HY, Dalinka MK, Spindler KP. Magnetic resonance imaging of the shoulder: sensitivity, specificity, and predictive value. *J Bone Joint Surg Am.* 1991;73(1):17–29.
62. Flannigan B, Kursunoglu-Brahme S, Snyder S, Karzel R, Del Pizzo W, Resnick D. MR arthrography of the shoulder: comparison with conventional MR imaging. *AJR Am J Roentgenol.* 1990;155(4):829–832
63. de Jesus JO, Parker L, Frangos AJ, Nazarian LN. Accuracy of MRI, MR arthrography, and ultrasound in the diagnosis of rotator cuff tears: a meta-analysis. *AJR Am J Roentgenol.* 2009;192(6):1701–1707.
64. Smith TO, Back T, Toms AP, Hing CB. Diagnostic accuracy of ultrasound for rotator cuff tears in adults: a systematic review and meta-analysis. *Clin Radiol.* 2011;66(11):1036–1048.
65. Crim J, Burks R, Manaster BJ, Hanrahan C, Hung M, Greis P. Temporal evolution of MRI findings after arthroscopic rotator cuff repair. *AJR Am J Roentgenol.* 2010;195(6):1361–1366.
66. Lee SC, Williams D, Endo Y. The repaired rotator cuff: MRI and ultrasound evaluation. *Curr Rev Musculoskelet Med.* 2018;11(1):92–101.
67. Collin P, Yoshida M, Delarue A, Lucas C, Jossaume T, Lädermann A; French Society for Shoulder and Elbow (SOFEC). Evaluating postoperative rotator cuff healing: prospective comparison of MRI and ultrasound. *Orthop Traumatol Surg Res.* 2015;101(6)(suppl):S265–S268.
68. Sugaya H, Maeda K, Matsuki K, Moriishi J. Repair integrity and functional outcome after arthroscopic double-row rotator cuff repair: a prospective outcome study. *J Bone Joint Surg Am.* 2007;89(5):953–960.

69. Yoshida M, Collin P, Josseaume T, et al. Post-operative rotator cuff integrity, based on Sugaya's classification, can reflect abduction muscle strength of the shoulder. *Knee Surg Sports Traumatol Arthrosc.* 2018;26(1):161–168.

70. Malavolta EA, Assunção JH, Ramos FF, et al. Serial structural MRI evaluation of arthroscopy rotator cuff repair: does Sugaya's classification correlate with the postoperative clinical outcomes? *Arch Orthop Trauma Surg.* 2016;136(6):791–797.

71. Charousset C, Grimberg J, Duranthon LD, Bellaïche L, Petrover D, Kalra K. The time for functional recovery after arthroscopic rotator cuff repair: correlation with tendon healing controlled by computed tomography arthrography. *Arthroscopy.* 2008;24(1):25–33.

72. Yang J Jr, Robbins M, Reilly J, Maerz T, Anderson K. The clinical effect of a rotator cuff retear: a meta-analysis of arthroscopic single-row and double-row repairs. *Am J Sports Med.* 2017;45(3):733–741.

73. Heuberer PR, Smolen D, Pauzenberger L, et al. Longitudinal long-term magnetic resonance imaging and clinical follow-up after single-row arthroscopic rotator cuff repair: clinical superiority of structural tendon integrity. *Am J Sports Med.* 2017;45(6):1283–1288.

74. Dodson CC, Kitay A, Verma NN, et al. The long-term outcome of recurrent defects after rotator cuff repair. *Am J Sports Med.* 2010;38(1):35–39.

75. Shamsudin A, Lam PH, Peters K, Rubenis I, Hackett L, Murrell GA. Revision versus primary arthroscopic rotator cuff repair: a 2-year analysis of outcomes in 360 patients. *Am J Sports Med.* 2015;43(3):557–564.

76. Lo IK, Burkhart SS. Arthroscopic revision of failed rotator cuff repairs: technique and results. *Arthroscopy.* 2004;20(3):250–267.

77. Piasecki DP, Verma NN, Nho SJ, et al. Outcomes after arthroscopic revision rotator cuff repair. *Am J Sports Med.* 2010;38(1):40–46.

78. Keener JD, Wei AS, Kim HM, et al. Revision arthroscopic rotator cuff repair: repair integrity and clinical outcome. *J Bone Joint Surg Am.* 2010;92(3):590–598.

79. Barber FA, Burns JP, Deutsch A, Labbé MR, Litchfield RB. A prospective, randomized evaluation of acellular human dermal matrix augmentation for arthroscopic rotator cuff repair. *Arthroscopy.* 2012;28(1):8–15.

80. McCarron JA, Milks RA, Mesiha M, et al. Reinforced fascia patch limits cyclic gapping of rotator cuff repairs in a human cadaveric model. *J Shoulder Elbow Surg.* 2012;21(12):1680–1686.

81. Mori D, Funakoshi N, Yamashita F. Arthroscopic surgery of irreparable large or massive rotator cuff tears with low-grade fatty degeneration of the infraspinatus: patch autograft procedure versus partial repair procedure. *Arthroscopy.* 2013;29(12):1911–1921.

82. Sano H, Mineta M, Kita A, Itoi E. Tendon patch grafting using the long head of the biceps for irreparable massive rotator cuff tears. *J Orthop Sci.* 2010;15(3):310–316.

83. Mihata T, Lee TQ, Watanabe C, et al. Clinical results of arthroscopic superior capsule reconstruction for irreparable rotator cuff tears. *Arthroscopy.* 2013;29(3):459–470.

84. Burkhart SS, Denard PJ, Adams CR, Brady PC, Hartzler RU. Arthroscopic superior capsular reconstruction for massive irreparable rotator cuff repair. *Arthrosc Tech.* 2016;5(6):e1407–e1418.

85. Pennington WT, Bartz BA, Pauli JM, Walker CE, Schmidt W. Arthroscopic superior capsular reconstruction with acellular dermal allograft for the treatment of massive irreparable rotator cuff tears: short-term clinical outcomes and the radiographic parameter of superior capsular distance. *Arthroscopy.* 2018;34(6):1764–1773.

86. Kelly BT, Williams RJ, Cordasco FA, et al. Differential patterns of muscle activation in patients with symptomatic and asymptomatic rotator cuff tears. *J Shoulder Elbow Surg.* 2005;14(2):165–171.

13

Complications of Management of Superior Labrum-Biceps Complex Injuries

Gabriella Ode, MD
and Answorth Allen, MD

INTRODUCTION

The term *SLAP lesion* (superior labrum anterior posterior) was first described by Andrews et al[1] in 1985 in a series of 73 throwing athletes. The etiology of SLAP lesions is multifactorial. They are commonly the result of throwing, overhead sports, heavy lifting, fall on an outstretched hand, and other types of acute or repetitive trauma.[2] Multiple classification systems have been developed to classify SLAP lesions. Snyder et al[3] first described 4 subtypes of SLAP injuries. Type I lesions involve fraying and degeneration of the superior labrum with a normal biceps tendon anchor. Type II lesions have pathologic detachment of the labrum and biceps anchor from the superior glenoid with or without fraying of the superior labrum. Type III SLAP lesions are described as a bucket-handle tear of the superior labrum with a normal biceps tendon anchor. Type IV is an extension of the bucket-handle tear into the biceps tendon, with the torn biceps tendon often displacing with the labral flap into the joint. Type II SLAP lesions are the most common type, accounting for 55% of all diagnosed lesions. Maffet et al[4] subsequently

Thompson TL, ed.
Arthroscopic Shoulder Surgery:
Complications and Management (pp 221-245).
© 2022 Taylor & Francis Group.

described a subclassification of type II SLAP lesions that accounted for previously unclassified extensions of type II lesions. Type V lesions are Bankart lesions that extend into the superior labrum. Type VI lesions are a type II SLAP lesion with an unstable anterior or posterior labral flap and a bucket-handle tear. Type VII lesions are a type II SLAP lesion with extension into the middle glenohumeral ligament, resulting in an incompetent capsulo-ligamentous complex. Powell et al[5] later expanded on this to describe type VIII lesions (type II lesion with posterior extension), type IX lesions (type II lesion with circumferential extension), and type X lesions (type II lesion with concomitant posteroinferior labral tear). Morgan et al[6] also classified type II SLAP lesions without associated anterior instability, Bankart lesion, or anterior inferior labral pathology into 3 subtypes: type II-A, an anterosuperior type II SLAP lesion; type II-B, a posterosuperior type II SLAP lesion; and type II-C, a combined anterior and posterior type II SLAP lesion. They evaluated 102 of these lesions arthroscopically and noted that anterior types (II-A) were slightly more common (37%), followed by posterior (31%) and combined anterior and posterior (31%). Regardless of the classification, the relevant issue for clinicians who are treating SLAP lesions is the stability of the biceps anchor and the presence of associated pathology.

EPIDEMIOLOGY

SLAP repairs are relatively common, accounting for approximately 6% of shoulder arthroscopies.[7,8] There have been generally accepted treatment guidelines for SLAP, depending on the subtype.[9,10] Type I lesions are treated with debridement of the degenerative labrum. Type II lesions can be treated with labral repair or biceps tenodesis/tenotomy. Type III and type IV lesions are treated with resection of the unstable bucket-handle labral fragment followed by biceps tenodesis or tenotomy if inspection of the biceps anchor reveals significant instability. The majority of literature on SLAP repairs is focused on management of type II SLAP repairs.[11-14]

REVIEW OF THE LITERATURE

Several studies have evaluated patient factors associated with poor outcomes following SLAP repair. The most commonly reported risk factors for poor outcomes were advanced age[13,15-17] and workers' compensation status.[12,15,17,18] Boileau et al[18] reported on 25 consecutive patients who underwent either SLAP repair (n = 10) with suture anchors or arthroscopic biceps tenodesis (n = 15). While the repair group had improvement in their

Constant score, only 20% were able to return to their previous level of activity compared to 87% of the biceps tenodesis patients. Additionally, 60% reported dissatisfaction with surgery due to persistent pain or inability to return to previous level of sports participation. Four patients with failed SLAP repairs underwent subsequent biceps tenodesis with resultant successful outcomes and full return to activity.

A recent systematic review on surgical treatment of SLAP injuries in patients older than 40 years with minimum 2-year outcomes demonstrated that patients over age 40 had significantly higher failure rates, decreased patient satisfaction, and increasing complications and reoperations than those who were younger than 40 years. Furthermore, postoperative stiffness and reoperation rates occurred at higher rates as patient age increased.[12] The combined literature demonstrated in this patient population that biceps tenotomy and tenodesis were reliable alternatives to SLAP repair in this patient population and should be considered both a primary treatment as well as a viable revision procedure.[12] Provencher et al[13] found a relative risk of failure of 3.45 in patients over age 36 years who underwent primary SLAP repair and concluded that reliable return to high-level activity was limited in patients over 36 who underwent SLAP repair. Overall, while both SLAP repair and biceps tenodesis can provide good to excellent outcomes,[19] appropriate patient selection is necessary to optimize outcomes.

Taylor et al[16] reviewed a national insurance database of more than 4700 patients who underwent arthroscopic SLAP repair and reported an overall 1.5% revision surgery rate. Regression analysis determined that risk factors for revision surgery included age older than 40 years, smoking, female sex, and obesity. However, a diagnosis of biceps tendinitis or long head of biceps tearing noted preoperatively or intraoperatively was the most significant risk factor noted, with odds ratios of 3.5 and 5.1, respectively.

ETIOLOGY

Some risk factors such as female sex, morbid obesity, and workers' compensation status cannot be mitigated. Patients should instead be informed of the presence for increased risk for revision surgery and worse outcomes due to these nonmodifiable patient characteristics. While age is not a modifiable risk factor for revision surgery, consideration should be given toward performing a biceps tenodesis instead of SLAP repair in patients over the age of 40 years who present with type II SLAP tears. Denard et al[17] reported higher rates of poor results in patients over the age of 40 years who underwent arthroscopic repair of type II SLAP lesions. Several studies have similarly recommended that SLAP repair should not be performed in individuals over age 40 years, and biceps tenodesis or tenotomy should be the preferred treatment in symptomatic lesions.[17,20] Tobacco use is another risk factor that can be modifiable. Cancienne et al[21] reported that tobacco use was associated with an increased rate of revision SLAP repair or conversion to biceps tenodesis as well as an increased rate of postoperative infection. Patients should be strongly advised against tobacco use before and after arthroscopic SLAP repair.

Various techniques for biceps tenodesis for management of isolated SLAP lesions or failed SLAP repair have been described.[22-25] These include open or arthroscopic approaches. The tenodesis can be placed proximal or distal to the bicipital groove. Different implants can be used for fixation such as suture only (soft tissue fixation), interference screws, suture anchors, and cortical buttons, among others.[26-30] Arthroscopic transfer of the biceps tendon to the conjoint tendon has also been described with good intermediate-term results.[31] Clinical studies have reported complication rates between 2% and 18% following biceps tenodesis.[32,33] A recent systematic review[34] of 7 level III clinical studies (n = 598 patients) comparing arthroscopic vs open biceps tenodesis demonstrated no significant difference between the 2 techniques in terms of patient-reported outcomes, patient satisfaction, and return to activity. The arthroscopic biceps tenodesis did have a slightly higher rate of complications related to fixation failure and postoperative stiffness. In another study of 6330 propensity-matched arthroscopic and open biceps tenodesis patients within the American College of Surgeons National Surgical Quality Improvement Program (ACS-NSQIP) database, there was a higher rate of adverse events following open biceps tenodesis (1.58% vs 0.95%), which included a higher rate of anemia-related transfusion (0.35% vs 0%).[35] In the case of failed biceps tenodesis, good results have been reported following either revision to biceps tenotomy or revision biceps tenodesis.[36,37]

SURGICAL COMPLICATIONS

After SLAP Repair

Postoperative Stiffness

Along with pain, postoperative stiffness is the most commonly reported cause of poor outcomes following type II SLAP repair.[9,12,38] Provencher et al[13] reported the outcomes of type II SLAP repairs in a military population and found significant decreases in shoulder forward flexion and abduction as well as an overall trend toward decreased postoperative range of motion in all patients. There was a 28% revision surgery rate in their patient cohort. Postoperative stiffness following SLAP repair can be caused by multiple factors. Tightening of the middle glenohumeral ligament, particularly in the setting of a closure of a sublabral foramen, has the unintended consequence of decreasing external rotation of the shoulder with the arm at the side.[14] Trans-rotator cuff approaches when the musculotendinous unit is violated during portal placement can also result in postoperative stiffness and pain.[39] If these portals are necessary, we would recommend access should be obtained through the muscle and not the tendon.

Another cause of postoperative stiffness is related to prolonged immobilization following arthroscopic repair. While surgical patients should have a period of immobilization to allow for healing, they should be directed on how to perform scapular stabilization exercises immediately postoperatively. Active motion can then be initiated within a pain-free range of motion after 2 weeks and then carefully progressed as tolerated. At 4 to 6 weeks, patients can begin more aggressive rehabilitation and progress as tolerated.

Persistent Pain

Persistent pain following SLAP repair can be multifactorial. Persistent pain may be the result of incorrect diagnosis of the SLAP lesion as the primary generator of pain in the shoulder. Many patients with SLAP lesions have concomitant pathology, including more distal biceps tendon lesions, partial- or full-thickness rotator cuff tears and impingement, glenohumeral internal rotation deficit, and acromioclavicular joint pathology.[14] Careful preoperative physical examination and adequate radiographic imaging are necessary to properly diagnose shoulder pathology. Pre/operative biceps tendon sheath injection using ultrasonography can be used to help distinguish intra-articular vs extra-articular biceps pathology.

Range of motion of the shoulder as compared to the uninjured side is paramount in order to rule out glenohumeral internal rotation deficit as a cause of pain similar to a SLAP lesion. At the time of surgery, visual inspection of the rotator cuff on both the articular and bursal side is important as well as inspection for impingement lesions and subacromial bursitis. Furthermore, thorough inspection of the biceps tendon both at the labral anchor and within the biceps tunnel is paramount to determining if concomitant biceps pathology exists that should be addressed. It is very difficult to evaluate the extra-articular portion of the biceps tendon arthroscopically. A subdeltoid approach can be used to open the biceps tendon sheath and inspect the tendon if there is suspicion of more distal biceps pathology. Extensive biceps tendon pathology and synovitis of the rotator interval are often encountered during reoperation following SLAP repair,[23] with some postulating improper diagnosis contributed to failure of the SLAP repair to relieve initial symptoms.[11]

Persistent pain can be the result of chondral injury after SLAP repair. Chondral injury can occur as the result of improper anchor placement, breakage or dislodging of implants, or biceps tendon abrasion from over-constraint of the biceps anchor. Park et al[40] reviewed a series of 11 patients with stable, healed SLAP tears who presented with knot-induced pain after arthroscopic fixation of unstable type II SLAP tears. Patients most commonly presented with sharp pain and clicking as well as tenderness in the bicipital groove. They noted that knots placed on the glenoid side of the SLAP lesion caused both glenoid cartilage damage and humeral head cartilage damage, as well as irritation and fraying of the articular side of the rotator cuff. These knots were most commonly placed in the 10-, 11-, and 1-o'clock positions of the labrum. All had pain relief and improvement in clinical outcomes with arthroscopic knot removal.[40]

Byram et al[41] evaluated humeral head abrasion associated with failed SLAP repairs. They found a humeral head lesion in 72% of patients with a failed SLAP repair and noted that this tended to occur in older patients and those with concomitant biceps tendinitis. They postulated that older patients with biceps tendinitis develop increased friction in the long head of the biceps during glenohumeral motion, and this friction limits the biceps motion, which may cause increased contact pressure on the humeral head. Ultimately, they suspected that SLAP repairs in this patient population overtension an already constrained biceps tendon, which leads to increased chondral wear on the humeral head and associated pain and joint stiffness, which contribute to failure of the repair.

Implant Failure

Implant failure is a complication of SLAP repair that is often associated with failure to heal of the SLAP lesions. Sassmannshausen et al[42] reported on 6 patients who had failed SLAP repair using poly-L-lactic acid bioabsorbable tacks. All patients presented with persistent postoperative pain, with magnetic resonance imaging (MRI) revealing a broken or dislodged tack and associated failure to heal of the SLAP lesion. In all cases, revision SLAP repair was performed with arthroscopic suture repair, and all patients had symptom relief at an average follow-up of 14 months. Katz et al[9] performed a descriptive analysis of 40 patients with poor outcomes following SLAP repair. Among these patients, 21 patients underwent revision surgery, of whom 4 of 21 (19%) had removal of loose suture material or prominent hardware.

Suprascapular Nerve Injury

Suprascapular nerve injury is a rare yet devastating complication of SLAP repair. There are reports of suprascapular nerve injury occurring during anchor insertion in SLAP repair. Yoo et al[43] presented a case report of an anchor inserted from the anterior glenoid rim through an anterosuperior portal, resulting in penetration of the spinoglenoid notch and subsequent suprascapular nerve injury. They postulated that an improper insertion angle and a starting point that was too posterior were the technical errors that led to the suprascapular nerve injury. Trusler et al[44] provided quantitative data on the angle of placement and location of anchors within the superior glenoid when performing repairs of type II SLAP lesions. From the axillary view, the angle formed with respect to the coronal axis should average 22 degrees for an anterosuperior anchor and 42 degrees for the posterosuperior anchor. Posterosuperior anchors with an insertion angle greater than 42 degrees can result in penetration through the glenoid into the spinoglenoid notch.

After Biceps Tenodesis

Popeye Sign

Popeye sign is a noticeable distal bulge of the muscle belly of the biceps that occurs in up to 5% of open biceps tenodesis and up to 15% of arthroscopic biceps tenodesis.[34] The presentation of a Popeye sign following biceps tenodesis is thought to be due to failure to restore the length-tension relationship of the biceps tendon or failure of fixation of the biceps tenodesis. Care must be taken to restore the normal anatomic length of the tendon at the level of fixation.

Previous anatomic studies have demonstrated that the mean biceps tendon length is approximately 25 mm from the origin to the humeral head articular margin, 74 mm to the upper pectoralis major, approximately 100 mm to the musculotendinous junction of the biceps tendon, and 120 mm proximal to the lower pectoralis major muscle.[45] Understanding these measurements, the optimal bone socket should be 25 mm from the articular margin for suprapectoral tenodesis. While subpectoral tenodesis fixation varies on the residual tendon following tenotomy, subpectoral tenodesis should always be performed at least 1 cm proximal to the lower border of the pectoralis major muscle with the elbow flexed to 90 degrees.

Persistent Anterior Shoulder Pain

Persistent anterior shoulder pain following biceps tenodesis is the most common complication, occurring in approximately 11% to 13% of patients.[46] McCrum et al[46] reported that persistent anterior shoulder pain following biceps tenodesis occurred more often after use of a soft tissue (suture-only) tenodesis technique and in patients who underwent biceps tenodesis for pain only instead of for structural issues. There was no difference in rates of anterior shoulder pain related to subpectoral vs suprapectoral techniques, anchor size following anchor fixation, and tunnel size following cortical button fixation.

Persistent anterior shoulder pain is usually localized to the bicipital groove and is typically attributed to mechanical failure of the biceps tenodesis, resulting in attenuations, tearing, or scarring of the biceps tendon distal to its fixation point.[47] Alternatively, persistent pain may be the result of failure to address associated shoulder pathology at the time of the initial surgery.[48] Some have argued that "hidden lesions," which are biceps tenosynovitis lesions that extend distally within the bicipital groove, are not addressed with suprapectoral tenodesis. An analysis of 36 retrieved biceps tendons following subpectoral tenodesis revealed that 80% had distal tearing that would have not been appropriately addressed with suprapectoral tenodesis.[49] Operative treatment in this setting involves revision biceps tenodesis or biceps tenotomy.

Postoperative Stiffness

A retrospective study of 249 patients who underwent open subpectoral vs arthroscopic suprapectoral biceps tenodesis revealed that arthroscopic suprapectoral tenodesis carried a higher rate of postoperative stiffness (17.9% vs 5.6%).[30] Risk factors for postoperative stiffness were female sex and smoking. It was postulated that a significantly more proximal location (32 mm from the top of humeral head vs 50 mm) correlated with postoperative stiffness in the suprapectoral group.

Brachial Plexus Palsy

Brachial plexus palsy is a rare complication,[50] but it is slightly more commonly reported in open subpectoral biceps tenodesis (~2% vs 0.2%). Most patients present with a transient neurapraxia that resolves within 3 months. During open techniques, care must be taken to avoid medial retraction during the exposure, which can place undue tension on the musculocutaneous nerve.

Fracture

Proximal humeral fracture is a rare complication after biceps tenodesis, occurring in 7.9 out of 10,000 cases.[51,52] Subpectoral tenodesis has a slightly higher incidence than suprapectoral tenodesis, with a reported incidence of 0.123% vs 0.085%.[46] Among reported fractures, most are torsional spiral fractures that have been successfully treated either nonoperatively with a functional brace or with operative plate fixation. A previous biomechanical study demonstrated that subpectoral biceps tenodesis performed with an interference screw imparted a higher risk of torsional humeral shaft fracture compared to the intact humerus. The size of the interference screw (6.25 mm vs 8.0 mm) did not appear to influence the fracture risk.[53] Other studies have not demonstrated a higher risk of fracture using interference fixation over cortical button or suture anchors.[51] Biomechanical studies have demonstrated that laterally eccentric malpositioned biceps tenodesis significantly weakened the humeral shaft (25%) compared to concentrically positioned biceps tenodesis.[54] Therefore, care should be taken to ensure that a concentric socket is made during subpectoral biceps tenodesis.

AUTHORS' PREFERRED TREATMENT

SLAP Repair

Our preferred approach for surgical management of SLAP lesions is dependent on the type of SLAP lesions. In accordance with previous literature, type I lesions are treated with arthroscopic debridement of the degenerative labrum in addition to addressing any concomitant glenohumeral or subacromial pathology encountered during diagnostic arthroscopy. Type II lesions are treated with labral repair or biceps tenodesis/tenotomy depending on the age of the patients, their physical demands and postsurgical needs, and presence of previously described nonmodifiable risk factors that could limit their ability to heal a labral repair (Case 1). For type II SLAP lesions, our preference is to perform a repair using a Neviaser portal through which a spinal needle is used to pass a nonabsorbable suture through the labrum, which is fixed with a knotless suture anchor. We avoid violation of the rotator cuff tendon during anchor placement.

Type III and type IV lesions are treated with resection of the unstable bucket-handle labral fragment followed by biceps tenodesis or tenotomy if inspection of the biceps anchor reveals significant instability (Case 2). If there is no significant pathologic involvement of the biceps anchor, then tenotomy/tenodesis is not performed. Following inspection of the unstable bucket-handle fragment, the remaining labrum is inspected for any instability. If there remains an unstable fragment following resection of the bucket-handle tear or if there is either anterior or posterior extension of the labral tear (types V to X), then a labral repair may be performed with or without biceps tenotomy/tenodesis to stabilize the labrum (Case 3).

Biceps Tenodesis

Biceps tenodesis is most commonly performed with either a supra-pectoral or subpectoral approach. Fixation options include use of anchors, interference screws, and unicortical or bicortical button fixation. If biceps tenodesis is to be performed, our preference is to perform an open sub-pectoral biceps tenodesis using cortical button fixation (Case 4). For this technique, biceps tenotomy is performed arthroscopically, and then a 3- to 4-cm incision is made just lateral to the axillary fold and just medial to the palpated pectoralis tendon with the arm in a slightly abducted position. Sharp dissection is taken down to the biceps fascia, which is incised in line with the humerus. Manual palpation through the longitudinal defect allows for localization of the biceps tendon within the bicipital groove. Once the tendon is identified, a large blunt Hohmann retractor is placed around the lateral border of the humerus for retraction of the pectoralis tendon. Placement of medial retractors is avoided to minimize risk of a transient neurapraxia on the brachial plexus. If better visualization is needed, then a blunt self-retaining retractor is placed superficially.

A right-angled clamp is inserted deep to the biceps tendon in the groove and used to deliver the tenotomized tendon. The tendon is further tenotomized approximately 20 to 25 mm proximal to the musculotendinous junction in order to maintain the optimal length-tension relationship after tenodesis. Heavy braided suture is whipstitched through the remaining tendon starting at the musculotendinous junction and exiting proximally. A bicortical drill hole is made approximately 15 mm from the inferior border of the pectoralis. A socket is made that corresponds to the diameter of the biceps tendon. We try to limit socket size to less than 6 mm to decrease the risk of a proximal humerus fracture.

Our preference is to use a distal biceps tendon cortical button as described by Snir et al,[26] which has a smaller-diameter drill hole than other manufactured proximal biceps buttons. The sutures are attached to the distal biceps button, which is passed through the posterior cortex and flipped. The tendon is then reduced into the socket. The residual sutures are tied in place with the elbow at 90 degrees of elbow flexion. In older patients, we avoid making sockets in the proximal humerus due to the potential increased risk of fracture. Our preference in this setting is an intramedullary unicortical cortical button for fixation.

CASE PRESENTATIONS

Case 1: Primary SLAP Repair (Type IIB)

History and Physical

The patient is a 30-year-old nonsmoking man who presents with 1 year of shoulder pain after sustaining a fall during snowboarding. He complained of mechanical symptoms as well as sensation of deep-seated shoulder pain. The patient is a nonsmoker and has no comorbid conditions. An outside MRI scan revealed a type II SLAP tear.

Physical Examination

- Range of motion full and symmetric
- Reproducible painful clicking on examination
- Positive O'Brien's test
- Negative apprehension/relocation
- Normal rotator cuff strength

Surgical Management

At examination under anesthesia, the patient had full range of motion of the right shoulder. Stability examination revealed a 1+ anterior drawer and trace inferior and posterior drawer. Using a standard posterior portal, diagnostic arthroscopy was performed. There was a complete detachment of the posterior superior labrum from the glenoid with a flap tear in the anterior portion of the labrum (Figure 13-1A). Additional diagnostic arthroscopy revealed a small partial-thickness articular tear of the supraspinatus. The subacromial space demonstrated no acromial spurring, subacromial bursitis, or bursal-sided rotator cuff tearing.

A decision was made to proceed with SLAP repair. An anterior portal was established through which the flap tear of the labrum was debrided (Figure 13-1B).

The undersurface tear of the supraspinatus tendon was also debrided (Figure 13-1C). The superior glenoid was debrided back to bleeding bone to create a good healing bed.

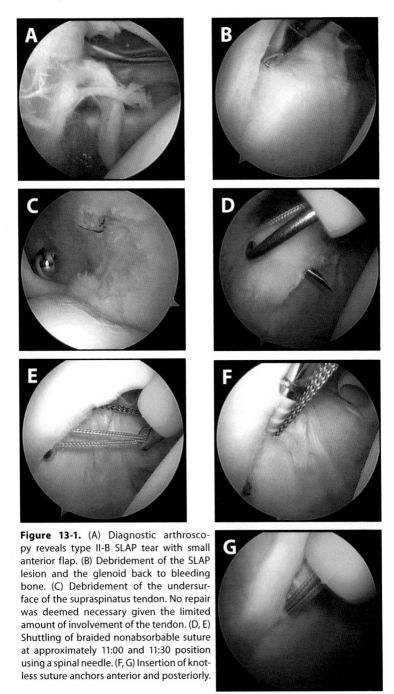

Figure 13-1. (A) Diagnostic arthroscopy reveals type II-B SLAP tear with small anterior flap. (B) Debridement of the SLAP lesion and the glenoid back to bleeding bone. (C) Debridement of the undersurface of the supraspinatus tendon. No repair was deemed necessary given the limited amount of involvement of the tendon. (D, E) Shuttling of braided nonabsorbable suture at approximately 11:00 and 11:30 position using a spinal needle. (F, G) Insertion of knotless suture anchors anterior and posteriorly.

Then, using a Neviaser portal, 2 sets of braided nonabsorbable sutures were shuttled through a spinal needle through the superior labrum at 11:00 and 11:30, respectively, taking care to avoid entrapment of the biceps anchor (Figures 13-1D and 13-1E). The 2 sutures were then placed in two 2.4-mm polyether ether ketone (PEEK) knotless anchors that were inserted to secure the biceps labral complex back to the glenoid (Figures 13-1F and 13-1G).

Following placement of the anchors, the labrum was probed and found to be stable. Further probing of the biceps anchor confirmed no restriction or overconstraint of the biceps tendon.

Case 2: Primary SLAP Repair (Type IV)

History and Physical

The patient is a 43-year-old right-hand–dominant man who works in high-rise construction and is very active with regard to boxing and weightlifting. He presented with 1 month of pain and weakness in his right shoulder in addition to mechanical symptoms. He had previously had mild symptoms that worsened after hitting a heavy bag during boxing training 3 weeks prior to presentation. Pain keeps him up at night. The pain is localized over the anterolateral aspect of his shoulder, and he has separate point tenderness over his acromioclavicular joint that preceded his current symptoms. A period of activity modification has not improved his symptoms; he is unable to exercise, and his symptoms are affecting his work.

Physical Examination and Radiographic Imaging

- Range of motion full and symmetric except for internal rotation—T8 spinal level on R vs T2 spinal level on L
- Minimal tenderness to palpation in the bicipital groove
- Moderate to severe acromioclavicular joint tenderness
- Positive O'Brien's test
- Positive Speed's test
- Pain with cross-body adduction
- Negative apprehension/relocation
- Normal rotator cuff strength
- Negative impingement signs
- MRI demonstrated complete detachment of the superior labrum extending into the biceps anchor (Figures 13-2A and 13-2B)

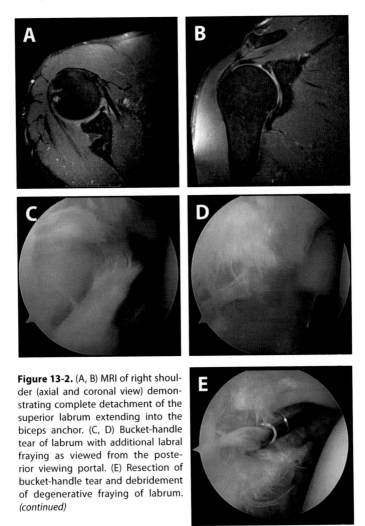

Figure 13-2. (A, B) MRI of right shoulder (axial and coronal view) demonstrating complete detachment of the superior labrum extending into the biceps anchor. (C, D) Bucket-handle tear of labrum with additional labral fraying as viewed from the posterior viewing portal. (E) Resection of bucket-handle tear and debridement of degenerative fraying of labrum. *(continued)*

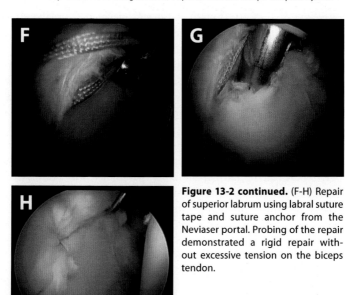

Figure 13-2 continued. (F-H) Repair of superior labrum using labral suture tape and suture anchor from the Neviaser portal. Probing of the repair demonstrated a rigid repair without excessive tension on the biceps tendon.

Surgical Management

On examination under anesthesia, the patient demonstrated full range of motion. Stability examination revealed grade 1 anterior drawer and trace posterior and inferior drawer.

Diagnostic arthroscopy through a standard posterior portal demonstrated a bucket-handle tear of the superior labrum with some degenerative tearing (type IV SLAP; Figures 13-2C and 13-2D).

Examination of the biceps tendon revealed mild tenosynovitis without any structural tearing. Additional diagnostic arthroscopy revealed mild articular surface tearing of the supraspinatus and infraspinatus with good overall tendon quality and no involvement of the bursal side. The distal clavicle appeared arthritic and osteolytic. Anteroinferior and anterolateral rotator interval portals were established. The bucket tear of the labrum was resected and the labrum was abraded back to a stable rim (Figure 13-2E).

The biceps tendon attachment point was elevated from the superior aspect of the glenoid but deemed repairable. A decision was made to proceed with SLAP repair without tenodesis of the biceps given the healthy appearance of the biceps tendon. The superior aspect of the glenoid was debrided back to bleeding bone. Using a Neviaser portal, a spinal needle was used to shuttle a simple stitch around the base of the biceps-labral complex using labral suture tape (Figure 13-2F). The tape was anchored with a 2.4-mm PEEK suture anchor at the 11:30 position to secure the labrum back to the glenoid (Figure 13-2G). Probing of the repair demonstrated a rigid repair without excessive tension on the biceps tendon (Figure 13-2H). Following the SLAP repair, all remaining shoulder pathology was addressed: the undersurface of the rotator cuff was debrided, the acromioclavicular joint was resected, and a complete subacromial bursectomy was performed.

Case 3: Primary SLAP Repair (Type VIII)

History and Physical

The patient is a 19-year-old female college softball player who complains of right shoulder pain. She had a remote history of trauma but subsequently developed pain after increasing workloads. A prior outside MRI scan showed evidence of a torn labrum. An ultrasound-guided glenohumeral injection allowed her to complete her softball season but did not provide long-term relief. Ultimately, she failed a prolonged course of supervised rehabilitation and was deemed a surgical candidate.

Physical Examination

- Range of motion full and symmetric
- 1+ sulcus sign
- Positive O'Brien's test
- Positive posterior stress test
- Negative apprehension/relocation
- Normal rotator cuff strength
- Negative impingement signs

Surgical Management

An examination under anesthesia was performed, revealing that the patient had 1+ anterior drawer, a 2+ posterior drawer, and trace inferior drawer. Diagnostic arthroscopy through a standard posterior viewing portal (Figures 13-3A and 13-3B) and then an anterosuperior viewing portal (Figures 13-3C and 13-3D) revealed complete detachment with fraying of the posterior labrum extending to 9:00 (classified as a type VIII). Superiorly, the labral detachment extended to 1:00.

The humeral head was centered slightly posteriorly associated with posterior capsular laxity (Figure 13-3E). There was some degenerative fraying of the articular side of the supraspinatus, which was later debrided (Figure 13-3F).

The glenohumeral cartilage appeared normal. Subacromial arthroscopy revealed no bursal-sided rotator cuff involvement or additional subacromial pathology.

To optimize viewing and working access to the posterior superior labrum, we would recommend creating an anterosuperior viewing portal, an anteroinferior working portal, and a lateral working portal. Through the anteroinferior portals, the labrum was debrided and elevated and the glenoid was debrided below the torn labrum (Figures 13-3G and 13-3H). Viewing from the anterosuperior portal, a suture passer loaded with polydioxanone suture was inserted in the posterior portal to perforate the posterior capsule and labrum from outside-in at the 9:00 position (Figures 13-3I through 13-3L). Setting the suture aside, a double-loaded 2.4-mm PEEK anchor with nonabsorbable braided suture was percutaneously inserted at the 9:30 position, and then the posterior labrum was repaired with a mattress suture configuration using the polydioxanone as a shuttling suture. This procedure was repeated with a second anchor placed at the 10:30 position.

The arthroscope was then placed back in the posterior viewing portal in preparation of the repair of the superior labrum. Through a Neviaser portal, a spinal needle was used to shuttle a nonabsorbable braided suture around the biceps-labral complex at the 11:30 position.

The suture was inserted into a 2.4-mm PEEK knotless suture anchor used to secure the biceps labral complex back to the glenoid, thus repairing the SLAP lesion (Figures 13-3M and 13-3N).

Further arthroscopic inspection revealed that the humeral head was recentered. The patient had a negative drive-through sign.

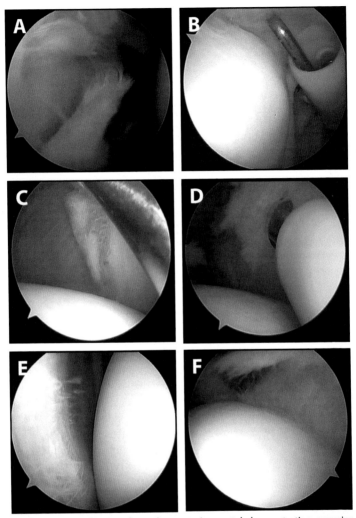

Figure 13-3. (A, B) View from the posterior portal demonstrating superior labral flap and extension of tear posteriorly. (C, D) Detachment of the posterior labrum and attenuation of the posterior capsule extending to 9:00 as viewed for the anterosuperior portal. (E, F) View from the posterior portal of the eccentric position of the humeral head posteriorly and undersurface fraying of a supraspinatus. *(continued)*

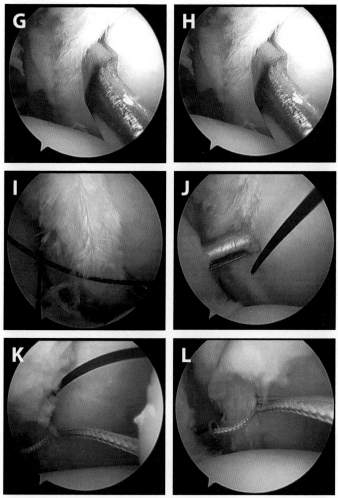

Figure 13-3 continued. (G, H) Elevation of the posterior labrum extending superiorly using an elevator. *Pearl—be sure that the elevator completely released the labrum all the way to the outer margin to ensure that the labrum is well mobilized enough to re-create a robust bumper. (I-L) Repair of the posterior labrum as viewed from the anterosuperior portal. *(continued)*

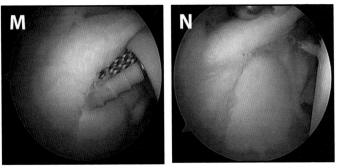

Figure 13-3 continued. (M, N) Repair of the superior labrum with PEEK anchor after shuttling suture with spinal needle. Final appearance of the repair.

Case 4: Open Subpectoral Biceps Tenodesis for Type II SLAP and Biceps Tendinopathy

History

The patient is a 50-year-old man who presents with 1 year of persistent left shoulder pain after lifting a heavy box at home. He complained of mechanical symptoms as well as a sensation of persistent deep-seated shoulder pain as well as intermittent sharp anterior shoulder pain. MRI scan (Figures 13-4A through 13-4D) revealed a type II SLAP tear (orange arrow) as well as biceps tendinopathy associated with increased fluid signal within the bicipital sheath (yellow arrow).

Physical Examination

- Range of motion full and symmetric
- Point tenderness at the bicipital groove
- Positive O'Brien's test
- Negative apprehension/relocation
- Normal rotator cuff strength

Surgical Management

At examination under anesthesia, the patient had full range of motion of the left shoulder. Using a standard posterior portal and an anterior working portal, diagnostic arthroscopy was performed. Arthroscopy confirmed the type II SLAP lesion associated with extensive tearing of the biceps tendon distal to the anchor insertion (Figure 13-4E).

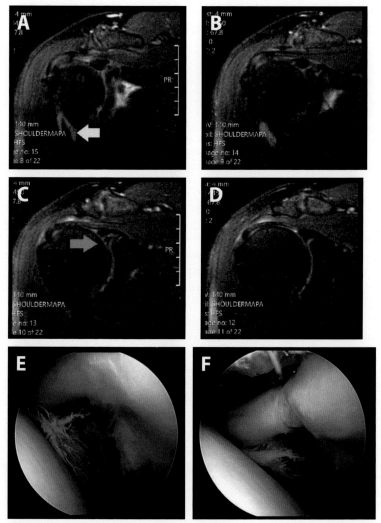

Figure 13-4. (A-D) MRI of shoulder demonstrates biceps tendinopathy associated with increased fluid signal within bicipital sheath (orange arrow) as well as an extensive degenerative SLAP tear (yellow arrow). (E) Extensive fraying of the biceps tendon distal to type II SLAP tear. (F) Arthroscopic tenotomy of the biceps using thermal ablation wand. *(continued)*

A decision was made to proceed with open biceps tenodesis to address both the SLAP lesion and the distal tearing of the biceps. The biceps tendon was tenotomized using a thermal ablation wand, and the frayed labrum was resected and debrided back to a stable rim (Figure 13-4F).

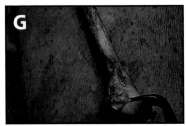 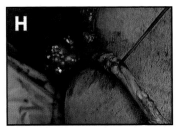

Figure 13-4 continued. (G) Retrieval of the biceps tendon through open anterior incision. Note extensive tearing of the biceps tendon distal to cauterized insertion. (H) Whipstitch of the biceps tendon starting at the musculotendinous junction and extending 20 mm proximally. The excess tendon after 20 mm will be cut.

The arthroscope was removed and fluid was drained from the shoulder. An approximately 3-cm anterior skin incision was made along the biceps deltoid junction. Dissection was carried down through the subcutaneous tissue, and the biceps fascia was incised. The long head of the biceps tendon was retrieved using a right angle clamp (Figure 13-4G).

A Krackow stitch was placed starting from the musculotendinous junction extending 20 mm proximally (Figure 13-4H).

The excess tendon was cut and removed. Bovie cautery was used to localize the docking point of the tendon within the bicipital groove. A bicortical drill hole was then made approximately 15 mm from the inferior border of the pectoralis. A 5-mm socket was made that corresponded to the diameter of the biceps tendon. The sutures were attached to the distal biceps button. The button was passed through the posterior cortex and flipped. The tendon was then reduced into the socket. The residual sutures were tied in place for additional fixation. This was accomplished with the elbow at 90 degrees of flexion. After thorough irrigation, the subcutaneous tissue, skin, and portals were closed and dressed and the patient was placed in a shoulder immobilizer for 3 weeks.

Conclusion

Management of SLAP lesions requires critical decision making, starting with the patients' history and physical examination. Careful diagnosis is essential to determine if patients will achieve optimal benefit from surgical treatment. Surgical management is contingent on both patient factors as well as the anatomy of the pathologic lesions. Thoughtful intraoperative decision making is necessary to determine if SLAP repair or biceps tenodesis will result in the most reliable recovery. Patients should be advised of the complications associated with SLAP repair or biceps tenodesis, and care must be taken to minimize these risks during surgery.

REFERENCES

1. Andrews JR, Carson WG, McLeod WD. Glenoid labrum tears related to the long head of the biceps. *Am J Sports Med.* 1985;13(5):337–341.

2. de Sa D, Arakgi ME, Lian J, Crum RJ, Lin A, Lesniak BP. Labral repair versus biceps tenodesis for primary surgical management of type II superior labrum anterior to posterior tears: a systematic review. *Arthroscopy.* 2019;35(6):1927–1938.

3. Snyder SJ, Banas MP, Karzel RP. An analysis of 140 injuries to the superior glenoid labrum. *J Shoulder Elbow Surg.* 1995;4(4):243–248.

4. Maffet MW, Gartsman GM, Moseley B. Superior labrum-biceps tendon complex lesions of the shoulder. *Am J Sports Med.* 1995;23(1):93–98.

5. Powell SE, Nord KD, Ryu R. The diagnosis, classification, and treatment of SLAP lesions. *Oper Techn Sports Med.* 2004;12:99–110.

6. Morgan CD, Burkhart SS, Palmeri M, Gillespie M. Type II SLAP lesions: three subtypes and their relationships to superior instability and rotator cuff tears. *Arthroscopy.* 1998;14(6):553–565.

7. Snyder SJ, Karzel RP, Del Pizzo W, Ferkel RD, Friedman MJ. SLAP lesions of the shoulder. *Arthroscopy.* 1990;6(4):274–279.

8. Handelberg F, Willems S, Shahabpour M, Huskin JP, Kuta J. SLAP lesions: a retrospective multicenter study. *Arthroscopy.* 1998;14(8):856–862.

9. Katz LM, Hsu S, Miller SL, et al. Poor outcomes after SLAP repair: descriptive analysis and prognosis. *Arthroscopy.* 2009;25(8):849–855.

10. Mileski RA, Snyder SJ. Superior labral lesions in the shoulder: pathoanatomy and surgical management. *J Am Acad Orthop Surg.* 1998;6(2):121–131.

11. Hester WA, O'Brien MJ, Heard WMR, Savoie FH. Current concepts in the evaluation and management of type II superior labral lesions of the shoulder. *Open Orthop J.* 2018;12(1):331–341.

12. Erickson J, Lavery K, Monica J, Gatt C, Dhawan A. Surgical treatment of symptomatic superior labrum anterior-posterior tears in patients older than 40 years: a systematic review. *Am J Sports Med.* 2015;43(5):1274–1282.

13. Provencher MT, McCormick F, Dewing C, McIntire S, Solomon D. A prospective analysis of 179 type 2 superior labrum anterior and posterior repairs: outcomes and factors associated with success and failure. *Am J Sports Med.* 2013;41(4):880–886.

14. Huri G, Hyun YS, Garbis NG, McFarland EG. Treatment of superior labrum anterior posterior lesions: a literature review. *Acta Orthop Traumatol Turc.* 2014;48(3):290–297.

15. Verma NN, Garretson R, Romeo AA. Outcome of arthroscopic repair of type II SLAP lesions in worker's compensation patients. *HSS J.* 2007;3(1):58–62.

16. Taylor SA, Degen RM, White AE, et al. Risk factors for revision surgery after superior labral anterior-posterior repair: a national perspective. *Am J Sports Med.* 2017;45(7):1640–1644.

17. Denard PJ, Lädermann A, Burkhart SS. Long-term outcome after arthroscopic repair of type II SLAP lesions: results according to age and workers' compensation status. *Arthroscopy.* 2012;28(4):451–457.

18. Boileau P, Parratte S, Chuinard C, Roussanne Y, Shia D, Bicknell R. Arthroscopic treatment of isolated type II SLAP lesions: biceps tenodesis as an alternative to reinsertion. *Am J Sports Med.* 2009;37(5):929–936.

19. Ek ETH, Shi LL, Tompson JD, Freehill MT, Warner JJP. Surgical treatment of isolated type II superior labrum anterior-posterior (SLAP) lesions: repair versus biceps tenodesis. *J Shoulder Elbow Surg.* 2014;23(7):1059–1065.

20. Weber SC, Martin DF, Seiler JG, Harrast JJ. Superior labrum anterior and posterior lesions of the shoulder: incidence rates, complications, and outcomes as reported by American Board of Orthopedic Surgery. Part II candidates. *Am J Sports Med.* 2012;40(7):1538-1543.
21. Cancienne JM, Brockmeier SF, Werner BC. Tobacco use is associated with increased rates of infection and revision surgery after primary superior labrum anterior and posterior repair. *J Shoulder Elbow Surg.* 2016;25(11):1764-1768.
22. Gupta AK, Bruce B, Klosterman EL, McCormick F, Harris J, Romeo AA. Subpectoral biceps tenodesis for failed type II SLAP repair. *Orthopedics.* 2013;36(6):e723-e728.
23. McCormick F, Nwachukwu BU, Solomon D, et al. The efficacy of biceps tenodesis in the treatment of failed superior labral anterior posterior repairs. *Am J Sports Med.* 2014;42(4):820-825.
24. Gottschalk MB, Karas SG, Ghattas TN, Burdette R. Subpectoral biceps tenodesis for the treatment of type II and IV superior labral anterior and posterior lesions. *Am J Sports Med.* 2014;42(9):2128-2135.
25. Gupta AK, Chalmers PN, Klosterman EL, et al. Subpectoral biceps tenodesis for bicipital tendonitis with SLAP tear. *Orthopedics.* 2015;38(1):e48-e53.
26. Snir N, Hamula M, Wolfson T, Laible C, Sherman O. Long head of the biceps tenodesis with cortical button technique. *Arthrosc Tech.* 2013;2(2):e95-e97.
27. Mazzocca AD, Rios CG, Romeo AA, Arciero RA. Subpectoral biceps tenodesis with interference screw fixation. *Arthroscopy.* 2005;21(7):896-896.e897.
28. Provencher MT, Leclere LE, Romeo AA. Subpectoral biceps tenodesis. *Sports Med Arthrosc.* 2008;16(3):170-176.
29. Mazzocca AD, Bicos J, Santangelo S, Romeo AA, Arciero RA. The biomechanical evaluation of four fixation techniques for proximal biceps tenodesis. *Arthroscopy.* 2005;21(11):1296-1306.
30. Werner BC, Pehlivan HC, Hart JM, et al. Increased incidence of postoperative stiffness after arthroscopic compared with open biceps tenodesis. *Arthroscopy.* 2014;30(9):1075-1084.
31. Taylor SA, Fabricant PD, Baret NJ, et al. Midterm clinical outcomes for arthroscopic subdeltoid transfer of the long head of the biceps tendon to the conjoint tendon. *Arthroscopy.* 2014;30(12):1574-1581.
32. Abtahi AM, Granger EK, Tashjian RZ. Complications after subpectoral biceps tenodesis using a dual suture anchor technique. *Int J Shoulder Surg.* 2014;8(2):47-50.
33. Nho SJ, Reiff SN, Verma NN, Slabaugh MA, Mazzocca AD, Romeo AA. Complications associated with subpectoral biceps tenodesis: low rates of incidence following surgery. *J Shoulder Elbow Surg.* 2010;19(5):764-768.
34. Hurley DJ, Hurley ET, Pauzenberger L, Lim Fat D, Mullett H. Open compared with arthroscopic biceps tenodesis: a systematic review. *JBJS Rev.* 2019;7(5):e4.
35. Gowd AK, Liu JN, Garcia GH, et al. Open biceps tenodesis associated with slightly greater rate of 30-day complications than arthroscopic: a propensity-matched analysis. *Arthroscopy.* 2019;35(4):1044-1049.
36. AlQahtani SM, Bicknell RT. Outcomes following long head of biceps tendon tenodesis. *Curr Rev Musculoskelet Med.* 2016;9(4):378-387.
37. Gregory JM, Harwood DP, Gochanour E, Sherman SL, Romeo AA. Clinical outcomes of revision biceps tenodesis. *Int J Shoulder Surg.* 2012;6(2):45-50.
38. Schröder CP, Skare O, Gjengedal E, Uppheim G, Reikerås O, Brox JI. Long-term results after SLAP repair: a 5-year follow-up study of 107 patients with comparison of patients aged over and under 40 years. *Arthroscopy.* 2012;28(11):1601-1607.

39. O'Brien SJ, Allen AA, Coleman SH, Drakos MC. The trans-rotator cuff approach to SLAP lesions: technical aspects for repair and a clinical follow-up of 31 patients at a minimum of 2 years. *Arthroscopy.* 2002;18(4):372–377.

40. Park JG, Cho NS, Kim JY, Song JH, Hong SJ, Rhee YG. Arthroscopic knot removal for failed superior labrum anterior-posterior repair secondary to knot-induced pain. *Am J Sports Med.* 2017;45(11):2563–2568.

41. Byram IR, Dunn WR, Kuhn JE. Humeral head abrasion: an association with failed superior labrum anterior posterior repairs. *J Shoulder Elbow Surg.* 2011;20(1):92–97.

42. Sassmannshausen G, Sukay M, Mair SD. Broken or dislodged poly-L-lactic acid bioabsorbable tacks in patients after SLAP lesion surgery. *Arthroscopy.* 2006;22(6):615–619.

43. Yoo JC, Lee YS, Ahn JH, Park JH, Kang HJ, Koh KH. Isolated suprascapular nerve injury below the spinoglenoid notch after SLAP repair. *J Shoulder Elbow Surg.* 2009;18(4):e27–e29.

44. Trusler ML, Bryan WJ, Ilahi OA. Anatomic and radiographic analysis of arthroscopic tack placement into the superior glenoid. *Arthroscopy.* 2002;18(4):366–371.

45. Denard PJ, Dai X, Hanypsiak BT, Burkhart SS. Anatomy of the biceps tendon: implications for restoring physiological length-tension relation during biceps tenodesis with interference screw fixation. *Arthroscopy.* 2012;28(10):1352–1358.

46. McCrum CL, Alluri RK, Batech M, Mirzayan R. Complications of biceps tenodesis based on location, fixation, and indication: a review of 1526 shoulders. *J Shoulder Elbow Surg.* 2019;28(3):461–469.

47. Heckman DS, Creighton RA, Romeo AA. Management of failed biceps tenodesis or tenotomy: causation and treatment. *Sports Med Arthrosc.* 2010;18(3):173–180.

48. Taylor SA, O'Brien SJ. "Hidden lesions" of the extra-articular biceps after subpectoral biceps tenodesis: letter to the editor. *Am J Sports Med.* 2015;43(3):NP3–NP4.

49. Moon SC, Cho NS, Rhee YG. Analysis of "hidden lesions" of the extra-articular biceps after subpectoral biceps tenodesis: the subpectoral portion as the optimal tenodesis site. *Am J Sports Med.* 2015;43(1):63–68.

50. Rhee PC, Spinner RJ, Bishop AT, Shin AY. Iatrogenic brachial plexus injuries associated with open subpectoral biceps tenodesis: a report of 4 cases. *Am J Sports Med.* 2013;41(9):2048–2053.

51. Overmann AL, Colantonio DF, Wheatley BM, Volk WR, Kilcoyne KG, Dickens JF. Incidence and characteristics of humeral shaft fractures after subpectoral biceps tenodesis. *Orthop J Sports Med.* 2019;7(3):2325967119833420.

52. Sears BW, Spencer EE, Getz CL. Humeral fracture following subpectoral biceps tenodesis in 2 active, healthy patients. *J Shoulder Elbow Surg.* 2011;20(6):e7–e11.

53. Beason DP, Shah JP, Duckett JW, Jost PW, Fleisig GS, Cain EL. Torsional fracture of the humerus after subpectoral biceps tenodesis with an interference screw: a biomechanical cadaveric study. *Clin Biomech (Bristol, Avon).* 2015;30(9):915–920.

54. Euler SA, Smith SD, Williams BT, Dornan GJ, Millett PJ, Wijdicks CA. Biomechanical analysis of subpectoral biceps tenodesis: effect of screw malpositioning on proximal humeral strength. *Am J Sports Med.* 2015;43(1):69–74.

14

Complications of Distal Clavicle Excision

Ferdinand J. Chan, MD
and Stephen J. Nicholas, MD

INTRODUCTION

Pain from the acromioclavicular joint is a common and at times debilitating pathology. The pathogenesis can be from primary or secondary (post-traumatic) osteoarthritis, distal clavicle osteolysis, or painful instability of the distal clavicle.

Initial conservative treatment to achieve pain-free shoulder range of motion and strength includes activity modification, anti-inflammatories, and physical therapy. If after 3 to 6 months of conservative management there is persistent pain, surgical intervention should be sought. Both open and arthroscopic distal clavicle excision has been met with largely successful outcomes.[1,2] High rates of good to excellent patient outcomes have been reported in long-term follow-up studies.[2,3]

Thompson TL, ed.
Arthroscopic Shoulder Surgery:
Complications and Management (pp 247-256).
© 2022 Taylor & Francis Group.

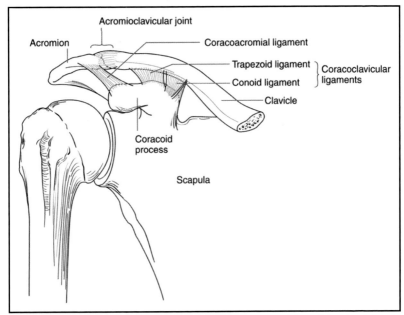

Figure 14-1. The normal acromioclavicular joint. Horizontal stability of the distal clavicle is provided by the acromioclavicular joint capsule while vertical stability is provided by the coracoclavicular ligaments. (Reproduced with permission from Rios CG, Arciero RA, Mazzocca AD. Anatomy of the clavicle and coracoid process for reconstruction of the coracoclavicular ligaments. *Am J Sports Med.* 2007;35:811–817.)

Complications and failure of the procedure to alleviate symptoms and disability are uncommon after both arthroscopic and open produces. However, they do occur and include diagnostic error, inadequate distal clavicle resection, acromioclavicular instability, heterotopic ossification, infection, distal clavicle fracture, scar formation, and stiffness.

ANATOMY

The acromioclavicular joint is a diarthrodial joint composed of the small convex facet on the lateral end of the clavicle and a small concave facet on the acromion of the scapula (Figure 14-1).[4] The acromioclavicular joint capsule is the primary static restraint against anteroposterior translation of the distal clavicle.[5] The superior ligament is rather thick and varies from 2 to 5.5 mm.[6] A biomechanical study with fresh frozen cadavers found that the thicker superior and posterior ligaments resist up to 56% and 25%, respectively, of the posteriorly directed forces.[5]

Vertical stability of the distal clavicle is provided by the coracoclavicular ligaments. The coracoclavicular ligament contains 2 structures: the trapezoid ligament, which is the anterolateral component, and the conoid portion, which is the posteromedial component.[4] The average distance from the lateral edge of the clavicle to the center of the trapezoid and conoid is 24.9 mm and 46.3 mm, respectively.[7] The average distance between the lateral clavicle edge to the lateral aspect of the trapezoid ligament is 15.3 mm (range, 11.0 to 22.8).[8] Increased superior-inferior translation is seen with transected coracoclavicular ligaments.[9]

COMPLICATIONS

Diagnostic Error

A meticulous history and physical examination are the first steps to prevent many so-called failures, which are likely misdiagnosing the origin of pain as from the acromioclavicular joint. The first step in evaluating a patient who is not improving after a distal clavicle resection is to reconsider whether the correct diagnosis was made initially. A typical patient presents with pain exacerbated by activities involving cross-arm activities, pushing, or overhead work.[10,11] Exercises such as bench press, pushups, and dips are especially painful.[11] A history of acromioclavicular separation or distal clavicle fracture may cause late symptomatic instability of the acromioclavicular joint.

On examination, tenderness to palpation of the acromioclavicular joint or lateral clavicle is often present. However, this test may be positive in some patients with subacromial impingement. Cross-body adduction reliably evokes pain.

If the diagnosis is still questionable after a thorough history and physical examination, a diagnostic injection can be performed. An injection directly into the acromioclavicular joint is perhaps the most reliable method to confirm the diagnosis. Complete pain relief is also prognostic for a successful outcome after distal clavicle resection.[10,12] Failure of pain relief or symptoms that persist after anesthetic injection should cue a clinician to an alternative or additional pathology, respectively.

INADEQUATE DISTAL CLAVICLE RESECTION

One of the most common technical causes of failure is inadequate resection. The location of incomplete resection is typically on the posterior or superior cortical ridge.[10,13-15] Inadequate resection is more common in arthroscopic cases compared to open procedures due to inadequate visualization of the whole distal clavicle. The advantages of an arthroscopic procedure include access of the glenohumeral joint, avoidance of violation of the deltotrapezial fascia, quicker recovery, and ability to address concomitant shoulder pathology. Patients with larger body habitus may present a technical challenge.

Patients with inadequate resection present postoperatively with similar symptoms as before surgery. The diagnosis can be confirmed with radiographic evaluation that includes an anteroposterior and Zanca view to visualize the acromioclavicular joint. A computed tomography scan with thin cuts of the joint or magnetic resonance imaging to evaluate for increased signal on T2 sequences and bone marrow edema of the distal clavicle may be necessary if plain radiographs are not revealing.[13] A second anesthetic injection into the joint may be necessary.

Several surgical techniques can help to enhance visualization during the procedure to ensure sufficient resection. Intermittent manual depression of the distal clavicle can assist with visualization when viewing from the lateral or posterior portals if a limited acromioplasty is done.[13,16] Use of a spinal needle directed inferiorly into the acromioclavicular joint can confirm that there is no remainder of the superior cortex that can at times blend in with the superior capsule.[13] Adequate resection confirmation should be performed from the anterior portal that is made in line with the acromioclavicular joint to allow direct visualization. With the arthroscope in the anterior portal, a burr from the posterior portal will reach the frequently missed posterior and superior aspects of the resection.

The amount resected can be estimated with the known dimensions of the arthroscopic burr. Alternatively, a spinal needle can be placed at the lateral aspect of the distal clavicle and another needle at the medial acromion to be measured.[1,10] The optimal minimal amount that is necessary to be resected can vary with each patient. Some authors demonstrated a minimum 5- to 10-mm resection is needed.[17-19] Studies also noted that resection of less than 11 mm would not violate any fibers of the trapezoid ligament in both sexes in 95% of the population.[8,20] We recommend performing a dynamic cross-arm adduction at the end of each case with the arthroscope in the posterior portal to guarantee no bony contact remains in this position.

If a revision surgery is needed, the same approach, whether open or arthroscopic, can be attempted again.

ACROMIOCLAVICULAR JOINT INSTABILITY

Joint instability secondary to overresection of the distal clavicle leads to complaints of pain with overhead activities. Physical examination demonstrates increased anterior and posterior translation of the clavicle if the posterosuperior capsule is violated.

In one study, patients' postoperative visual analog pain scales correlated with the magnitude of anteroposterior translation.[21] However, neither the amount of translation nor the postoperative pain score correlated with the joint space seen on postoperative standard anteroposterior or Zanca radiographs.[21] This lack of correlation makes the optimal resection amount difficult to be determined. One study found that half their patients had increased horizontal clavicular motion with an average of 19 mm of bone resection.[22] Another study found that patients who had a resection amount less than 10 mm had less pain than those who had had a larger amount.[23] A biomechanical study done by Branch et al[17] concluded that if only 5 mm of the distal clavicle was resected, there was not increased range of motion of the scapula with reference to the clavicle, and there was no bone-to-bone contact in rotation postoperatively. Therefore, the optimal resection amount is likely between 5 and 10 mm.

Iatrogenic symptomatic instability of the acromioclavicular joint is initially treated conservatively. This includes activity modification, physical therapy, and corticosteroid injection. The Weaver-Dunn procedure has fallen out of favor secondary to its unacceptable failure rate to adequately stabilize the acromioclavicular joint.[24,25] The mainstay of surgical management is coracoclavicular ligament reconstruction. In both mechanical and clinical studies, Nicholas et al[26-29] have shown the semitendinosus allograft is a strong and biologic option for reconstruction of the coracoclavicular ligaments.

HETEROTOPIC OSSIFICATION

Heterotopic ossification is a less common complication after distal clavicle resection. Incidences in literature range from 2% to 16%.[1,18,30] Heterotopic ossification has been reported after both open and arthroscopic distal clavicle resection, which makes the theory that this results from spilled marrow contents unlikely since there is continuous suction and irrigation with arthroscopy.

Recurrent symptomatic shoulder pain due to heterotopic ossification requires a large amount of bone formation in the acromioclavicular interval.[31] These patients are typically males with hypertrophic osteoarthritis of the acromioclavicular joint and have some form of pulmonary ailment.[31] On the other hand, partial ossification of the coracoclavicular ligaments is an asymptomatic finding.

A repeat trial of conservative management can be undertaken if symptomatic heterotopic ossification formation has occurred. Surgical excision is reserved for those with continued pain. It is recommended that heterotopic ossification prophylaxis should be started on revision patients with either indomethacin or 5 Gy of radiation treatment.[31] No reports of recurrence have been seen after revision surgery with prophylaxis.

INFECTION

Infection is a risk of any surgery and occurs in distal clavicle excision at a rate of 4% to 10% (7% deep and 3% superficial in one study and only one superficial infection in another cohort) in open cases.[18,19] No cases of infection after arthroscopic procedure have been reported in the literature. Continuous wound drainage as well as persistent pain should alert the surgeon of a possible infection.

Superficial infections usually resolve with a short course of oral antibiotics ranging from 5 to 7 days. Deep infections should be tackled with surgical debridement and intravenous antibiotics.

DISTAL CLAVICLE FRACTURE

This rare complication is included to stress the importance of visualization during distal clavicle resection. In a case report, an iatrogenic fracture of the distal clavicle was caused after misidentification of the acromioclavicular joint (Figure 14-2).[32] This led to burring of clavicle 3 cm medial to the distal end of the clavicle. The case was further complicated by development of adhesive capsulitis and symptomatic callus formation that required a second surgery.

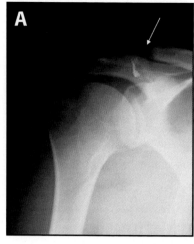

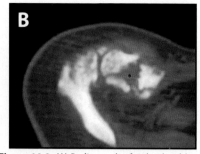

Figure 14-2. (A) Radiograph of right shoulder with arrow showing fracture at the distal end of the clavicle. (B) Computed tomography scan with asterisk showing comminuted fracture at the distal aspect of the clavicle. (Reproduced with permission from Ghodadra N, Lee GH, Kung P, Busfield BT, Kharazzi FD. Distal clavicle fracture as a complication of arthroscopic distal clavicle resection. *Arthroscopy.* 2009;25:929–933.)

Achieving adequate visualization of the acromioclavicular joint is paramount for a successful outcome. If identification of the acromioclavicular joint is not certain when viewing from the posterior portal, the surgeon can switch the arthroscope to the lateral portal. Cleaning of the undersurface of the acromion with a radiofrequency device should be done from a lateral to medial direction to easily identify the acromioclavicular joint.[32] Last, palpation of the distal clavicle and providing an inferiorly directed force will aid in arthroscopic identification of the distal clavicle.

SCAR FORMATION

When an open surgery instead of arthroscopic distal clavicle excision is elected, scar hypertrophy and scar sensitivity can result. Scar hypertrophy and sensitivity have been reported in 14% and 55% of patients.[18] Postoperative scars are located in a readily visibly area and become a cosmetic issue if scar hypertrophy occurs. This can be minimized by using a bra strap incision instead of a longitudinal incision. Patients also report significantly more satisfaction with the appearance of their scars with an incision following the orientation of the Langer lines of the skin.[33]

STIFFNESS

Postoperative stiffness of the shoulder ranges from 0% to 29%.[16,18,23] This appears more likely after open procedures compared to arthroscopic procedures. Infection, heterotopic ossification, and lack of formal postoperative physical therapy are often related to postoperative stiffness.[18]

Treatment is conservative in the short term, including anti-inflammatories in the form of an intra-articular corticosteroid injection or a methylprednisolone dose pack as well as physical therapy program for range of motion.[13] However, if this fails and there is continued pain and loss of motion, a formal lysis of adhesion and manipulation under anesthesia should be undertaken.

OTHER COMPLICATIONS

Other complications after distal clavicle resection include biceps tendinitis in the immediate postoperative period that resolved with conservative care,[1] reoperation 4 months after index procedure for bursal scarring causing painful popping,[1] persistent pain from missed superior labrum anterior posterior lesions,[34] and reossification and solid ankyloses across the acromioclavicular joint requiring a repeat operation.[35]

REFERENCES

1. Snyder SJ, Banas MP, Karzel RP. The arthroscopic Mumford procedure: an analysis of results. *Arthroscopy.* 1995;11:157–164.
2. Robertson WJ, Griffith MH, Carroll K, O'Donnell T, Gill TJ. Arthroscopic versus open distal clavicle excision: a comparative assessment at intermediate-term follow-up. *Am J Sports Med.* 2011;39:2415–2420.
3. Rabalais RD, McCarty E. Surgical treatment of symptomatic acromioclavicular joint problems: a systematic review. *Clin Orthop Relat Res.* 2007;455:30–37.
4. Culham E, Peat M. Functional anatomy of the shoulder complex. *J Orthop Sports Phys Ther.* 1993;18:342–350.
5. Klimkiewicz JJ, Williams GR, Sher JS, Karduna A, Des Jardins J, Iannotti JP. The acromioclavicular capsule as a restraint to posterior translation of the clavicle: a biomechanical analysis. *J Shoulder Elbow Surg.* 1999;8:119–124.
6. Salter EG Jr, Nasca RJ, Shelley BS. Anatomical observations on the acromioclavicular joint and supporting ligaments. *Am J Sports Med.* 1987;15:199–206.
7. Rios CG, Arciero RA, Mazzocca AD. Anatomy of the clavicle and coracoid process for reconstruction of the coracoclavicular ligaments. *Am J Sports Med.* 2007;35:811–817.
8. Harris RI, Vu DH, Sonnabend DH, Goldberg JA, Walsh WR. Anatomic variance of the coracoclavicular ligaments. *J Shoulder Elbow Surg.* 2001;10:585–588.

9. Dawson PA, Adamson GJ, Pink MM, et al. Relative contribution of acromioclavicular joint capsule and coracoclavicular ligaments to acromioclavicular stability. *J Shoulder Elbow Surg.* 2009;18:237–244.

10. Shaffer BS. Painful conditions of the acromioclavicular joint. *J Am Acad Orthop Surg.* 1999;7:176–188.

11. Cahill BR. Osteolysis of the distal part of the clavicle in male athletes. *J Bone Joint Surg Am.* 1982;64:1053–1058.

12. Worcester JN Jr, Green DP. Osteoarthritis of the acromioclavicular joint. *Clin Orthop Relat Res.* 1968;58:69–73.

13. Strauss EJ, Barker JU, McGill K, Verma NN. The evaluation and management of failed distal clavicle excision. *Sports Med Arthrosc Rev.* 2010;18:213–219.

14. Jerosch J, Steinbeck J, Schroder M, Castro WH. Arthroscopic resection of the acromioclavicular joint (ARAC). *Knee Surg Sports Traumatol Arthrosc.* 1993;1:209–215.

15. Tolin BS, Snyder SJ. Our technique for the arthroscopic Mumford procedure. *Orthop Clin North Am.* 1993;24:143–151.

16. Martin SD, Baumgarten TE, Andrews JR. Arthroscopic resection of the distal aspect of the clavicle with concomitant subacromial decompression. *J Bone Joint Surg Am.* 2001;83:328–335.

17. Branch TP, Burdette HL, Shahriari AS, Carter FM II, Hutton WC. The role of the acromioclavicular ligaments and the effect of distal clavicle resection. *Am J Sports Med.* 1996;24:293–297.

18. Chronopoulos E, Gill HS, Freehill MT, Petersen SA, McFarland EG. Complications after open distal clavicle excision. *Clin Orthop Relat Res.* 2008;466:646–651.

19. Gartsman GM. Arthroscopic resection of the acromioclavicular joint. *Am J Sports Med.* 1993;21:71–77.

20. Renfree KJ, Wright TW. Anatomy and biomechanics of the acromioclavicular and sternoclavicular joints. *Clin Sports Med.* 2003;22:219–237.

21. Blazar PE, Iannotti JP, Williams GR. Anteroposterior instability of the distal clavicle after distal clavicle resection. *Clin Orthop Relat Res.* 1998;348:114–120.

22. Cook FF, Tibone JE. The Mumford procedure in athletes: an objective analysis of function. *Am J Sports Med.* 1988;16:97–100.

23. Eskola A, Santavirta S, Viljakka HT, Wirta J, Partio TE, Hoikka V. The results of operative resection of the lateral end of the clavicle. *J Bone Joint Surg Am.* 1996;78:584–587.

24. Millett PJ, Horan MP, Warth RJ. Two-year outcomes after primary anatomic coracoclavicular ligament reconstruction. *Arthroscopy.* 2015;31:1962–1973.

25. Moatshe G, Kruckeberg BM, Chahla J, et al. Acromioclavicular and coracoclavicular ligament reconstruction for acromioclavicular joint instability: a systematic review of clinical and radiographic outcomes. *Arthroscopy.* 2018;34:1979–1995.e8.

26. Lee SJ, Nicholas SJ, Akizuki KH, McHugh MP, Kremenic IJ, Ben-Avi S. Reconstruction of the coracoclavicular ligaments with tendon grafts: a comparative biomechanical study. *Am J Sports Med.* 2003;31:648–655.

27. Nicholas SJ, Lee SJ, Mullaney MJ, Tyler TF, McHugh MP. Clinical outcomes of coracoclavicular ligament reconstructions using tendon grafts. *Am J Sports Med.* 2007;35:1912–1917.

28. Lee SJ, Keefer EP, McHugh MP, et al. Cyclical loading of coracoclavicular ligament reconstructions: a comparative biomechanical study. *Am J Sports Med.* 2008;36:1990–1997.

29. Kowalsky MS, Kremenic IJ, Orishimo KF, McHugh MP, Nicholas SJ, Lee SJ. The effect of distal clavicle excision on in situ graft forces in coracoclavicular ligament reconstruction. *Am J Sports Med.* 2010;38:2313–2319.

30. Charron KM, Schepsis AA, Voloshin I. Arthroscopic distal clavicle resection in athletes: a prospective comparison of the direct and indirect approach. *Am J Sports Med.* 2007;35:53–58.

31. Berg EE, Ciullo JV. Heterotopic ossification after acromioplasty and distal clavicle resection. *J Shoulder Elbow Surg.* 1995;4:188–193.

32. Ghodadra N, Lee GH, Kung P, Busfield BT, Kharazzi FD. Distal clavicle fracture as a complication of arthroscopic distal clavicle resection. *Arthroscopy.* 2009;25:929–933.

33. Shukla DR, Rubenstein WJ, Barnes LA, et al. The influence of incision type on patient satisfaction after plate fixation of clavicle fractures. *Orthop J Sports Med.* 2017;5:2325967117712235.

34. Berg EE, Ciullo JV. The SLAP lesion: a cause of failure after distal clavicle resection. *Arthroscopy.* 1997;13:85–89.

35. Tytherleigh-Strong G, Gill J, Sforza G, Copeland S, Levy O. Reossification and fusion across the acromioclavicular joint after arthroscopic acromioplasty and distal clavicle resection. *Arthroscopy.* 2001;17:E36.

Financial Disclosures

Dr. Benjamin Albertson has not disclosed any relevant financial relationships.

Dr. Answorth Allen has no financial or proprietary interest in the materials presented herein.

Dr. Akhil Andrews has not disclosed any relevant financial relationships.

Dr. Craig Bennett has a consulting agreement with Arthrex Inc.

Dr. Alexander R. M. Bitzer has no financial or proprietary interest in the materials presented herein.

Dr. James E. Carpenter has no financial or proprietary interest in the materials presented herein.

Dr. Ferdinand J. Chan has not disclosed any relevant financial relationships.

Dr. Filippo Familiari has not disclosed any relevant financial relationships.

Dr. Gazi Huri has no financial or proprietary interest in the materials presented herein.

Dr. Timothy S. Johnson has no financial or proprietary interest in the materials presented herein.

Dr. Ibrahim M. Khaleel has no financial or proprietary interest in the materials presented herein.

Dr. Stephanie L. Logterman has no financial or proprietary interest in the materials presented herein.

Dr. Eric C. McCarty has not disclosed any relevant financial relationships.

Dr. Edward G. McFarland has not disclosed any relevant financial relationships.

Dr. Prashant Meshram has no financial or proprietary interest in the materials presented herein.

Jerome Colin Murray has no financial or proprietary interest in the materials presented herein.

Dr. Abbas Naqvi has no financial or proprietary interest in the materials presented herein.

Dr. Thomas X. Nguyen has no financial or proprietary interest in the materials presented herein.

Dr. Stephen J. Nicholas reports consulting for Arthrex and Zimmer.

Dr. Jane H. O'Connor is a KCI/Acelity research grant recipient and consultant.

Dr. Gabriella Ode has no financial or proprietary interest in the materials presented herein.

Dr. Emmanuel N. Osadebey has no financial or proprietary interest in the materials presented herein.

Dr. Benjamin Packard has not disclosed any relevant financial relationships.

Dr. Rajeev Pandarinath has not disclosed any relevant financial relationships.

Dr. Marc E. Rankin has not disclosed any relevant financial relationships.

Dr. Dustin L. Richter receives fellowship funding support from Arthrex.

Dr. Jorge Rojas has not disclosed any relevant financial relationships.

Dr. Christopher G. Salib has no financial or proprietary interest in the materials presented herein.

Dr. Robert C. Schenck Jr receives fellowship funding support from Arthrex.

Dr. Christopher Shultz has not disclosed any relevant financial relationships.

Dr. Seth Stake has no financial or proprietary interest in the materials presented herein.

Dr. Taylor Swansen has not disclosed any relevant financial relationships.

Dr. Terry L. Thompson has no financial or proprietary interest in the materials presented herein.

Dr. Daniel C. Wascher receives fellowship funding support from Arthrex.

Dr. Rolanda A. Willacy has not disclosed any relevant financial relationships.

Dr. Robert H. Wilson has no financial or proprietary interest in the materials presented herein.

INDEX

impaction, 60
loose/prominent anchors, 60
loosening, 60-61
trephination, 61
epidemiology, 46
literature review, 46-55
surgical techniques, 57-59
general anchor insertion concepts, 57
labral instability, 58-59
rotator cuff repair, 57-58
suture anchor design rationale, 46-49
suture–anchor implant interface, modes of failure, 48
workup for loose anchors, 55-56
distal clavicle excision complications, 247-256
acromioclavicular joint instability, 251
anatomy, 248-249
biceps tendinitis, 254
bursal scarring, 254
distal clavicle fracture, 252-253
heterotopic ossification, 251-252
inadequate distal clavicle resection, 249-250
infection, 252
reossification, 254
scar formation, 253
solid ankyloses, 254
stiffness, 254
drilling anchor, 60
dystonia, 142

enzymatic capsulotomy, postarthroscopic arthrofibrosis, 127

Evans, James A., 133
extracorporeal shock wave therapy, postarthroscopic arthrofibrosis, 125
extravasation of fluid, 21-32
etiology, 22-27
anatomy-based etiology, 24
factors prognosticating, 24-26
fluid pressure, 27
patient positioning, 26
procedural-based etiology, 24
regional block, 26
potential complications, 28-31
airway compromise, 29
arterial, 30
brain death, 30-31
cerebral edema, 30-31
chest, 28
midarm, 28
neck, 28
rhabdomyolysis, 29-30

glenohumeral chondrolysis, postarthroscopic, 153-160
diagnosis, 156-158
epidemiology, 154
etiology, 154-155
nonoperative treatment, 158
operative treatment, 158
pathophysiology, 155-156
patient factors, 154
postoperative factors, 155
prevention, 159
signs/symptoms, 156
surgical factors, 154-155
treatment, 158-159

Printed in the United States
by Baker & Taylor Publisher Services